Denton A. Cooley, M.D.

W9-DFE-232

Diagnostic Techniques
and Assessment Procedures
in Vascular Surgery

Diagnostic Techniques and Assessment Procedures in Vascular Surgery

Edited by

Roger M. Greenhalgh, M.A., M.D., M.Chir., F.R.C.S.

Professor of Surgery
Charing Cross & Westminster Medical School
Department of Surgery
Charing Cross Hospital
London, England

Grune & Stratton
(Harcourt Brace Jovanovich, Publishers)
London   Orlando   San Diego   New York
Toronto   Montreal   Sydney   Tokyo

British Library Cataloguing in Publication Data

Diagnostic techniques and assessment procedures
    in vascular surgery.
    1. Blood-vessels — Diseases — Diagnosis
    I. Greenhalgh, Roger M. (Roger Malcolm)
    616.1'3075   RC691.5
    ISBN 0-8089-1721-8

Library of Congress Catalog Card Number 85-047773

© **1985 BY GRUNE & STRATTON, LTD.**
All rights reserved. No part of this publication
may be reproduced or transmitted in any form or
by any means, electronic or mechanical, including
photocopy, recording, or any information storage
and retrieval system, without permission in
writing from the publisher.

GRUNE & STRATTON, LTD.
24/28 Oval Road
London NW1 7DX

United States edition published by
GRUNE & STRATTON, INC.
Orlando, Florida 32887

International Standard Book Number 0-8089-1721-8
Printed in the United States of America
85 86 87 88   10 9 8 7 6 5 4 3 2 1

Acknowledgements

I should like to acknowledge my gratitude to all of the authors who have produced the chapters in record time. I am grateful to them for turning their attention to the problem of vascular diagnostic techniques and assessment procedures in this very practical way.

I am especially grateful to Mrs. Alison George for illustrating most of this book and to Miss Jill Wallace for co-ordinating the authors and the editor! We would not have had the chapter from Maroso et al, which was submitted in German, if it had not been for the kind and expert translation into English by my wife, Mrs. Karin Greenhalgh.

The contents of this book were quite difficult to put together and I was grateful for the help of a number of my colleagues who assisted me with this and also made recommendations about which author should be invited to do the chapter. I am most grateful to the following who contributed in this way: Mr. Roger Baird; Prof. Peter Bell; Prof. Norman Browse; Mr. David Charlesworth; Mr. Crawford Jamieson; Miss Averil Mansfield; Mr. Charles McCollum; and Prof. Andrew Nicolaides

Contents

CEREBRAL REVASCULARISATION

AORTIC ANEURYSMS AND RENAL ISCHAEMIA

VASCULAR AND MICROVASCULAR RECONSTRUCTION

AMPUTATION LEVELS

UPPER LIMB ISCHAEMIA

ARTERIO-VENOUS MALFORMATIONS

VENOUS

PRACTICAL DEVELOPMENTS

Contributors

M.I. ALDOORI, F.R.C.S.
Research Fellow in Surgery
Department of Surgery
Bristol Royal Infirmary
Bristol, England

DAVID J. ALLISON, B.Sc.,M.D.,
F.R.C.S.
Director, Department of Diagnostic
    Radiology
Royal Postgraduate Medical School
Hammersmith Hospital
London, England

M.R. ANDRESS, M.B.,Ch.B.,F.R.C.R.,
D.M.R.D.
Consultant Radiologist
Royal Victoria Hospital
Boscombe, Bournemouth
Dorset, England

ENRICO ASCER, M.D.
Assistant Professor of Surgery
Albert Einstein College of Medicine
Head, Vascular Surgery Laboratory
Montefiore Medical Center
New York, USA

ROGER N. BAIRD, Ch.M.,F.R.C.S.
Consultant Surgeon
Department of Surgery
Bristol Royal Infirmary
Bristol, England

ANDREAS P. BARABAS, M.D.,
F.R.C.S.
Consultant Surgeon
West Suffolk Hospital
Bury St. Edmunds
Suffolk, England

S. BASTIANELLO
Department of Neurological Sciences
Section of Neuroradiology
University of Rome
Rome, Italy

PETER R.F. BELL, M.D.,F.R.C.S.
Department of Surgery
University of Leicester
Leicester, England

P. BERGERON
Department of Cardio Vascular Surgery
Hopital Saint-Joseph
Marseilles, France

GIORGIO BIASI, M.D.
Clinical Chirurgica 2°
University of Milan
Pad. Zonda, Policlinico
Milano, Italy

L. BOZZAO
Department of Neurological Sciences
Section of Neuroradiology
University of Rome
Rome, Italy

ALLAN D. CALLOW, M.D.,Ph.D.
Tufts New England Medical Center
Boston, Massachusetts, USA

DAVID CHARLESWORTH, D.Sc.,
M.D.,F.R.C.S
Reader in Surgery
University of Manchester
Manchester, England

SUSAN E.A. COLE, B.Sc.
Senior Medical Physicist
Department of Medical Physics
Bristol Royal Infirmary
Bristol, England

DENTON A. COOLEY, M.D.
Surgeon-in-Chief
Texas Heart Institute
Houston, Texas, USA
Clinical Professor of Surgery
University of Texas Health Science
   Center
Houston, Texas, USA

NATHAN P. COUCH, M.D.
Assistant Professor of Surgery
Brigham and Women's Hospital
Boston, Massachusetts, USA

ROBERT COURBIER
Department of Cardio Vascular Surgery
Hopital Saint-Joseph
Marseilles, France

JOHN J. CRANLEY, M.D.
Director of Surgery
Director of Medical Education
Director of Peripheral Vascular Research
   Laboratory
Good Samaritan Hospital
Cincinnati, Ohio, USA
Clinical Professor of Surgery
University of Cincinnati Medical Center
Cincinnati, Ohio, USA

SIMON G. DARKE, M.D.,F.R.C.S.
Consultant Surgeon
Royal Victoria Hospital
Boscombe, Bournemouth
Dorset, England

WILLIAM K. EHRENFELD, M.D.
Professor of Surgery
Co-Chief Vascular Surgery
Department of Surgery
University of California
San Francisco, California, USA

H. EHRINGER
The First Medical University Clinic
Vienna, Austria

B.C. EIKELBOOM, M.D.,Ph.D.
Department of Surgery
St. Antonius Ziekenhius
Nieuwegan, Utrecht, The Netherlands

L.M. FANTOZZI
Department of Neurological Sciences
Section of Neuroradiology
University of Rome
Rome, Italy

M. FERDANI
Department of Cardio Vascular Surgery
Hopital Saint-Joseph
Marseilles, France

PAOLO FIORANI
Head, Department of Vascular Surgery
University of Rome
Rome, Italy

LARRY D. FLANAGAN, M.D.
Kachelmacher Fellow in Vascular
   Diseases
Good Samaritan Hospital
Cincinnati, Ohio, USA

D. PRESTON FLANIGAN, M.D.
Associate Professor of Surgery
Chief, Division of Vascular Surgery
Department of Surgery
University of Illinois at Chicago
Chicago, Illinois, USA

M. FORMICHI
Department of Cardio Vascular Surgery
Hopital Saint-Joseph
Marseilles, France

IAN L. GREEN, M.B.,B.S.
Research Fellow
Charing Cross & Westminster Medical
    School
Department of Surgery
Charing Cross Hospital
London, England

ROGER M. GREENHALGH, M.A.,
M.D.,M.Chir.,F.R.C.S.
Professor of Surgery
Charing Cross & Westminster Medical
    School
Department of Surgery
Charing Cross Hospital
London, England

GORDON HEARD, M.Ch.,F.R.C.S.
Consultant Surgeon
University Hospital of Wales
Cardiff, Wales

BRIAN P. HEATHER, M.S.,F.R.C.S.
Senior Registrar
Department of Surgery
Charing Cross Hospital
London, England

ANNE P. HEMINGWAY, B.Sc.,
M.R.C.P.,F.R.C.R
Senior Lecturer and Consultant in Charge
    of Vascular Studies
Department of Diagnostic Radiology
Royal Postgraduate Medical School
Hammersmith Hospital
London, England

HERBERT B. HECHTMAN, M.D.
Associate Professor of Surgery
Harvard Medical School
Surgeon
Brigham and Women's Hospital
Boston, Massachusetts, USA

P. HOLSTEIN
Department of Clinical Physiology
Bispebjerg Hospital
Copenhagen, Denmark

EDWARD HOUSLEY, F.R.C.P.E.,
F.R.C.P.
Consultant Physician
Physician in Charge of the Peripheral
    Vascular Clinic
Royal Infirmary
Edinburgh, Scotland

J.M. JAUSSERAN
Department of Cardio Vascular Surgery
Hopital Saint-Joseph
Marseilles, France

W.D. JEANS, F.R.C.R.
Consultant Radiologist
Department of Radiology
Bristol Royal Infirmary
Bristol, England

B.M. JONES
Honorary Lecturer
Charing Cross & Westminster Medical
    School
Department of Surgery
Charing Cross Hospital
London, England

HORST KNIEMEYER, M.D.
Associate Professor
Department of Vascular Surgery and
    Kidney Transplantation
University of Dusseldorf
Dusseldorf, West Germany

WOLFGANG KOX, M.D.
Director Intensive Care
Department of Anaesthesia
Charing Cross Hospital
London, England

NIELS A. LASSEN
Department of Clinical Physiology
Bispebjerg Hospital
Copenhagen, Denmark

H. LOEPRECHT, M.D.
Krankenhauszweckverband Augsburg
I. Chirurgische
Steglinstrasse
Augsburg, West Germany

J.W. LUDWIG, M.D., Ph.D.
Department of Radiology
St. Antonius Ziekenhius
Nieuwegein, Utrecht, The Netherlands

R. MacFARLANE, M.A.,M.B.,
B.Chir.,S.H.O.
West Suffolk Hospital
Bury St. Edmunds
Suffolk, England

JOHN A. MANNICK, M.D.
Mosley Professor of Surgery
Harvard Medical School
Surgeon-in-Chief
Brigham and Women's Hospital
Boston, Massachusetts, USA

AVERIL O. MANSFIELD, Ch.M.,
F.R.C.S.
Consultant Surgeon
St. Mary's Hospital, London
Senior Lecturer in Vascular Surgery
Royal Postgraduate Medical School
London, England

L. MAROSI
The First Surgical University Clinic
Vienna, Austria

ADRIAN MARSTON, D.M., M.Ch.,
F.R.C.S.
Consultant Surgeon
The Middlesex Hospital
London, England

CHARLES N. McCOLLUM, M.D.,
F.R.C.S.
Senior Lecturer in Surgery
Charing Cross & Westminster Medical
    School
Charing Cross Hospital
London, England

PETER T. McCOLLUM, F.R.C.S.I.
Research Fellow
Vascular Laboratory
Ninewells Hospital
Dundee, Scotland

SERGIO MIANI, M.D.
Clinica Chirurgica 2°
University of Milan
Pad. Zonda, Policlinico
Milano, Italy

RICHARD D. MILES, Ph.D.
Assistant Professor
Department of Surgery
Southern Illinois University School of
    Medicine
Springfield, Illinois, USA

J. MONNIG, M.D.
Krankenhauszweckverband Augsburg
I. Chirurgische Klinik
Stenglinstrasse
Augsburg, West Germany

DERMOT J. MOORE, M.B.,F.R.C.S.I.
Research Fellow
Section of Peripheral Vascular Surgery
Southern Illinois University School of
    Medicine
Springfield, Illinois, USA

JOHN G. MOSLEY, B.Sc.,M.D.,
M.R.C.P., F.R.C.S.
Senior Surgical Registrar
The Middlesex Hospital
London, England

KEN A. MYERS,
M.S.,F.A.C.S.,F.R.A.C.S.
Head of Department of Vascular Surgery
Prince Henry's Hospital
Melbourne, Australia
Senior Lecturer, Department of Surgery
Monash University
Melbourne, Australia

DAVID NEGUS, M.A., D.M.,M.Ch.,
F.R.C.S
Surgeon
Lewisham Hospital
Teacher in Surgery
The United Dental and Medical Schools
    of Guy's and St. Thomas'
London, England

ANDREW N. NICOLAIDES, M.S., F.R.C.S.,F.R.C.S.E.
Professor of Vascular Surgery
Academic Surgical Unit and Irvine
    Laboratory for Cardiovascular
    Investigation and Research
St. Mary's Hospital Medical School
London, England

EVAGORAS P. NICOLAIDES, B.Sc., M.A.,M.B.,B.Ch.
Research Fellow
Academic Surgical Unit and Irvine
    Laboratory for Cardiovascular
    Investigation and Research
St. Mary's Hospital
London, England

LARS NORGREN, M.D.,Ph.D.
Associate Professor of Surgery
Head, Section of Vascular Surgery
Department of Surgery
Lund University
Lund, Sweden

SIMON D. PARVIN, F.R.C.S.
Department of Surgery
University of Leicester
Leicester, England

PIERRE PERONNEAU, Ph.D.
Maitre de Recherche
Instrumentation et Dynamique
    Cardiovasculaire
Hopital Broussais
Paris, France

PAOLO PIGNOLI, M.D.
Clinica Chirurgica 2°
University of Milan
Pad. Zonda, Policlinico
Milano, Italy

G.R. PISTOLESE
Department of Vascular Surgery
University of Rome
Rome, Italy

F. PIZA
The First Surgical University Clinic
Vienna, Austria

M. RASURA
Department of Neurological Sciences
University of Rome
Rome, Italy

M. REGGI
Department of Cardio Vascular Surgery
Hopital Saint-Joseph
Marseilles, France

LINDA M. REILLY, M.D.
Vascular Fellow
Department of Surgery
University of California
San Francisco, California, USA

JEREMY O. ROBERTS
Lecturer
Charing Cross & Westminster Medical
    School
Department of Surgery
Charing Cross Hospital
London, England

UGO RUBERTI, M.D.
Professor of Surgery
Clinica Chirurgica 2°
University of Milan
Pad. Zonda, Policlinico
Milano, Italy

A-MAJEED SALMASI, M.D.,Ph.D.
Research Fellow
Academic Surgical Unit and Irvine
    Laboratory for Cardiovascular
    Investigation and Research
St. Mary's Hospital Medical School
London, England

WILHELM SANDMANN, M.D.
Professor of Surgery
Director of the Department of Vascular
    Surgery and Kidney Transplantation
University of Dusseldorf
Dusseldorf, West Germany

E. SBARIGIA
Department of Vascular Surgery
University of Rome
Rome, Italy

DONALD SILVER, M.D.
Professor and Chairman
Department of Surgery
University of Missouri-Columbia
Columbia, Missouri, USA

TANSUKH N. SONECHA, M.B.,
M.R.C.P.,D.T.M.&H.
Senior Research Fellow
Academic Surgical Unit and Irvine
    Laboratory for Cardiovascular
    Investigation and Research
St. Mary's Hospital Medical School
London, England

VANCE A. SPENCE, Ph.D
Principal Physicist
Vascular Laboratory
Nineweels Hospital
Dundee, Scotland

DAVID S. SUMNER, M.D.
Professor of Surgery and Chief
Section of Peripheral Vascular Surgery
Southern Illinois University School of
    Medicine
Springfield, Illinois, USA

A.J. TAAMS, M.D.
Department of Radiology
St. Antonius Ziekenhuis
Nieuwegein, Utrecht, The Netherlands

C. TEEUWEN, M.D.
Department of Radiology
St. Antonius Ziekenhuis
Nieuwegein, Utrecht, The Netherlands

C.C. van SCHAIK, M.D.
Department of Radiology
St. Antonius Ziekenhuis
Nieuwegein, Utrecht, The Netherlands

FRANK J. VEITH, M.D.
Professor of Surgery
Albert Einstein College of Medicine
Chief, Division of Vascular Surgery
Montefiore Medical Center
New York, USA

M. VENTURA
Department of Vascular Surgery
University of Rome
Rome, Italy

O. WAGNER
The First Surgical University Clinic
Vienna, Austria

H. WEBER, M.D.
Krankenhauszweckverband Augsburg
I. Chirurgische Klinik
Stenglinstrasse
Augsburg, West Germany

ANTHONY D. WHITTEMORE, M.D.
Assistant Professor of Surgery
Harvard Medical School
Surgeon
Brigham and Women's Hospital
Boston, Massachusetts, USA

JOHN P. WOODCOCK, B.Sc.,M.Phil,
Ph.D.,F.I.N.S.T.P.
Professor in Bioengineering
Department of Medical Physics and
    Bioengineering
University Hospital of Wales
Cardiff, Wales

JAMES S.T. YAO, M.D., Ph.D.
Professor of Surgery
Northwestern University Medical School
Director, Blood Flow Laboratory
Northwestern Memorial Hospital
Chicago, Illinois, USA

Roger M. Greenhalgh

1

Introduction

This book is concerned with the application of research and investigations to the benefit of the patient. The literature is full of reports of investigations that are valuable for research matters but may never be useful to the practising clinician. These chapters are specifically orientated towards clinical practice. The authors have been encouraged to say which tests they find particularly helpful and to identify those investigations that just add to the world literature without benefitting our patients that have vascular disease.

Before any vascular reconstruction can begin, it is important to know that the blood will clot properly and that it will behave in such a way that the surface of vessels and graft materials can heal properly. The essential haematological investigations are therefore considered first. Radiolabelling of cells is presently rapidly moving from the field of research to become an essential aspect of clinical practice and the use of isotopes is also becoming extremely valuable in assessing cardiac function. The noninvasive assessment of coronary vessels is an area that has lagged behind the noninvasive assessment of carotid and peripheral arteries but there is a great demand for a really reliable test to be used as a screen for coronary angiography. These matters are fully discussed in the section on "Principles of Investigation." For optimum results, vascular surgeons are increasingly using sophisticated cardiovascular monitoring; the details of how this is done is included in this section. The principles of Doppler ultrasound, ultrasonic imaging, and digital subtraction angiography complete this section.

Investigations concerning the timing of cerebral revascularisation are becoming more sophisticated each year, and in this full part of the book the essential investigations that are employed before, during, and after carotid surgery are documented.

Sudden death from leaking of abdominal aortic aneurysm is still a major problem, but population screening for this condition is in its infancy. It should be possible with the new imaging techniques at our disposal to design population studies to provide the information we require. The value of cardiovascular monitoring is also underlined in this section and the effect of surgery for renal ischaemia is discussed.

DIAGNOSTIC TECHNIQUES AND ASSESSMENT
PROCEDURES IN VASCULAR SURGERY

© 1985 Grune & Stratton
ISBN 0-8089-1721-8 All rights reserved

In the next section a full range of preoperative assessment for lower limb ischaemia is covered and an interesting new test for the evaluation of the aorto-iliac segment is included. Most advances in this area concern tests that are being used at the time of operation. These concern assessment of peripheral resistance and hydraulic impedance. Vascular endoscopy has not become accepted in all parts of the world but it has been in regular usage in Germany in particular and is fully described here. The discovery of arterio-venous fistulae after in-situ vein bypass is described and thorough perioperative assessment for microvascular anastomoses is also discussed.

In practice, the levels for amputation for severe ischaemia are almost always determined by clinical assessment but the possible place of transcutaneous oxymetry and regional blood flow and blood pressure measurements predicting amputation wound healing are described. Problems in the upper limb concern hyperhidrosis, Raynauds phenomenon, and ischaemia from major vessel arterial disease. Essential investigations in these spheres are considered in the upper limb section. The detection and management of arterio-venous malformations have undergone great advances in the last 5 years, not least because of the ability to embolise the malformations from within. This has proved to be inordinately better than removing the malformations by surgery.

In the venous section, the value of venography and the application and the assessment of the deep venous system using noninvasive techniques is considered along with the novel use of Duplex scanning to detect venous thrombosis in the extremities.

The book concludes with a chapter by one of the great cardiovascular pioneer surgeons—Denton Cooley—and he discusses the development of vascular prostheses to meet the surgeon's requirements. In this chapter investigations and research and effort come together to show how management of our patients can be improved. It also becomes clear that many advances are only possible with total cooperation with the manufacturing industries. Surgical technique alone is not enough.

PART I

Principles of Investigation

Donald Silver

2

Haematological Aspects and Heparin

The only weapon with which the unconscious patient can immediately retaliate upon the incompetent surgeon is haemorrhage. If he bleeds to death, it may be presumed that the surgeon is to blame, whereas if he dies of infection, or shock, or from an unphysiological operative performance, the surgeon's incompetence may not be so evident.[1]

William Stewart Halsted

The hemostatic process arrests hemorrhage at the site of vascular injury. The careful, meticulous surgeon aids the hemostatic process with precise, sharp dissection and prompt control with hemostat, clip, cautery, or ligature of the severed vessels. Occasionally, the surgeon encounters bleeding that is caused by a defect(s) in the hemostatic process and cannot be controlled mechanically. This chapter will attempt to help the surgeon identify those patients who are bleeding, or likely to bleed, from congenital or acquired deficiencies of the hemostatic process. It must be emphasized, however, that bleeding is more often due to local, controllable causes than to defects in the hemostatic process. The chapter will also review the pharmacology and complications of heparin therapy.

HEMOSTASIS

Three complex, interrelated mechanisms acting in concert usually control bleeding from small disrupted vessels. These mechanisms are vessel wall contractions, platelet adherence and aggregation, and the formation of a fibrin clot. Early, or primary, hemostasis is achieved by vasoconstriction and the formation of platelet aggregates (the platelet plug). Later, or secondary, hemostasis reinforces and secures the platelet plug by incorporating it into a resilient fibrin clot. The resultant thrombus of platelets, fibrin and trapped cellular elements maintains hemostasis until vascular repair, or obliteration by scarring, has occurred. The thrombus is gradually dissolved by the fibrinolytic process or replaced by the process of organization.

DIAGNOSTIC TECHNIQUES AND ASSESSMENT
PROCEDURES IN VASCULAR SURGERY

© 1985 Grune & Stratton
ISBN 0-8089-1721-8 All rights reserved

Vessel Wall

The smooth muscle in small arteries and veins contracts when the vessels are injured and reduces or stops blood flow through the injured areas so that the formation of platelet aggregates and fibrin clots are enhanced. The vasoconstriction, which is less effective in larger arteries or veins, has neurogenic and myogenic components and may also be humorally induced, e.g., by thromboxane A_2 that is released from adherent platelets.

The blood vessels contain, in addition to smooth muscle, endothelial and supporting structures to maintain the integrity of the vascular bed. A number of congenital and acquired disorders (Table 2-1) that effect vascular integrity have been recognized. These disorders may contribute to formidable hemorrhage in the surgical or trauma patient. Although such bleeding is less common than that associated with defects of the other components of hemostasis, it is frequently difficult to recognize and manage.[2]

Table 2-1
Vascular Disorders

Hereditary
  Ehlors-Danlos Syndrome
  Marfan's Syndrome
  Hereditary Hemorrhagic Telangectasia
  Pseudoxanthoma Elasticum
  Osteogenesis Imperfecta

Acquired*
  Purpura (varied causes)
  Inflammatory
  Drug Induced
  Amyloidosis
  Diabetes
  Macroglobulinemia

* Most common and more likely to be associated with hemorrhage.

Platelets

Platelets are small, anuclear, disc-shaped cells that are produced by megakaryocytes. The circulating life for platelets is approximately 10 days with there usually being 200,000–400,000 platelets/mm^3 in human blood. The platelet is a very compact, complex "bundle" of energy (ATP, ADP, etc.), bioactive amines (serotonin, histamine, and catecholamines), coagulation proteins (fibrinogen, factor V, and factor VIII), procoagulants (platelet factor 3 [PF3]), and anticoagulants (platelet factor 4 [PF4]). Platelets have the ability to synthesize fatty acids (peroxy- and hydroxy- fatty acids) and phospholipids (prostaglandins i.e., thromboxane A_2, PGE_2, $PGF_{2\alpha}$ etc.).

Platelets normally do not adhere to each other or to normal vascular endothelium. Prostacyclin (PGI_2) produced by endothelial cells helps prevent this adhesion. Within seconds after injury, however, platelets begin to adhere to the injured vessel especially to exposed basement membrane and collagen. The rate of growth of the platelet plug is determined by the number of available platelets and the rate of blood flow, which at high rates may dislodge or disrupt the adherent platelets.

After adhesion, platelets undergo a change in shape and secrete bioactive substances such as ADP, ATP, and serotonin. The ADP, serotonin, epinephrine, thrombin, and thromboxane A_2 cause additional changes in the platelet surface that are conducive to adhesion of platelets to each other, i.e., platelet aggregation. This aggregation leads to the formation of the platelet plug.

Platelets supply procoagulant activity as PF3 and release coagulation factors, i.e., fibrinogen and factors V and VIII, during the early stages of aggregation. PF3 participates in the activation of factor X and the conversion of prothrombin to thrombin. The fibrin network formed by activation of the coagulation system helps stabilize the platelet hemostatic plug. Contraction of platelet microfilaments, in conjunction with activated factor XIII, leads to clot retraction. Platelet factor IV, released during aggregation, has heparin neutralizing activity.

Bleeding disorders may be caused by too few or too many platelets or by platelets with congenital or acquired storage or release disorders. Vascular integrity depends upon the presence of an undetermined platelet factor(s). Increased vascular fragility and permeability with extravascular accumulation of fluid and blood cells, i.e., petechiae, accompany severe, prolonged thrombocytopenia especially when the platelet count is in the $20,000/mm^3$ range. Bleeding may be associated with platelet counts less than $30,000/mm^3$ but rarely occurs in the presence of greater than $100,000/mm^3$ of normal platelets unless there are defects in the vasculature or coagulation mechanism. Surgery associated with limited blood loss can frequently be accomplished safely in patients with platelet counts as low as $30,000/mm^3$. An excessive number of platelets is more often associated with thrombosis than with bleeding but patients with sustained thrombocytosis may have bleeding. The platelet count in these patients is often above $1,000,000/mm^3$ and may be greater than $10,000,000/mm^3$. The bleeding is usually from the mucous membranes or gastrointestinal tract.

Qualitative platelet disorders should be suspected when bleeding occurs in the presence of normal tests of coagulation and normal platelet counts. The qualitative platelet disorders contribute to spontaneous bleeding less frequently than do the quantitative disorders. Abnormal platelet function is rarely the cause of significant bleeding but may exacerbate existing bleeding, e.g., after trauma or during surgery. Although qualitative platelet disorders maybe congenital, they are more often acquired. Many of the qualitative defects are caused by drugs that adversely affect platelet adhesion, release and/or aggregation, e.g., aspirin, dipyridamole, ibuprofen, antihistamines, etc.

Coagulation

The initial control of hemorrhage by vasoconstriction and the platelet plug is usually followed by the formation of a fibrin clot that maintains the hemostasis. Blood coagulation is the end result of a series of complex interrelated enzymatic reactions that involve the plasma coagulation factors. Twelve clotting factors have been identified and are numbered I–XIII; the original factor VI has subsequently been found not to be a true coagulation factor. Table 2-2 lists synonyms, plasma concentrations, and half lives of the coagulation factors.

Table 2-2

Coagulation Factors*

Factor	Synonym	Plasma half-life (hours)	Plasma concentration (mg/dl)	Vitamin K dependent
I	Fibrogen	90	200–400	No
II	Prothrombin	65	10	Yes
III	Tissue thromboplastin		0	No
IV	Calcium ion		4–5	No
V	Proaccelerin	15	1	No
VII	Proconvertin	6	0.05	Yes
VIII	Antihemophiliac factor A	12	1–2	No
IX	Antihemophiliac factor B (Christmas factor)	25	0.3	Yes
X	Stuart-Prower factor	40	1	Yes
XI	Plasma thromboplastin antecedent	45	0.5	No
XII	Hageman factor	50	3	No
XIII	Fibrin stabilizing factor	120	1–2	No

* All protein clotting factors, with the exception of factors III and VIII are synthesized in the liver. High-molecular weight kininogen and prekallikrein are involved in the initial phases of the intrinsic pathway and are considered by some to be coagulations factors.

The activation of factor X leads to the final pathway of coagulation, which includes the conversion of prothrombin to thrombin and the subsequent conversion of fibrinogen to fibrin. Factor X activation may occur through the activation of the intrinsic or extrinsic, or both, pathways of coagulation (Fig. 2-1). Injured tissues release tissue thromboplastin into the blood to form a complex with factor VII and calcium to activate factor X (the extrinsic system). The prothrombin time tests the efficiency of this system. The intrinsic coagulation sequence begins when factor XII is activated through contact with foreign surfaces, e.g., collagen or basement membrane. Activated XII activates the sequence of events that culminates in activation of factor X. The partial thromboplastin time is a good monitor of the extrinsic pathway. The initial fibrin is soluble. However, cross linking, by covalent bonds, of the fibrin polymer by activated factor XIII increases the stability of the clot and reduces its solubility. The two pathways are not distinct but are linked by the activation of factor IX by activated factor VII. It should be apparent that surgery and other forms of trauma can activate either, or both, pathways.

Disorders of coagulation may be caused by congenital or acquired deficiencies of the coagulation factors, inadequate replacement of coagulation factors during times of bleeding or consumption of coagulation factors by clotting at a faster rate than they can be replaced. Congenital deficiencies have been described for all of the clotting factors, excluding factors III and IV (Table 2-3). A deficiency may be characterized by reduced production of the clotting factor or by the production of a clotting factor that is antigentically similar but without procoagulant activity due to structural alterations. The congenital clotting disorders usually involve a single factor deficiency while the acquired deficiency disorders frequently have deficiencies of several factors. A patient with a congenital deficiency of a clotting factor may bleed only when stressed by surgery or trauma since only 5–10% of normal factor activity is needed to maintain hemostasis under normal conditions.

The most common congenital bleeding disorders, hemophilia and Christmas disease (hemophilia A and hemophilia B) are caused by deficient or defective production of factors VIII and IX respectively. The true incidence of hemophilia A is difficult to ascertain, but it is estimated that there are 3500–4000 patients with classical hemophilia in the United Kingdom and 15,000–20,000 in the United States.[3] The frequency of Christmas disease is 1/6–1/10 that of classic hemophilia, while von Willebrand's disease, another relatively common congenital disorder of hemostasis, has an incidence of 1/3–1/6 that of classic hemophilia. Patients with von Willebrand's disease have reduced levels of factor VIII-coagulant activity and the von Willebrand factor (produced by endothelial cells), which has an important role in the initial adherence of platelets to a surface and the subsequent aggregation process.

Acquired disorders of coagulation may be due to deficient production, deficient replacement, or excessive consumption of coagulation factors, or to anticoagulant therapy. All coagulation factors with the exception of tissue thromboplastin and factor VIII are made in the liver. Consequently, impaired hepatic function can lead to significant decreases in coagulation factor concentrations. Patients with vitamin K deficiency may have insufficient amounts of this cofactor for the synthesis of factors II, VII, IX, and X. Massive blood transfusions, e.g., 25 units per 24 hours or 5–6 units per hour to normal patients, and lesser amounts to patients with depressions of their coagulation proteins, may cause bleeding through dilution of the clot-

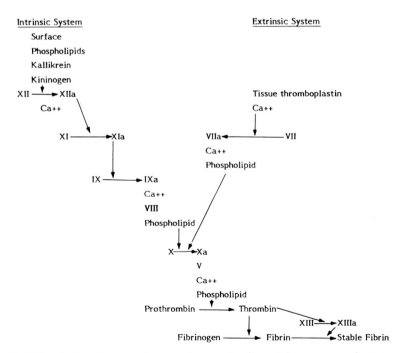

Fig. 2-1. Both pathways of coagulation are "activated" by surgery or by trauma.

Table 2-3
Congenital Coagulation Disorders

Deficiency	Manifestations	Inheritance	Incidence per 100,000 live births
Factor I	Serious neonatal and early bleeding	Autosomal recessive, both sexes	<0.05
Factor II	Serious neonatal and early bleeding	Autosomal recessive, both sexes	<0.05
Factor V	Mild, excessive bleeding early in life	Highly penetrant autosomal recessive affecting both sexes	0.1
Factor VII	Mild to moderate bleeding or purpura	Autosomal recessive, both sexes	Homozygous form, 0.25; heterozygous more common but may not cause bleeding
Factor VIII	Bleeding during infancy. Excessive bleeding following minor trauma, dental procedures, and minor	Sex-lined recessive with males as bleeders, females as carriers	4.0 Most common factor deficiency
Factor IX	Excessive bleeding following trauma or surgery	Sex-lined recessive with males as bleeders, females as carriers	1.0
Factor X	Mild bleeding in later life	Autosomal recessive, both sexes	Homozygous, 0.25; heterozygous, 20
Factor XI	Excessive bleeding following trauma or surgery. Bleeding may be delayed	Autosomal recessive, both sexes	0.1
Factor XII	Rarely associated with significant bleeding	Autosomal recessive, both sexes	0.1
Factor XIII	Neonatal bleeding is common with cord hemorrhage, echymoses, and hematomas	Autosomal recessive, both sexes	<0.05
von Willebrand's disease	Spontaneous, G.I. bleeding and easy bruisability	Autosomal dominant, both sexes	0.5–1.0

ting factors—especially the labile factors, V and VIII. A dilutional thrombocytopenia also frequently occurs with the transfusion of large volumes of bank blood. An increasing number of patients are receiving coumarins or heparin to reduce the incidence of recurrent deep venous thrombosis and/or pulmonary embolism and are prone to bleed from drug induced alterations of their coagulation mechanism.

Intravascular coagulation is usually controlled by the dilutional effect of the blood and the naturally occurring inhibitors. Usually, consumption of the coagulation factors by the clotting process does not exceed their rate of production and hemostasis remains intact. Occasionally, however, the rate of intravascular coagulation is excessive, e.g., with sepsis, amniotic fluid embolism, and incompatible blood transfusions so that the coagulation factors are consumed more rapidly than they can be produced. The depletion of fibrinogen, prothrombin, and factor V, VIII, IX, X, XII, and XIII, and platelets that occurs during a consumptive coagulopathy is frequently associated with bleeding.

Fibrinolysis

The fibrinolytic system exists to restore and maintain the patency of blood vessels and other structures that are at risk of being occluded by fibrin. Plasminogen, the inactive precursor of plasmin, circulates bound to fibrinogen and remains bound to fibrin. Plasminogen is converted to plasmin by a variety of activators. Plasmin preferentially digests fibrin but also digests fibrinogen, other coagulation factors, and plasma proteins. Fibrinolysis occurs whenever the plasmin produced exceeds the available antiplasmins. Excessive activation of plasminogen occurs most often as a response to diffuse intravascular clotting but may also occur with profound hypotension or hypoxemia, electric shock, extensive trauma,[4] or infusions of fibrinolytic activators, e.g., urokinase or streptokinase. The hyperfibrinolysis that occurs in response to a diffuse intravascular coagulation is called secondary fibrinolysis and occurs much more commonly than does a primary hyperfibrinolysis. Primary hyperfibrinolysis is an uncommon cause of bleeding. During surgery, hyperfibrinolysis may cause clots to lyse and may impair clotting by digesting the coagulation proteins. Intraoperative fibrinolysis is suspected when there is diffuse intraoperative bleeding, especially when there is bleeding from previously "dry" areas.

DIAGNOSIS

History

The clinical history is invaluable for detecting latent, and for defining active, hemorrhagic disorders. The family history should alert the physician to the possibility of an inherited bleeding disorder and should help distinguish a congenital disorder from an acquired one. The type of hemostatic disorder may be suspected from the pattern of inheritance. Hemophilia A and hemophilia B, two common disorders, have a X-linked recessive pattern of inheritance with the males being affected and the females transmitting the disease. Deficiencies of the other coagulation factors are less common, being transmitted as recessive disorders. The autosomal dominant disorders, e.g., hereditary hemorrhagic telangectasia, von Willebrand's disease, and others, afflict 50% of the members of the involved family.

The ages of onset of bleeding disorders are important. When excessive bleeding occurs with umbilical cord separation, with circumcision, with the minor trauma of childhood, or menses, an inherited bleeding diathesis should be suspected. Most of the acquired hemorrhagic disorders occur later in life, frequently in association with other disorders, e.g., hepatic or renal disease. It is useful to question patients about bleeding after tooth extractions, tonsillectomy, minor trauma, and surgical procedures. Excessive bleeding after any of these conditions requires careful laboratory evaluation while the absence of excessive blood loss makes it unlikely that the patient has an inherited bleeding disorder.

The type and sites of bleeding provide insight into the etiology of the bleeding. Petechiae are usually associated with platelet or vascular abnormalities, e.g., thrombocytopenia, von Willebrand's disease, and functional disorders of platelets while ecchymoses may occur with any of the bleeding disorders. The bleeding associated with platelet or vascular disorders is eventually, even hours later, controlled while the bleeding associated with coagulation defects is poorly controlled and is associated with hemarthroses, hematuria, retroperitoneal hematomas, and hematomas of the abdominal viscera. Congenital factor defects are usually the cause of hemarthroses.

Nose bleeds in young normotensive individuals are frequently associated with thrombocytopenia, von Willebrand's disease, or hereditary hemorrhagic telangectasia. Umbilical cord bleeding occurs in infants with factors XIII, VII, or I deficiency while excessive bleeding with circumcision may indicate the presence of hemophilia. Gastrointestinal bleeding may occur with many of the bleeding disorders and especially with excessive anticoagulation, thrombocytopenia, thrombocythemia, and von Willebrand's disease. Menorrhagia may be associated with any of the bleeding disorders. Bleeding from multiple sites, needle punctures, gastrointestinal tract, and areas of trauma may be caused by excessive anticoagulation, hyperfibrinolysis, or intravascular consumptive coagulation with a secondary hyperfibrinolysis.

The use of anticoagulants and/or drugs that alter platelet function may affect hemostasis and be responsible for bleeding. Hemorrhagic diatheses may be caused or aggrevated by liver or renal insufficiency, leukemia and collagen or vascular disorders.

Physical Examination

The physical examination should include an inspection for the presence and the distribution of petechiae, purpura, ecchymoses, hemangiomas, tumors, jaundice, hematomas, and hemarthroses. Ecchymoses occurring in combination with hematuria and gastrointestinal hemorrhage suggest the presence of an acquired coagulation defect. Hemarthroses and expanding hematomas are common sequlae of congenital coagulation factor deficiencies. Hemangiomas of skin and mucous membranes may help establish the diagnosis of hereditary hemorrhagic telangectasia.

The physical examination is useful in detecting disorders that accompany, or cause, coagulation problems. The large spleen may be responsible for the thrombocytopenia. The malignancy with secondary lymphadenopathy and/or hepatosplenomegaly may reduce clotting factor and platelet synthesis and/or accelerate their consumption through accelerated intravascular coagulation. Hepatic insuffiency may be associated with decreased production of coagulation factors, qualitative platelet disorders, and increased fibrinolytic activity. Several disorders are associated with "circulating anticoagulants," e.g., systemic lupus erythematous, malignancies, and some collagen disorders.[5] Bleeding from significant reductions of factors II, VII, IX, and X may occur during starvation, periods of intestinal sterilization, and in patients with altered fat absorption.

Laboratory Tests

"Screening tests" and, when indicated, specific tests are utilized in the laboratory evaluation of "bleeders" and "potential bleeders." The screening tests are utilized preoperatively for the majority of surgical patients who do not have a history or a family history of excessive bleeding and for whom the physical examination does not indicate the presence of hemostatic defect. A history and physical examination that do not suggest a bleeding disorder and normal results from the screening battery offer the surgeon a high level of assurance that the patient is hemostatically competent preoperatively.

The most commonly utilized screening tests include the prothrombin time (PT), partial thromboplastin time (PTT), thrombin time (TT), platelet count, and template bleeding time (Table 2-4). The PT is a measure of clotting initiated by the extrinsic pathway of coagulation. It is prolonged by deficiencies of factors I, II, V, VII, and X and by inhibitors of coagulation, e.g., heparin. The PT is especially sensitive to reductions of factors VII, V, and X. The PTT measures the plasma's intrinsic coagulation activity and is prolonged by deficiencies or inhibitors to the clotting factors of the intrinsic pathway. The PTT does not detect deficiencies of factor VII or XIII. The TT measures the ability of thrombin to convert fibrinogen to fibrin and is prolonged in the presence of low fibrinogen, abnormal fibrinogen, heparin, and fibrin, and fibrinogen degradation products. The platelet count will detect quantitative deficiencies of platelets. Spontaneous or excessive bleeding is unusual when more than $30,000/mm^3$ of normally active platelets are available. The template bleeding time measures the interactions of platelet and the vessel wall, i.e., the formation of the hemostatic plug.[6] The bleeding time is prolonged by quantitative and/or qualitative deficiencies of platelets, decreases of coagulation factors I and V and von Willebrand's factor and by vessel wall abnormalities. Tests of fibrinolysis are not done routinely preoperatively because primary hyperfibrinolysis is extremely rare and secondary hyperfibrinolysis usually accompanies intravascular coagulation.

The screening tests help the surgeon to detect, preoperatively, most patients with hemostatic defects. When the screening tests are abnormal, specific factor assays and tests for circulating inhibitors, platelet function, fibrinolytic activity, and fibrin solubility may be required to determine, and correct, specific defects of hemostasis.

The nonmechanical intraoperative bleeding encountered by surgeons is much more likely to be caused by acquired defects of the hemostatic mechanisms than congenital ones. The acquired defects include the thrombocytopenia and/or factor deficiency, especially V and VIII, that occurs during the replacement of brisk blood

Table 2-4
Screening Tests

Test	Function	Interpretation
Prothrombin time	Assays integrity of extrinsic system, especially factors I, II, V, VII, and X	Prolonged by reductions of vitamin K dependent factors (II, V, VII and X) and fibrinogen. A prolonged PT and a normal PTT indicate factor VII deficiency
Partial thromboplastin time	Tests for deficiency of all protein coagulation factors except factor VII	*Prolonged by reduction of any factor except VII, and by von Willebrand's disease
Thrombin time	Tests the conversion of prothrombin to thrombin	Prolonged by low fibrinogen, heparin, and fibrin and degradation products
Platelet count	Normal 200,000–400,000/mm^3	Spontaneous bleeding unlikely if $> 30,000$/mm^3. 50,000 to 100,000/mm^3 required to contain bleeding
Template bleeding time	Normal bleeding time four to ten minutes	Prolonged in afibrinogenemia, von Willebrand's disease, thrombocytopenia, and qualitative platelet defects

* A prolonged PTT in a non-bleeder suggests factor XII or high molecular-weight kininogen deficiency, or the presence of heparin.

loss with large quantities of older bank blood. The other common causes of acquired surgical bleeding are the bleeding associated with a consumptive coagulopathy and the accompanying secondary hyperfibrinolysis.[7] The acquired bleeding usually occurs in patients with major trauma and/or major surgery. The intravascular coagulation that accompanies gram negative sepsis, large aneurysms, giant hemangiomas, AV fistulae, major trauma, retained fetus and so forth may not consume the coagulation factors sufficiently to cause bleeding preoperatively. However, surgery may increase the consumption of the factors, which will only be partially replaced with the older bank blood, and bleeding will ensue.

Intraoperative, nonmechanical bleeding seems to have two major forms. The surgeon may note that all incised surfaces bleed excessively and continuously and no clots are forming. This type of bleeding represents platelet and/or factor(s) deficiency. On the other hand, the surgeon may notice that previously "dry" surfaces are bleeding and that incised surfaces continue to bleed. This type of bleeding suggests the presence of hyperfibrinolysis, usually in addition to platelet and factor(s) deficiency.

The initial evaluation of intraoperative bleeding includes the PT, PTT, platelet count, fibrinogen assay, and whole blood or euglobulin lysis times (Table 2-5). A

Table 2-5
Evaluation of Intraoperative Bleeding

	PT	PTT	Platelets	Lysis Times	Fibrinogen
Platelet Deficiency	N*	N	L*	N	N
Factor(s) Deficiency	P or N	P*	N	N	N or L
Consumptive coagulopathy	P	P	L	N	L
with increased lysis	P	P	L	S*	L
Primary Hyperfibrinolysis	P	P	N	S	L

* N = normal; L = low; P = prolonged; S = shortened.

normal platelet count and shortened lysis times with prolongation of the PT and PTT, and reduced fibrinogen suggest that the bleeding is from hyperfibrinolysis. A low platelet count, prolonged PT and PTT and reduced fibrinogen with an accelerated lysis suggest that the bleeding is from intravascular consumption of the coagulation factors and a secondary hyperfibrinolysis. A low platelet count with the rest of the results being nearly normal indicates the need for platelet transfusions, while a prolonged PT and/or PTT suggest the need for factor(s) replacement. There is usually not time during intraoperative bleeding to test for specific coagulation factor deficiencies. Therefore, all factors are replaced with fresh frozen plasma and/or cryoprecipate until hemostasis is secured or the PT and PTT become less than 1.5 times the control times. If hyperfibrinolysis persists after the intravascular coagulation is controlled, or if the hyperfibrinolysis is primary, a fibrinolytic inhibitor, epislonaminocaproic acid, may be required to control bleeding.

Summary

Congenital disorders of hemostasis can be detected preoperatively by careful history, physical examination, and a battery of screening, and frequently specific, tests. The identification of the disorder allows the surgeon to correct the deficiency preoperatively and to plan an operation that will minimize blood loss. The factor replacement is continued postoperatively until wound healing is complete. Acquired disorders of hemostasis may occur intraoperatively and require coordinated efforts between the surgeon, coagulation lab, and blood bank for identification and correction of the disorders. Platelet transfusions and transfusions of fresh frozen plasma will correct most acquired disorders of hemostasis. Occasionally, when bleeding is from excessive fibrinolytic activity, fibrinolytic inhibitors are also required.

HEPARIN

Heparin was discovered by McLean in 1916[8] and was entered into clinical trials in 1935.[9] By 1960,[10] its important role in the management of venous thromboembolism had been established. The ability of heparin, given intravenously, to promptly prevent the coagulation of blood during surgery, even during times of cessation of blood flow, has allowed cardiovascular surgeons to develop and perform a variety of complex operations without worrying about intravascular coagulation. Heparin has such a prominent role in the management of vascular disorders, with over one trillion units of heparin utilized yearly, that it behooves the vascular surgeon to be familiar with its pharmacology and complications.

Pharmacology

Heparin is a highly sulfated mucopolysaccharide, a linear anionic poly-electrolyte, which occurs in all animals above the horseshoe crab. Heparin is composed of alternating residues of uronic acid and glucosamine. The uronic acids and the glucosamine residues exist as a variety of moieties, causing heparin to exhibit considerable polydispersity in molecular size, charge, and activity. Even "purified" commercial heparin, which is usually extracted from the lung or intestinal mucosa, contains polysaccharide chains with molecular weights that vary from 3000 to 40,000 daltons. It appears that 85% of the anticoagulant activity of commercial heparin resides in one-third of the heparin mass.[11]

Heparin has no anticoagulant activity of its own. It requires the presence of antithrombin III (AT-III), a serine protease inhibitor, for its anticoagulant effect. Heparin accelerates the neutralization by AT-III of thrombin and other activated coagulation proteins that are also serine proteases. The heparin-ATIII complex inactivates thrombin quite rapidly. After the heparin-ATIII complex combines with thrombin or other serine proteases, the heparin is released to combine with another AT-III molecule. Activated factor X is the clotting factor most sensitive to inactivation by the heparin-ATIII complex. Inhibition of one unit of activated factor X prevents the potential generation of more than fifty units of thrombin; this amplifying action is responsible for the "mini-dose" heparin effect in thromboembolism prophylaxis.[12]

Clinical Applications

Heparin utilization by the vascular surgeon falls into four major categories: (1) prophylaxis for venous thromboembolism; (2) management of venous thromboembolism; (3) prevention of intravascular thrombosis during vascular reconstruction; and (4) maintenance of patency of indwelling arterial and venous monitoring and infusion lines.

Numerous studies have demonstrated the effectiveness of low dose heparin (5000–10,000 units every 12 hours or 5000 units every 8 hours) in reducing the incidence of venous thrombosis in all types of patients.[13] When utilized in surgical patients, the first 5000 units of heparin is given 2 hours preoperatively. Studies have shown that the incidence of venous thrombosis may be reduced from 30 to 50% in untreated patients to 6 to 12% in treated patients.[13,14] Intraoperative blood loss has not been increased significantly by the heparin.

Heparin's role in the management of patients with deep venous thrombosis and/or pulmonary embolism is well established. The heparin serves to stop the clotting process and clot propagation, to allow and enhance thrombolysis[15] and to reduce the incidence of recurrences. Large amounts of heparin are required during the early management of the deep venous thrombosis or pulmonary embolism to stop the intravascular coagulation. Initial "loading" doses of heparin of 400 units/kg are given intravenously and are followed by a continuous infusion of sufficient amounts (usually 800–1200 units/hour) to keep the PTT at 2–2½ times the control. Bleeding rarely occurs when the PTT remains at this level. The doses are reduced in the postmenopausal female because of her tendency to bleed while anticoagulated. The intravenous heparin is continued for 10–14 days and is followed by self-administered subcutaneous heparin, 5000 units every 8 hours for 3 months, or by warfarin therapy, which keeps the PTT twice the control for 3 months. Of course, other measures are instituted to reduce recurrences, e.g., elastic stockings, avoiding positions of stasis and so forth.

Heparin is used to prevent intravascular coagulation during vascular surgical procedures. The heparin may be infused into the involved vascular system before, or immediately after, clamps are applied. However, most often heparin is given, prior to clamp application, intravenously in sufficient amounts to produce a temporarily incoagulable state. The amount of heparin required varies according to the procedure and the patient's size. The author utilizes 5000–6000 units of heparin intravenously for a carotid endarterectomy. Seven thousand units of heparin with an additional 1000 units at the end of each hour that clamps are in place are utilized for extended surgical procedures, e.g., aorto-femoro-popliteal bypass. The short, 90 minute half life of heparin and the fact that, if mechanical hemostasis is secured, bleeding will not occur negate the need for heparin neutralization in most cases.

The vascular surgeon should be aware that many other health care professionals also use heparin. Radiologists and cardiologists use heparin during their catheterization procedures. Small continuous amounts of heparin are utilized by intensive care nurses to maintain patency of in dwelling arterial and venous lines. Heparin may be added by pharmacists to infusates that promote vascular irritation or thrombosis, e.g., parenteral nutrition. It is important that the surgeon read the label of all solutions given to his patients; he will be surprised at the number of solutions that contain heparin.

Complications

Most failures of heparin therapy are iatrogenic and are related to the use of heparin in patients with contraindications to anticoagulation, to the utilization of insufficient amounts of heparin, to delaying the beginning of prophylactic regimens, and to using heparin in patients with heparin sensitivities and/or congenital deficiencies of antithrombin III. If patients with ATIII deficiencies and heparin antibodies are excluded, most failures of heparin therapy will be related to the administration of insufficient amounts of heparin or to utilizing heparin for improper reasons, e.g., venous obstruction by tumor rather than thrombosis.

Hemorrhage is the most common complication of heparin therapy. It occurs in 7–10% of patients receiving heparin and varies according to the dose, mode of administration, and indication for treatment. The postmenopausal patient is most sensitive to heparin and is the patient most likely to bleed. Therefore, she requires smaller doses and careful monitoring. The author has rarely seen heparin cause bleeding in patients whose PTTs were less than 80 seconds. However, bleeding is not uncommon in patients whose PTTs are greater than 100 seconds for more than 24 hours. If bleeding is caused by heparin, it is usually controlled by merely stopping the administration of heparin. If the bleeding is excessive, the circulating heparin can be neutralized with protamine sulfate. The amount of protamine required can be calculated from the results of a protamine titration test. If the protamine titration test cannot be done $1-1\frac{1}{2}$ mg protamine are usually given to neutralize 100 units of heparin. One usually utilizes half the calculated amount of protamine, which is given slowly to reduce the risk of hypotension and brachycardia. If bleeding continues, additional small amounts of protamine may be given slowly at 5–10 minute intervals.

Despite attempts to purify heparin, sensitivity reactions continue with 2–5% of patients having mild reactions such as bronchial constriction, lacrimation, urticaria, and rhinitis. Anaphylaxis with circulatory collapse is a very rare complication of heparin therapy. Osteoporosis and alopecia have been noted in patients receiving heparin for greater than 6 months. The alopecia usually resolves after cessation of the heparin. The incidence of alopecia is higher when oral anticoagulants are also administered.

Thrombocytopenia

Clinically insignificant thrombocytopenia was first noted in animals in 1941[16] and subsequently in humans. A heparin induced thrombocytopenia that is associated with serious thrombosis and hemorrhage was described in 1973.[17] The heparin induced thrombocytopenia occurs in the absence of excessive intravascular coagulation and appears to be caused by a heparin induced antiplatelet antibody, which, in the presence of heparin, causes platelet aggregation with thrombocytopenia and thrombohemorrhagic complications. The heparin induced thrombocytopenia occurs in 0.6–9% of patients receiving heparin and is independent of source, amount, or route of heparin administration.[18,19] Recent experiences suggest that about 2% of our patients receiving heparin are at risk for developing this disorder.

The heparin induced thrombocytopenia usually occurs after 5–15 days of initial heparin therapy (mean 8.8 days) or after 1–9 days (mean 5 days) of recurrent heparin therapy.[18] The disorder is heralded by falling platelet counts and increased heparin resistance that is manifested by requiring increasing amounts of heparin to maintain a stable PTT. If the disorder is not recognized and, if heparin is continued, platelet aggregation with thrombosis and/or hemorrhage will occur. The heparin thrombocytopenia has been associated with a 23% mortality and an 84% morbidity.[18]

Over 100 cases of heparin induced thrombocytopenia have been studied by the author and his associates. In order to reduce the serious complications of this disorder, it is recommended that all patients receiving initial heparin therapy have platelet counts daily after day four of heparin therapy and all patients receiving recurrent heparin therapy have daily platelet counts. Any patient who develops new thrombosis, whose platelet count falls below 100,000/mm^3, or whose heparin requirements increase should have platelet aggregation testing. If the aggregation testing is positive, heparin therapy *must* be discontinued. At the time heparin is discontinued, the author usually institutes aspirin (300 mg, twice a day) and persantine (50 mg, four times a day) therapy and coumadin anticoagulation if the need for anticoagulation persists. The thrombohemorrhagic complications will continue until heparin is discontinued.

SUMMARY

Heparin is used daily by vascular surgeons in the operative and nonoperative management of their patients. When used in sufficient amounts and for proper indications, heparin has great therapeutic benefit. The most serious complication of heparin therapy, the heparin induced thrombocytopenia syndrome, requires platelet monitoring in all patients receiving heparin and aggregation testing in any patient with new thrombosis or a falling platelet count. The complications of heparin can usually be managed by stopping the infusion, treating the symptoms, and interfering, when indicated, with the coagulation process with other anticoagulants. If the vascular surgeon is knowledgeable about the pharmacology and complications of heparin, he will be able to utilize heparin in his practice with confidence.

REFERENCES

1. Halsted WS: The effect of ligation of the common iliac artery on the circulation and function of lower extremity. Report of the cure of iliofemoral aneurism by the application of an aluminum band to that vessel. Johns Hopkins Hospital Bulletin 23:191, 1912
2. Bick RL: Vascular disorders associated with thrombohemorrhagic phenomena. Seminars in Thrombosis and Hemostasis 5:167, 1979
3. U.S. Department of Health, Education and Welfare, (NIH) 77-1274, 1980, Study to Evaluate Supply-Demand Relationships for AHF and PTC through 1980
4. Kapsch DN, Metzler M, Harrington M, et al: Fibrinolytic response to trauma. Surgery 95:473, 1984
5. Margolius A Jr, Jackson DP, Ratnoff OD: Circulating anticoagulants: A study of 40 cases and a review of the literature. Medicine 40:145, 1961
6. Mielke CH Jr, Kaneshiro MM, Maher IA, et al: The standardized normal ivy bleeding time and its prolongation by aspirin. Blood 34:204, 1969
7. Spero JA, Lewis JH, Hasiba U: Dessiminated intravascular coagulation. Findings in 346 patients. Thrombosis and Haemostasis 43:28, 1980
8. McLean J: The thromboplastic action of cephalin. American Journal Physiology 41:250, 1916
9. McLean J: The discovery of heparin. Circulation 19:75, 1959
10. Barritt DW, Jordan SC: Anticoagulant drugs in the treatment of pulmonary embolism. A controlled trial. Lancet 1:1309, 1960
11. Lam LH, Silbert JE, Rosenberg RD: The separation of active and inactive forms of heparin. Biochemical Biophysical Research Communication 69:570, 1976
12. Yin ET, Wessler S, Stoll PJ: Identity of plasma-activated factor X inhibitor with antithrombin III and heparin cofactor. Journal of Biological Chemistry 246:3712, 1971
13. Kakkar VV: Prevention of venous thromboembolism. Clinics in Haematology 10:543, 1981
14. Rosenow EC III, Osmundson PJ, Brown ML: Pulmonary embolism. Mayo Clinical Proceedings 56:161, 1981
15. Silver D, Hall JH: Effect of heparin on the fibrinolytic system. Surgical Forum 17:11, 1966
16. Copley AL, Robb TP: The effect of heparin on the platelet count in dogs and mice. American Journal of Physiology 133:P248, 1941

17. Rhodes GR, Dixon RH, Silver D: Heparin induced thrombocytopenia with thrombotic and hemorrhagic manifestations. Surgical Gynecology and Obstetics 136:409, 1973
18. Silver D, Kapsch DN, Tsoi E: Heparin-induced thrombocytopenia thrombosis and hemorrhage. Annuals of Surgery 198:301, 1983
19. Ansell J, Slepchuk N Jr, Kumar R, et al: Heparin induced thrombocytopenia: a prospective study. Thrombosis and Haemostasis 43:61, 1980

Charles N. McCollum

3

The Value of Radiolabelled Cells

Vascular disease exerts a wide range of crippling and life-threatening effects, usually as a result of occlusion or embolisation. In the vast majority of cases both effects are the result of the formation of a thrombus on diseased intima which may detach as emboli or continue to accumulate, ultimately resulting in occlusions. The vascular surgeon also must deal with aneurysmal disease where weakness of the arterial wall is the main concern. Even where this is the case, the redundant lumen is usually occupied by thrombus although in these cases thromboembolic complications, although not rare, are surprisingly infrequent.

The same processes are perhaps even more important in the cause of failure following arterial reconstruction. This is particularly true as all reconstructions involve areas of trauma to the intima, and most result in the loss of endothelium over extensive areas. As a result the process of thrombus formation is initiated by contact activation and platelet adhesions. Over the years many attempts have been made to measure these phenomena because of the important implications in the evaluation and development of procedures, prostheses, and medications for use in this field. These methods of evaluation were initially inprecise; researchers depended predominantly on the measurement of secondary phenomena such as platelet release factors or changes in platelet survival measured by ^{51}Cr-labelled platelets. More recently, labelling techniques have improved such that the isotope ^{111}Indium can be used as a stable label for platelets. This isotope has many advantages: it has a half life of 2.81 days, thus permitting the study of in vivo phenomena over a one-week period, and it has high energy gamma emmissions that produce quality images on a gamma camera. As a result, radiolabelled cells have been used in a variety of applications in surgical research, and their potential role in the field of clinical diagnosis is becoming apparent. In this chapter we shall consider the value of radiolabelled platelets and leucocytes, emphasising the clinical applications as they are relevant to the vascular surgeon.

DIAGNOSTIC TECHNIQUES AND ASSESSMENT
PROCEDURES IN VASCULAR SURGERY
© 1985 Grune & Stratton
ISBN 0-8089-1721-8 All rights reserved

RADIOLABELLED PLATELETS

[111]Indium was first reported as a platelet label by Thackur et al in 1976.[1] The technique has now been improved for use in labelling platelets from small volumes of venous blood by incubating the platelets with Indium oxine in a plasma-free suspension.[2] Using these techniques, the dose of isotope that can safely be administered is limited by splenic irradiation at 7.4 mGy/MBq (27.4 rad/mCi),[3] a splenic dose very similar to that we have observed in our patients. This permits the safe administration of approximately 200 μCi for routine diagnostic or research purposes, although the clinician may need to administer higher doses in individual patients. Radiolabelled platelets may be used for the detection of arterial and venous thrombi, and as a result, their main clinical application is in the detection of deep-vein thrombosis and the source of both arterial and venous emboli. In discussing their value in these fields it is relevant to examine how these cells have been used in the measurement of thrombus formation on prosthetic surfaces where their kinetics are now fairly well understood.

Measurements of Vascular Graft Thrombogenicity

It is well recognized that platelets are intimately involved in the process that leads to thrombosis of prosthetic vascular grafts. Furthermore it seems likely that they are of equal importance in the early period after the implantation of saphenous vein grafts. As the failure rate in femoropopliteal grafts is relatively high, any technique that purports to measure the rate of thrombus formation is eagerly evaluated. The clinical relevance of ^{111}In-platelet deposition on vascular grafts was assessed in a series of 67 femoropopliteal bypass patients.[4] Autologous Indium-labelled platelets were injected on the seventh day after graft insertion and the radioactivity of the graft and the opposite thigh (as a reference) was measured daily for one week. Platelet uptake was expressed as the daily increase in the rate of radioactivity graft over reference and called thrombogenicity index (TI). The TI for Dacron® grafts was significantly greater than that for PTFE, and both prosthetic grafts accumulated platelets much faster than vein (Fig. 3-1). The clinically more significant findings relate to the relationship between TI and subsequent graft patency. All patients were followed for one year and the patency of the graft at 12 months was compared with the TI that had been measured one week after surgery. It was found that in the grafts that subsequently occluded the mean ($\pm$ SEM) TI were 0.19 ± 0.018, compared with 0.07 ± 0.009 in those patients whose grafts remained patent. The importance of these results are illustrated in Figure 3-2 where the patency by life table is plotted for those grafts with a platelet uptake in the lower half of the range (TI less than the median) and compared to those with platelet uptake in the upper half of the range (TI greater than median). At 12 months the cumulative patency of those grafts with a TI greater than the median was 90% compared with 39% when the rate of platelet deposition was in the upper half of the range ($P < 0.001$). These results emphasize the significance of measuring the rate of platelet deposition, particularly as neither the indication for surgery, the position of the distal anastomosis above or below the knee, nor the state of the run-off vessels on angiography significantly influenced patency by life table in this series.

The clinical application of such a technique may be the use of radiolabelled

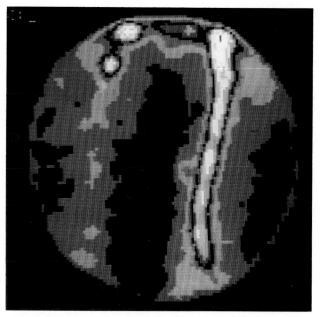

Fig. 3-1. The left femoropopliteal graft using poly-
tetrafluorethylene is imaged five days after the injection of
autologous ^{111}In platelets and demonstrates the accumulation
of platelets in the thrombus on its luminal surface.

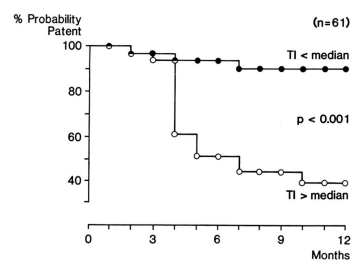

Fig. 3-2. The TI was measured in 61 patients using ^{111}In-platelets one week after surgery
and was related to subsequent graft patency plotted by life table. Those grafts with a TI in the
upper half of the range had a cumulative patency of only 39% compared with 90% in those
with a TI below the median.

platelets shortly after the insertion of a bypass graft to assess the risk of failure. It could be argued that patients with a high TI should receive platelet inhibitory drugs, a course that may not be indicated in those with a low TI. While this approach is logical, the technique is unlikely to gain wide application as most hospitals do not have, and are unlikely to get, adequate facilities for the routine labelling of blood cells. The realistic value of this technique is more for the evaluation of new prosthetic materials or potential antithrombotic drugs. It is hoped that with these initial assessments, clinical trials will only be required for those materials or drugs that can be shown to be at least as good as the current alternatives.

Locating the Source of Emboli

The vascular surgeon is often confronted with a patient with an ischaemic lesion but no evidence of significant occlusive arterial disease. It is usually presumed that there is either thrombosis or arteritis affecting the small distal vessels or that an embolus has lodged in these vessels arising from the heart or disease of the arterial tree at some proximal site. Echography has been used to detect sources within the heart on the assumption that some residual thrombus or filling defect will still be present. The assessment of potential sources of emboli in the large arteries has been particularly difficult. There was no method for detecting a thrombogenic lesion and the demonstration of anatomical disease does not necessarily indicate that this is the source of emboli. We have now investigated 11 patients with clinical signs strongly suggestive of embolization to the legs. Among these patients, six lesions were found to accumulate radiolabelled platelets and were imaged on the gamma camera. These included two small popliteal aneurysms, localized uptake in the superficial femoral and common iliac in two individuals, and uptake related to the distal anastomosis of an axillofemoral and an aortofemoral graft in two patients. Specific applications for the detection of sources of emboli are particularly related to the diagnosis of aneurysm, carotid disease, and deep venous thrombosis. Each of these topics is now discussed in turn.

Aneurysms

As a diseased artery dilates, blood flow within its lumen becomes turbulent and often relatively stagnant near the arterial wall. As a result thrombus is usually deposited and the lumen is reduced to the size of the nonaneurysmal arteries proximal and distally. As the flow surface is not endothelialized, an aneurysm will image using radiolabelled platelets and can therefore be detected by this means. Clearly, abdominal aortic aneurysms are more easily assessed by palpation or ultrasound examination. As radiolabelled cell scintigraphy is not going to give clarity of image sufficient to assess the anatomical extent of an aneurysm, its main value is merely in detecting smaller aneurysms such as those affecting the popliteal or subclavian arteries. Usually, these aneurysms cause symptom by virtue of distal embolization and the request for Indium platelet studies is based on the desire to find a proximal source.

To date we have imaged over 20 aneurysms, either to detect the source of emboli or incidentally during radiolabelled platelet investigations for other reasons. During a study on platelet uptake in aneurysms we have found that 10 of 11 confirmed aneurysms were imaged using radiolabelled platelets (Fig. 3-3). The radioac-

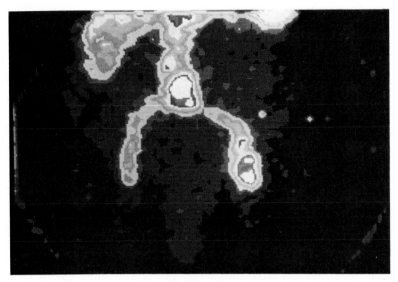

Fig. 3-3. The gamma image in this patient demonstrates accumulation of radiolabelled cells in an abdominal aneurysm.

tivity over the aneurysm was nearly double that over the adjacent normal artery. In general, larger aneurysms of the aorta had a greater ratio of radioactivity to normal arteries than the smaller false or popliteal aneurysms with (mean aneurysm uptake ratio, 2.02 compared with 1.41, respectively). The dilemma in managing patients with popliteal aneurysms is deciding whether these aneurysms require repair. Where distal embolization has occurred and ischaemic symptoms resulted, then repair is urgent as the limb is known to be threatened. However, we often find popliteal aneurysms in the vascular clinic while following up patients with other arterial disease, particularly following aortic aneurysm surgery. In these cases it is far from clear whether surgery is required as the prognosis for aneurysms of different size is uncertain. Currently we tend to repair the large aneurysms and follow the small ones. It is possible that it may be more logical to investigate the thrombogenicity and repair only those that are more active in taking up radiolabelled platelets.

Carotid Disease

Extracranial arterial disease is thought to be the cause of both transient cerebral ischaemia and stroke in more than half the affected patients. The incidence of this major arterial disease, particularly affecting the origin of the internal carotid, is still higher in patients with cerebral infarction which can now be precisely distinguished from intracerebral haemorrhage by computerized tomography. Despite this knowledge and considerable advances in noninvasive techniques for the detection of stenoses in the carotid artery, we still cannot identify the pathophysiology of individual events of cerebral ischaemia. In some cases, a tight stenosis of the carotid will impair blood flow and produce symptoms by depriving the brain of blood. Alternatively, artheromatous disease or ulcerated plaques may promote thrombosis and distal embolization to produce identical symptoms. Finally, and to add further confusion, many critical stenoses may be causing symptoms not by blood starvation but

Table 3-1
111-In Images Related to Angiographic Findings in
18 Patients with Carotid Disease

	Angiogram			
[111]In Images	Stenosis >80%	Atheromatous Plaque	Normal or Minimal Disease	Total
Positive	5	11	5	21
Negative	5	1	8	14
Total	10	12	13	35

Note. Data are no. of patients. Sensitivity was 73% (16 of 22), and specificity was 61% (8 of 13).

rather by promoting the formation of emboli in the turbulence distal to the stenosis. Whereas the clinician has excellent tools[5] for the evaluation of stenoses impairing blood flow, there have been no techniques enabling thrombogenicity to be evaluated.

Radiolabelled platelets were used in the assessment of 25 patients with unilateral transient cerebral ischaemia.[6] Following the injection of autologous ^{111}In-platelets, gamma images were taken over a period of two to five days (Fig. 3-4). These images were reported by a physicist who was not familiar with the patient's clinical details and the results were compared with angiography and Doppler assessment of the degree of stenosis. Twenty-two lesions were seen on angiography and were divided into stenosis of more than 80% luminal diameter or artheromatous ulcers (Table 3-1). Radiolabelled platelet uptake to produce positive images occurred in 11 of the 12 atheromatous plaques and 5 of the 10 stenoses. Interestingly, platelet uptake was also reported in 5 of the 13 arteries classified as normal or minimal disease on angiography. As Doppler ultrasound reliably detects stenoses of this grade, there was only one patient with significant carotid disease on angi-

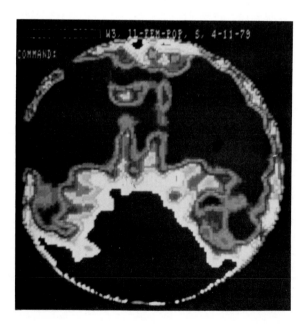

Fig. 3-4. This patient had experienced transient left hemiparesis on several occasions in less than one month prior to this gamma image taken 48 hours after injection of autologous radiolabelled platelets. Their accumulation at the right carotid bifurcation is obvious. This "hot spot" was removed at carotid endarterectomy.

ography that was not detected by the combination of the two relatively noninvasive tests (ultrasound and radiolabelled platelet imaging). Therefore, it could be argued that this combination of investigations may be used in the initial assessment of patients with carotid disease. However, it is probably more realistic to accept that the main value of the test is in determining the source of cerebral emboli in those patients where no important stenosis is detected by Doppler imaging or duplex scanning. This approach is particularly pertinent as it is in these patients, (that is, without critical stenosis), that platelet inhibitory drug therapy may be all that is required.

A further potential use for radiolabelled cells is to evaluate the risk of stroke in individual patients. It is conceivable that distinguishing patients with thrombogenic stenoses from those with nonactive stenoses and patients with ulcerated plaques that attract platelets from those that do not may help in the prediction of stroke risk in patients already evaluated by duplex or Doppler imaging systems. This principle is being studied but of necessity we must await follow up for three years before we can assess whether these techniques have any predicted value. It is to be hoped that we will have an earlier clue from the assessment of radiolabelled platelet uptake following carotid endarterectomy and subsequent clinical events.[8] Although again this association can only be made once follow-up has been completed in an adequate number of patients for at least 12 months.

Deep Vein Thrombosis

It is well recognized that the diagnosis of deep vein thrombosis on the basis of clinical signs is both difficult and frequently incorrect. This is particularly true following pulmonary emboli where there may be little or no signs of venous thrombosis in either leg. The plethora of diagnostic techniques available, including Doppler flow, impedence plethysmography, thermography, and various isotope methods, demonstrate that none is entirely satisfactory. The main drawbacks are that the techniques that depend on measuring flow disturbance will only detect occlusion of major veins. I^{125}-fibrinogen has been widely used as a research method for detecting deep vein thrombosis but has little value in clinical diagnosis as the isotope must be circulating while the thrombus is forming. Furthermore it is excreted in the bladder and is a poor gamma emitter, effectively preventing useful imaging, particularly in the pelvis.

As there must always be a surface contact between the thrombus and flowing blood, platelet deposition can be anticipated. This approach has been investigated with sufficient numbers of patients to confirm its value.[8,9] The sensitivity and specificity reported by Fenech et al were 95% and 100% respectively,[9] but a number of false-negative images were obtained in the series by Grimly et al which included patients already on heparin for up to three weeks after the venous thrombosis.[8] It is reasonable to conclude that this technique is of particular value in patients where the thrombus is recent or is still extending. Clinically, the most exciting application is in the detection of the source of pulmonary emboli, Figure 3-5 demonstrates the radiolabelled platelet and venography findings in a patient (age, 68 years) with right heart failure due to multiple small pulmonary emboli. The gamma image clearly shows dramatic radiolabelled platelet uptake on a small tongue of thrombus extending from the left profunda femoral into the common femoral vein. The image of the chest also shows a recent embolus lodged in the apex of the right lobe of the lung.

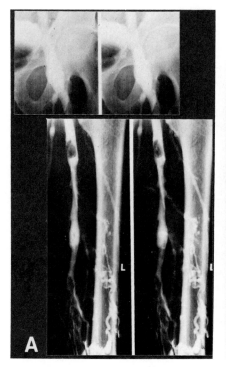
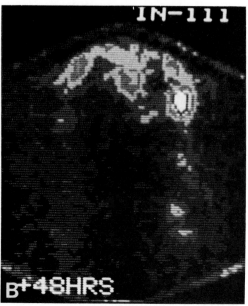

Fig. 3-5. Multiple pulmonary emboli were thought to be the cause of unremitting right heart failure in this patient. The radiolabelled platelet study demonstrates marked localized uptake in the left upper thigh (B). On venography a tongue of thrombus is seen emerging from the profunda femoris into the common femoral vein (A).

Where the clinician has access to radiolabelled platelet techniques the investigation of deep vein thrombosis may be his predominant indication. The reasons for this are that the technique is accurate for the detection of recent thrombi and is very much less invasive than venography. It is possible that it would be more precise in the detection of small thrombi than venography and certainly more sensitive at detecting those areas of a thrombus that are actively extending or behaving as a source of emboli. For these reasons we usually use ^{111}In-platelets as our primary investigation in deep vein thrombosis. It must be remembered, however, that this technique will not distinguish the "free floating" nonocclusive thrombi that may detach to produce massive pulmonary emboli from the relatively innocuous totally occluding and well-adherent thrombi. For this reason patients with clinical evidence of extensive iliac and pelvic thrombi should have early venography as protective measures, such as vena caval filtration, as necessary.

RADIOLABELLED LEUCOCYTES

The most important single cause of mortality in patients with postoperative sepsis is delay in diagnosis. All the difficulties inherent in locating an abscess are particularly prevalent in the postoperative period. It is to be hoped that septic complications should be extremely rare following vascular surgery but they do occur and are particularly lethal due to the occasional involvement of prosthetic grafts. I feel that radiolabelled leucocytes are a considerable advance in the diagnosis of occult sepsis and I will discuss their application with particular reference to vascular surgeons.

Postoperative Sepsis

Following abdominal surgery, septic fossae are easily missed by ultrasound and computerized tomography. This is particularly true where the abscess is located in the retroperitoneum or between loops of bowel where the presence of gas and fluid confuse the picture. Gallium scanning is insensitive due to the normal uptake of this isotope in the intestine and it administers a relatively large dose of radiation. [111]In labelled leucocytes were first developed in 1976 and the earliest reports of their clinical value appeared in 1979.[10,11] Again, the labelling technique is relatively simple and involves the separation of leucocytes by sedimentation in the presence of Dextran or Haemaccel. The leucocytes are then incubated with Indium oxine for 90 seconds. These cells are then resuspended in the patient's own plasma and administered intravenously.

The best results are obtained if careful attention is paid to the timing of gamma images. At four hours leucocyte uptake in sites of inflammation will be apparent. A delayed image at 24 hours is essential for the detection of an abscess as cell migration into pus takes longer. By using images at both 4 and 24 hours it is possible to distinguish a collection of pus from other sources of inflammation in almost every case. Again, the critical organ with respect to the dose of radiation is the spleen and we do not think that it should be necessary to inject more than 200 μCi of ^{111}In in the performance of this investigation. In the Queen Elizabeth Hospital, Birmingham and Charing Cross Hospital, London we have performed over 150 ^{111}In-leucocyte studies in the search for occult sepsis. Of 53 abscesses subsequently confirmed by the drainage of pus, the diagnosis was accurately reported with the abscess located in 50

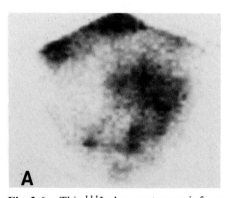
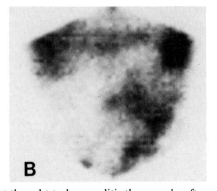

Fig. 3-6. This ^{111}In-leucocyte scan is from a patient thought to have colitis three weeks after repair of a ruptured aortic aneurysm. The massive left retroperitoneal haematoma had become infected and is clearly imaged at 24 hours (A). At 72 hours the radioactivity has moved into the colon (B) demonstrating that the source of both infection and diarrhoea was the rupture of the haematoma into the large bowel.

(sensitivity, 94%). In only one case was a false-positive diagnosis of abscess made giving the test a specificity of 99% and an overall accuracy of 97%. An example of the value of this technique to the vascular surgeon can be seen from the images in a 68-year-old man who was thought to have acute colitis two weeks after the repair of a ruptured abdominal aneurysm with a massive left retroperitoneal haematoma (Fig. 3-6). At 24 hours after the injection of radiolabelled cells the region of the haematoma was obviously radioactive suggesting that it had become infected. One day later the radioactivity had moved into the colon suggesting that the haematoma ruptured into the colon, became infected, and discharged via the colon. Clearly the Dacron graft repair would be infected in this case and had to be removed with subsequent axillobifemoral bypass.

Infected Prosthetic Grafts

The high morbidity and mortality associated with infected grafts makes this among the most feared complications in vascular surgery. Again delay in diagnosis contributes to the poor results of repair. The potential application of ^{111}In-leucocytes in the diagnosis is therefore quite obvious. This approach was studied in six animals receiving intravenous staphylococci following graft implantation.[12] In this study all six infected grafts were easily detected by eight weeks following graft implantation. Unfortunately this is a highly artificial circumstance with gross purulent infection around the graft. We would expect Indium leucocytes to detect this with precision, but in most cases of clinical graft infection the problem is chronic with low-grade infection and very little pus. The problem is further aggravated by the inevitable contamination of the leucocyte preparation by platelets. As prosthetic grafts in humans rarely ever endothelialize, this platelet contamination is likely to produce uptake of radioactivity in the graft whether or not there is infection. The use of purified leucocytes using density gradient columns does not entirely overcome this problem and we are currently searching for alternative methods of labelling leucocytes or macrophages in these patients. Nevertheless, despite these problems it is possible to gain useful information, and we have successfully detected the extent of graft involvement in four of six patients studied. An example is given in Figure 3-7 where the left limb of a patient with an aortobicarotid bypass accumulated marked radioactivity following the administration of radiolabelled leucocytes, indicating the need for graft excision.

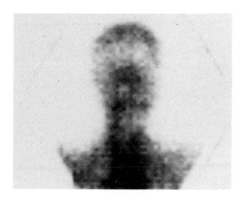

Fig. 3-7. This patient developed a sinus over the left limb of the aortobicarotid bypass. The gamma image shows uptake of radiolabelled leucocytes on both limbs of this Dacron graft confirming infection and the need to remove the graft.

Mycotic Emboli

Most vascular surgeons will be familiar with the awful and self-inflicted arterial and venous pathologies seen in drug addicts. Where the infected vascular puncture involves the artery, the clinical signs of mycotic aneurysm with bacteriologic support and plain roentgenograms is all that is required to proceed to definitive treatment. With venous puncture however, the site of the puncture may be undetectable by inspection and palpation. The patient presents with septicaemia or pneumonia that may initially be attributed to aspiration. In two young men we have recently confirmed the diagnosis of lung abscess and identified the source of septic emboli by gamma imaging following the administration of ^{111}In-leucocytes (Fig. 3-8). Equally important is the ability to exclude such pathology and in one further patient this diagnosis was refuted and the lung pathology identified as inflammation due to aspiration during drug-induced stupor.

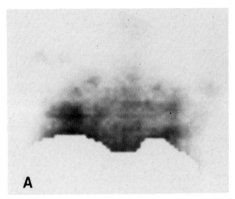 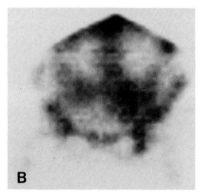

Fig. 3-8. The gamma image of the lungs following ^{111}In leucocytes demonstrates multiple abscesses (A). The source of the mycotic emboli was not apparent on clinical examination but this drug addict was known to inject both groins, and considerable radioactivity is seen in the region of the left common femoral and external iliac vein (B).

It must be accepted that the techniques and facilities required for the radiolabelling of blood cells are unlikely to be available in most district general hospitals. This is particularly true as their main application prior to the last two to three years has been in research. Where there is access to these techniques their value is proven in the diagnosis of deep vein thrombosis and in the detection and localization of occult sepsis. For the vascular surgeon the most obvious and exciting potential is the use of ^{111}In-platelets in the detection in the source of emboli, whether arterial or venous. We eagerly await the results of studies to determine whether platelet uptake on atheromatous carotid disease is a significant risk factor for future stroke.

REFERENCES

1. Thakur ML, Welch MJ, Joist JH, et al: Indium 111 labelled platelets: Studies on preparation and evaluation of in vitro and in vivo functions. Thromb Res 9:345, 1976
2. Hawker RJ, Hawker LM, Wilkinson AR: Indium (111-In) labelled human platelets: Optimal method. Clin Sci 58:243, 1980

3. Van Reenan OR, Lotter MG, Minnaar PC, et al: Radiation dose from human platelets labelled with indium 111. Br J Radiol 53:790, 1980

4. Goldman M, Hall C, Dykes J, et al: Does 111 Indium-platelet deposition predict patency in prosthetic arterial grafts? Br J Surg 70:635, 1983

5. Lane IF, Poskitt KR, Sinclair M, et al: The diagnosis of true and false aneurysms with 111 Indium labelled platelets, In Vascular Surgery, Orlando, Grune & Stratton, 1985 (in press)

6. Goldman M, Leung JO, Aukland A, et al: 111-Indium platelet imaging, Doppler spectral analysis and angiography compared in patients with transient cerebral ischaemia. Stroke 14:752, 1983

7. Lusby RJ, Ferrell LD, Englestad BL, et al: Vessel wall and indium 111 labelled platelet response to carotid endarterectomy. Surgery 93:424, 1983

8. Grimly RP, Rafiqi E, Hawker RJ, et al: Imaging of 111 In-labelled platelets: A new method for the diagnosis of deep vein thrombosis. Br J Surg 68:714, 1981

9. Fenech A, Hussey JK, Smith FW, et al: Diagnosis of deep vein thrombosis using autologous indium-111 labelled platelets. Br Med J 282:1020, 1981

10. Thakur ML, Coleman RE, Mayhall G, et al: Preparation and evaluation of 111 In labelled leucocytes as an abscess imaging agent in dogs. Radiology 119:731, 1976

11. Ascher NL, Ahrenholz DH, Simmons RL, et al: Indium 111 autologous tagged leucocytes in the diagnosis of intraperitoneal sepsis. Arch Surg 114:386, 1979

12. Serota AI, Williams RA, Rose JG, et al: Uptake of radiolabelled leucocytes in prosthetic graft infection. Surgery 90:35, 1981

John G. Mosley
and Adrian Marston

4

Radionuclide Angiocardiography

Patients who require aortic surgery for occlusive or aneurysmal disease invariably have widespread arterial disease. Unfortunately, during aortic surgery, major haemodynamic changes are inevitable; for instance, the systemic vascular resistance increases by nearly 50% during aortic cross clamping.[1] Therefore, it is not surprising that myocardial failure accounts for 50% of the deaths following abdominal aortic surgery.

Preoperative myocardial function can be assessed by a number of methods including right heart catheterization, echocardiography, digital subtraction angiography, and nuclear magnetic resonance tomography. In this chapter, the evaluation of noninvasive global ventricular function by radionuclide angiocardography is described.

The most accurate indicator of left ventricular function has been found to be the ejection fraction (LVEF). This method relates stroke volume to end diastolic volume.[2,3] The LVEF corresponds closely to the cardiac index, measured directly by right heart catheterization, and both indices are accurate predictors of mortality in patients undergoing open-heart surgery[4] and abdominal aortic surgery.[1]

The left ventricular blood pool can be imaged using radionuclides either during the initial transit of a peripherally injected radionuclide bolus through the central circulation, or when a blood pool tracer has reached equilibrium concentration. The great attraction of radionuclides is that, assuming complete mixing of tracer with blood, detected activity is proportional to volume. Ejection fraction can be calculated without any of the assumptions about the shape of the left ventricle inherent when derived from contrast angiocardiography or echocardiography.[5]

During a first-pass study there is good separation of the ventricles with very low levels of background activity; however, the high count rates encountered and the limited opportunity for data collection place severe demands on conventional single-crystal gamma cameras, although this is much less of a problem with multi-crystal cameras and probe systems. The assumption that the tracer is completely mixed with blood may be untrue. A significant streaming of labelled and unlabelled red cells can adversely affect the accuracy of the LVEF estimation.

DIAGNOSTIC TECHNIQUES AND ASSESSMENT
PROCEDURES IN VASCULAR SURGERY

© 1985 Grune & Stratton
ISBN 0-8089-1721-8 All rights reserved

We have favoured the equilibration of a radionuclide because tracer mixing is, by definition, complete. Count rates are much more suitable for conventional gamma cameras than those encountered during first-pass studies and several estimations can be made for as long as the tracer remains in the blood, usually for several hours. Data collection does, however, take several minutes, and during this time a steady state is assumed. Therefore, such conditions as atrial fibrillation completely preclude equilibrium studies, while frequent extrasystoles can present problems. Background activity is relatively high and the presence of tracer in both ventricles simultaneously necessitates imaging in the left anterior oblique position with a head up tilt to obtain separate images of the ventricles.

METHOD

Stannous fluoride pyrophosphate is administered intravenously. This facilitates the subsequent uptake of the radionuclide by the red cells. A 40 mL sample of autologous blood is labelled with 740 mBq ^{99m}TcO and reinjected. The patient is placed in front of a gamma camera at 20 degrees of head up tilt (Fig. 4-1). The camera is positioned over the heart and rotated to 45 degrees for a left anterior oblique projection to maximize the separation of the ventricles. When the patient is comfortable and at rest, a radionuclide ventriculogram is carried out with an IGE 400T Informatek Simis III computer system. The camera is linked to an ECG monitor and each 16 frame cycle is triggered by the R wave (Fig. 4-2). Sixteen frames are taken during each cardiac cycle with 320,000 counts per frame. Each study takes four to five minutes.

The LVEF is determined from the count changes over the left ventricle in diastole and systole after background activity has been subtracted. The left ventricular activity is calculated graphically for an average cardiac cycle (Fig. 4-3). The LVEF is

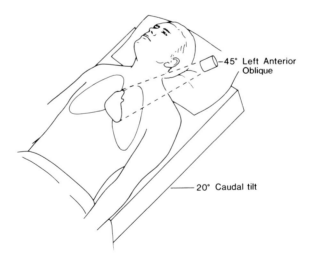

Fig. 4-1. The patient is positioned on a couch tilted to 20° head up and the gamma camera is placed at 45° left anterior projection focused to the region of the heart.

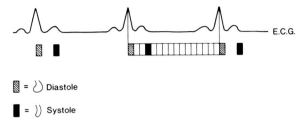

§ = 🌢 Diastole

█ = 🌢 Systole

Fig. 4-2. Resting ECG with R wave triggering each series of 16 frames per cardiac cycle. The initial and late frames show activity from the left ventricle in diastole.

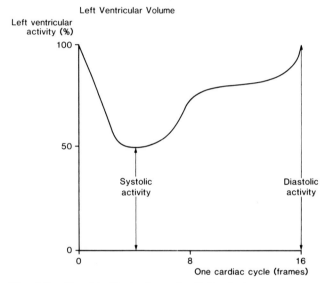

Fig. 4-3. Graphic illustration of activity during an average cardiac cycle. The horizontal axis indicates the 16 frames and the vertical axis indicates the activity expressed as a percentage of maximum activity at end diastole.

then calculated from the graph where the diastolic activity is taken as the maximum activity and the systolic activity as the minimum.

$$LVEF = \frac{Diastolic\ activity - Systolic\ activity}{Diastolic\ activity}$$

The normal range is 0.5–0.7; hence, normally the left ventricle ejects between 50%–70% of its diastolic volume at each systole.

RESULTS

A consecutive series of 41 patients (age, 54–76 years) undergoing abdominal aortic surgery were studied using this technique. Twenty-four of the operations were for aortic aneurysms, 14 were for aortic occlusion, and three were for occlusion of

Table 4-1
LVEF and Postoperative Mortality

		Ischaemic	Postoperative Deaths	
EF	No. of Patients	ECG	Cardiac	Noncardiac
0–0.3	4	3	3*	0
0.31–0.6	27	19	1	3
0.61	10	4	0	0

* $P < 0.001$ by sign test.

the mesenteric arteries. There were 37 men and four women. The patients postoperative progress was followed and there were four deaths due to myocardial failure related to the LVEF (Table 4-1).

Three of the four deaths from cardiac failure occurred in the group of four patients whose preoperative LVEF was <0.3. A high proportion of our patients had an ischaemic E.C.G., though one patient who died on the second postoperative day from myocardial failure had a normal E.C.G. despite an LVEF of 0.27. There were three postoperative deaths due to causes unrelated to myocardial failure.

Radionuclide angiocardiography is a simple technique that accurately predicts those patients most at risk of myocardial failure and has enabled us to take preoperative measures to maximize the myocardial performance of patients whose LVEF is below 0.4 prior to undertaking major aortic surgery.

REFERENCES

1. Fiser WP, Thompson BW, Thompson AR, et al: Nuclear cardiac ejection fraction and cardiac index in abdominal aortic surgery. Surgery 94:736, 1983
2. Cohn PF, Gorling R, Cohn LH, et al: Left ventricular ejection fraction as a prognostic guide in surgical treatment of coronary and valvular heart disease. Am J Cardiol 34:136, 1974
3. Jones RH, Douglas JM, Reiych SK, et al: Non-invasive radionuclide assessment of cardiac function in patients with peripheral vascular disease. Surgery 85:59, 1979
4. Oldham HN, Kong Y, Bartel AG, et al: Risk factors in coronary artery bypass surgery. Arch Surg 105:918, 1972
5. Walton S: Non-invasive evaluation of right ventricular function. J R Soc Med 76:337, 1983

Andrew N. Nicolaides, Tansukh N. Sonecha,
Evagoras P. Nicolaides, and A-Majeed Salmasi

5

The Assessment of Cardiac Function in Patients with Peripheral Vascular Disease

The management of cardiac disease has improved dramatically during the last 15 years as a result of advances in diagnosis, monitoring, and therapy. In particular, the advent of aortocoronary bypass has revolutionized the treatment of ischaemic heart disease. The perioperative mortality of this operation is now less than 2% and the five-year survival greater than 90%.[1–5] However, despite advances in vascular surgical and anaesthetic techniques and the availability of intensive care units for postoperative care, the same degree of success has not been attained in patients undergoing peripheral vascular reconstructive surgery. The disparity is striking. The perioperative mortality in these patients is of the order of 2%–5% and the three-year mortality is 30%–40%, the majority of deaths being the result of myocardial infarction.[6–16] This rate is due to the fact that presence of concomitant coronary artery disease (CAD) has often been overlooked by the vascular surgeon, and the cardiac status of the patient has been less than adequately evaluated before peripheral vascular reconstructive procedures. The reasons for this are briefly outlined below.

The best indicator of risk (coronary death) is the severity and distribution of coronary atheroma (whether it affects one, two, or three coronary arteries) and the left ventricular function. Traditionally, accurate localization and quantification has been obtained by coronary angiography and left ventriculography. However, because of practical, logistic, and financial implications, clinicians have been reluctant to use such invasive techniques for routine preoperative evaluation and thus have been unable to detect covert CAD which cannot always be diagnosed by the history, clinical examination, the stethoscope, the resting electrocardiogram, and chest roentgenogram.

It is only during the last 10 years that coronary surgery has been shown to diminish morbidity and mortality. The older generation of vascular surgeons have either not been fully aware of the indications and benefits of coronary reconstructions or are working in an environment where cardiologists with facilities to investigate their patients fully are not available.

DIAGNOSTIC TECHNIQUES AND ASSESSMENT
PROCEDURES IN VASCULAR SURGERY © 1985 Grune & Stratton
ISBN 0-8089-1721-8 All rights reserved

37

Another reason has been the relative lack of simple cardiac noninvasive techniques. Localization and quantification of peripheral vascular disease in the 1950s and 1960s were obtained by angiography. The 1970s saw the introduction of noninvasive tests and the proliferation of noninvasive vascular laboratories that revolutionalized the investigation of vascular patients. Today, only patients selected with the view to peripheral vascular reconstruction on the basis of history, clinical examination, and noninvasive screening are admitted to hospital for angiography. Unfortunately, the development of simple and accurate noninvasive tests to assess myocardial ischaemia and left ventricular function have not kept pace with the advances in the noninvasive assessment of peripheral vascular problems.

Despite the situations described above, the attitude of vascular surgeons is now changing. They are becoming aware of the benefits of coronary surgery and the importance of an accurate assessment of the patient's cardiac status. In addition, a number of cardiac noninvasive investigations are now becoming available and the demand for simple, inexpensive screening tests is being fulfilled.

The purpose of this chapter is to outline the recent information about the incidence of both overt and occult cardiac disease in patients with peripheral vascular disease; the new noninvasive tests used to select the high risk patients for further invasive cardiac investigations; the benefit of coronary reconstruction in such patients; and finally to discuss the implications and impact current thinking may have on vascular practice during the next decade.

Prevalence of Ischaemic Heart Disease in Patients with Peripheral Vascular Disease

The patient with peripheral vascular disease, whether lower-limb atherosclerotic, extracranial cerebrovascular, or aneurysmal arterial disease is particularly likely to have concomitant coronary disease. This is because atherosclerosis is a systemic disorder that may affect several blood vessels in different organs simultaneously. Although the patient may present with symptoms such as claudication, transient ischaemic attacks (TIAs), or angina indicating disease predominantly in one area, it does not follow that other areas are free from atheroma. The prevalence of coronary disease in patients with claudication varies from 25% to 90% depending on the patient selection and diagnostic method used.[17-25]

In a series of 531 patients considered for carotid endarterectomy, the history and clinical examination revealed a 56% incidence of coronary artery disease; when additional criteria were used from ECG at rest the incidence was found to be 66%.[17] In another series of 1000 patients, CAD was clinically suspected in 52% of 263 patients presenting with abdominal aortic aneurysm, 56% of 381 with lower limb ischaemia, and 57% of 169 with cerebrovascular disease.[18] However, when routine coronary angiography was performed, in all 1000 patients only 18% were found to have normal coronary arteries.

A carefully taken history may reveal that the patient had a myocardial infarct in the past. Some patients may recall having angina which disappeared when claudication developed or when the claudication distance became shorter; they might even say that the angina is "cured." Although these findings are good indicators of the presence of CAD, they are relatively crude or even poor indicators of risk (see below). At one end of the spectrum is the patient who had an infarct several years earlier as a result of disease in only one coronary artery, with a well-developed collateral circulation; the risk in such a patient is low. At the other end of the spectrum is the patient who had claudication for years, is now well adapted to a life style requiring relatively little exercise, and who has developed severe stenoses in all three coronary arteries (left anterior descending, circumflex, and right) or even in the left main stem. Although the latter may have no symptoms referable to the heart and his resting ECG may be normal, he would be at high risk of myocardial infarction.

The inability of clinical criteria to identify the presence of severe CAD particularly in such patients who do not take exercise because they are limited by claudication and the impracticability of routine coronary angiography has prompted several centres to investigate the efficacy of ECG stress testing. Treadmill, bicycle ergometry, or even arm ergometry have been used.[19-25] The incidence of a positive effort test has varied from 24% in asymptomatic patients with a normal ECG at rest to 88% in patients with an abnormal ECG at rest (Table 5-1).

Table 5-1
Clinical Findings in Patients with Lower Limb Ischaemia

Clinical Findings	Incidence of Positive ECG Stress Test	Reference Number
No cardiac symptoms and normal ECG at rest	24%	19
No cardiac symptoms	33%	20
History of cardiac disease	44%	21
Symptoms of cardiac disease	66%	20
Abnormal ECG at rest	88%	19

We have studied 100 consecutive patients presenting with claudication who were referred to our noninvasive vascular laboratory for ankle pressure measurements before and after standard exercise on a horizontal treadmill at 4 km per hour. This was part of the routine assessment of the severity of lower-limb ischaemia. We used conventional 12-lead ECG monitoring during the exercise. A total of 62% had ECG evidence of ischaemic heart disease. During the exercise test 20% developed severe myocardial ischaemia and yet only three patients developed angina.[24]

We now use routine electrocardiographic chest wall mapping during bicycle ergometry to screen all our patients with peripheral arterial disease (see below).[26] This test can detect not only the presence of myocardial ischaemia but also the extent of the disease whether in one, two or three coronary territories (see below).

Indicators of Risk and the Effect of Aorto-coronary Bypass on Risk

The clinical spectrum of atherosclerotic CAD is extremely broad and the risk of myocardial infarction or death varies depending on whether the patient is asymptomatic, had prior myocardial infarction (uncomplicated or complicated, recent or remote), stable angina, unstable angina, or whether he has already undergone aorto-coronary bypass grafting. It has already been indicated that absence of cardiac symptoms does not mean absence of coronary disease. This is especially so in patients whose exercise tolerance is limited by claudication. Established "risk factors" for long-term development of CAD such as smoking, hyperlipidaemia, left ventricular hypertrophy, and glucose intolerance do not predict perioperative myocardinal infarction.[27] On the other hand, age, history of previous myocardial infarction, presence of congestive cardiac failure, or premature ventricular contractions are factors that correlate with life-threatening and fatal complications.[27]

In patients with previous myocardial infarction undergoing major noncardiac surgery, the more recent the infarction the greater the perioperative morbidity and mortality. Major surgery performed during an episode of acute myocardial infarction carries a mortality of 90%; if performed within six months or less after myocardial infarction the cardiac mortality is 23%. With infarction occurring more than six months before noncardiac surgery, the risk gradually declines and eventually levels off at about 2.5%.[27]

While, the operative risks in patients with myocardial infarction are well defined, the risk in patients with angina pectoris are ill defined. A variable surgical mortality from 0 to 17% has been reported in patients with angina undergoing noncardiac operations.[28] Most studies have not commented on the type of angina pectoris present despite the fact that the prognosis is different in different categories. Patients with stable angina with a normal ECG at rest and after exercise have the same operative risk as patients of the same age without angina; patients with stable angina and ischaemic changes on the ECG have a moderate risk, and patients with angina at rest or unstable angina constitute a major risk.

It has already been stated that the perioperative mortality in patients having major vascular operations is in the region of 3%–5% and cardiac causes account for the majority of deaths.[12–15] We now know that the distribution and severity of coronary atheroma are the most important determinants of cardiac morbidity and mortality available, provided left ventricular function is good. We also know that patients with good results after aortocoronary bypass (that is, relief of angina and good left ventricular function) have a life expectancy close to the general population of the same age[15] and can undergo major operations without increased risk.[29–31]

Of 873 patients with known CAD who underwent noncardiac surgery at Emory University Hospital in 1976, 48 had an acute myocardial infarction within three months of operation. In contrast, of 53 patients who had aortocoronary bypass prior to noncardiac surgery only one of them had a perioperative myocardial infarct.[32]

In another series 358 patients with prior myocardial revascularization underwent subsequent major noncoronary surgery. The subsequent operation was vascular in 232 patients with 1.3% mortality, general surgical in 113 with 0.9% mortality, and thoracic in 43 with no deaths.[33]

It seems that successful revascularization of the myocardium before subsequent surgery reduces operative morbidity and mortality; however, the risk of the bypass procedure should be included in the overall mortality and morbidity.

Another benefit from aortocoronary bypass is the improvement in long-term survival. A number of reports suggest that an overall five-year actuarial survival of 90% may be expected for cardiac patients who had myocardial revascularization.[3–5] In 77 patients who presented with TIAs and ischaemic heart disease and had carotid endarterectomy, a 20% three-year mortality was observed. In contrast, only a 3.5%

mortality was observed at three years in 135 patients who presented with TIAs and ischaemic heart disease and subsequently had carotid endarterectomy and aortocoronary bypass.[34] Similarly, Bernstein et al reported a 5% mortality in patients who had carotid endarterectomy and aortocoronary bypass surgery, but in those who had carotid endarterectomy only or carotid endarterectomy plus peripheral vascular surgery without aortocoronary reconstruction the mortality was 23% and 31%, respectively.[35]

Because of the above, we feel that in 1985 a mortality of 30%–40% at three years in patients with peripheral vascular disease is unacceptable. We also believe, as stated by Hertzer[36] that "referral of a patient for peripheral vascular reconstructive surgery is the golden moment for the diagnosis of associated coronary artery disease; such a moment may never occur again in his life time."

In patients over the age of 70, the risk of coronary artery bypass graft surgery is high. Although there is an increase in the incidence of inoperable CAD with advancing age, surgically correctable coronary lesions occur with similar frequency in all age groups of patients with peripheral vascular disease. It is the younger patient with arteriopathy who would benefit from the investigations for detection and effective therapy of his coronary artery disease.

Current Practice (Fig. 5-1)

When confronted with a patient with peripheral arterial disease, we ask the following questions: (1) Is there any covert cardiac disease in a patient with no known heart disease, and (2) what is the diagnosis and what is the severity of the disease in patients with covert, known, or symptomatic cardiac disease?

Correct answers to the above two questions are an essential prerequisite for determining (1) the cardiac risk of patients undergoing vascular reconstructions; (2) whether underlying occult or asymptomatic disease will become unmasked after vascular reconstruction and produce symptoms; (3) the patient's life expectancy; (4) whether it will be in the patient's interest (that is, in terms not only of operative risk, but also of duration and quality of life) to consider a cardiac operation prior to vascular reconstruction, and (5) what measures should be taken to minimize the risk of cardiac complications if cardiac function is compromized and a cardiac operation cannot be considered because of advanced age, an inoperable cardiac situation, or lack of time as in the case of a threatened limb or a vascular emergency.

To be able to answer such questions, some teams have used routine cardiac catheterization with coronary angiography and left ventriculography as described by Dr Hertzer. We have followed a different approach and developed noninvasive tests that would demonstrate the presence of covert CAD, indicate its extent (one, two, or three vessel disease), and assess left ventricular function, so that only selected high-risk patients would be subjected to invasive investigations.

ECG Chest Wall Mapping Stress Test

The details and validation of this test have been described elsewhere.[26] In our initial study chest wall mapping of ST segment changes, inverted U waves and Q waves using 16 electrocardiographic electrodes was performed at rest, during, and after bicycle ergometry in 150 patients presenting with chest pain suggestive of

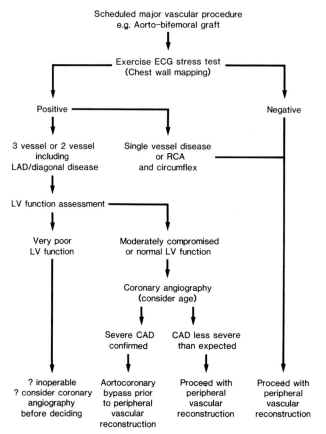

Fig. 5-1.   Outline of current practice when confronted with a
patient with peripheral arterial disease.

angina. All patients underwent coronary angiography. The principle of this test is
based on the observation that ECG changes obtained with an electrode at a point
on the chest wall reflect changes in the myocardium immediately deep to that point.
The position of the leads was such that they would reflect changes in the three main
coronary artery territories, providing spatial information. Electrodes were placed in
four vertical rows of four. Four were just to the right of the sternum providing
information about the right coronary territory; four were just to the left of the
sternum and four along the anterior axillary line providing information about the
LAD/Diagonal territory; four were on the back 6 cm medial to the posterior axillary line providing information about the circumflex coronary territory. By using
multiple criteria (ST segment depression, Q waves at rest, and the appearance of
inverted U waves) the accuracy was improved. The presence or absence of appreciable CAD ($>50\%$ stenosis) was detected with a sensitivity of 98% and a specificity of 88%. The identification of lesions in individual coronary arteries was also
possible: there was a sensitivity of 98% and a specificity of 88% for lesions of the
left anterior descending or main diagonal artery; a sensitivity of 71% and a specificity of 85% for lesions of the right coronary artery; and a sensitivity of 86% and a
specificity of 80% for lesions of the circumflex artery. The absence of appreciable

CAD and the presence of single, double, or triple vessel disease was predicted correctly in 70% of patients. Errors occurred in 25% of patients because the disease was missed or falsely diagnosed in one coronary artery. Errors in more than one vessel occurred in only 5% of patients. Left main-stem coronary disease present in 11 patients was in every case demonstrated as disease of LAD/Diagonal and circumflex territories.

Subsequently, we applied this test in claudicants. We have found that although these patients cannot exercise adequately on a treadmill, they can do better on a bicycle and on average increase their heart rate to 82% of the expected maximum producing a valid test. We have found that one third of patients with claudication and no known cardiac disease have a positive effort test and in one third of the latter the test reveals the presence of three-vessel coronary disease. Patients with three-vessel disease and patients with two-vessel disease including LAD/Diagonal disease are selected for coronary angiography and left ventriculography (Fig. 5-1).

Ambulatory ST segment (Holter) Monitoring

Spontaneous or exertional chest pain, if accompanied by ST segment shift on a frequency modulated system may help to substantiate the diagnosis of CAD. The frequency and magnitude of ST segment shift, with or without pain may indicate the severity of the underlying CAD. The monitoring can be done while the patient is at home or at work without the need for hospitalization. Exercise ECG stress test and ambulatory ST segment (Holter) monitoring should be regarded as complimentary to each other.[37-41]

2-D Echocardiography

In the presence of CAD, the assessment of LV function is as important as the information concerning the anatomical distribution of coronary artery lesions in arriving at a decision regarding the optimum management. There are several noninvasive methods of evaluation of the LV status and 2-D echocardiography is one of the least invasive methods.[42-44]

Extensive tomographic sampling of LV dimensions, shape, and regional wall motion study permits the detection of segmental dysfunction, ventricular aneurysm, and the estimation of LV ejection fraction. The other cardiac chambers and great vessels can also be assessed together with morphology and mobility of heart valves. These features are important in identification of underlying cardiac disorders such as mitral valve disease, mural thrombus, bacterial endocarditis, atrial myxoma, or cardiomyopathy as a source of peripheral arterial embolization.

Stroke Volume Exercise-Induced Changes Detected by Transcutaneous Aortovelography

A still better indication of LV function is the determination of change in stroke volume in response to exercise. Although this is difficult to do with 2-D echocardiography it can be easily measured with transcutaneous aortovelography (TAV).[45-49] This is a new, noninvasive test we have developed for the assessment of left ventricular function.[45] A 2 MHz continuous-wave Doppler probe is applied at the suprasternal notch and directed in such a way that the beam insonates the aortic arch tangentially. The position of the probe is adjusted so that the maximum signal is obtained which is processed by frequency analysis and displayed as a sonogram (frequency v time). The area under the maximum frequency envelope is directly proportional to stroke volume, and any changes in stroke volume as a result of exercise can be measured with an error of less than 5%.[46] The technique has been validated by comparison to simultaneous invasive measurements performed during cardiac catheterization.[47–49] In our initial clinical study[45] we used TAV to determine changes in stroke volume on exercise in two groups of individuals. Group I consisted of 20 normal volunteers and 14 patients with atypical chest pain, who had normal left ventricular function and coronary arteriograms. Group II consisted of 44 patients who had >50% stenosis in one, two, or three coronary arteries. Aortic velocity was recorded before and immediately after maximum tolerated supine exercise using a bicycle ergometer. An increase in the average area (stroke volume) under the aortic velocity per time curve exceeding 5% (range, 7%–40%) was shown by all the subjects in group I and 16 in group II who had an ejection fraction >60% calculated from the left ventriculogram. In 22 patients from Group II with ejection fraction <60%, the average area (stroke volume) decreased by 5% to 36%. The increase in cardiac output in these patients was the result of increase in heart rate rather than increase in stroke volume.

We are now using this test to assess left ventricular function in patients with peripheral vascular disease. It provides information about the effect of exercise and we believe it is quantitatively superior to 2-D echocardiography which is performed at rest. It is also less invasive, simpler, and less expensive than the currently available radionuclide methods using a gated blood pool technique.

Thallium-201 Myocardial Perfusion Scan

In patients in whom the simple noninvasive tests such as exercise ECG stress test, ambulatory Holter monitoring, TAV, and 2-D echocardiography have failed to explain atypical cardiac symptoms, thallium myocardial perfusion scan and radionuclide cine angiography may help elucidate the problem further without resorting to coronary angiography and contrast left ventriculography.[50–53] In our current practice we have found that only an extremely small number of patients with peripheral vascular disease fall into this category.

Thallium-201 distributes uniformly throughout the left ventricular myocardium. During myocardial ischaemia, such as induced by exercise, if a poorly perfused region is not exposed to the isotope, it is detected as a "cold spot." Subsequently, when a redistribution image is obtained after a suitable interval following exercise, this cold spot disappears provided the myocardial ischaemia is reversible.

This test may be useful (1) when the result of the exercise ECG stress test is equivocal or inconclusive, (2) when the ECG changes on exercise cannot be interpreted because of a conduction abnormality, (3) when the specificity of the conventional stress test is reduced in the presence of left ventricular hypertrophy, cardiomyopathy, drug therapy, etc, and (4) to ascertain as to what extent the myocardial ischaemia is reversible, before deciding about the need for coronary artery bypass surgery.

Thallium-201 myocardial perfusion scan is considerably more expensive than an exercise ECG stress test and should not be used as a substitute for conventional exercise electrocardiography.

Radionuclide Cine Angiography (RCA)

The blood pool is labelled with a gamma-emitting tracer, such as ^{99}Tcm. The images are collected over successive cardiac cycles to acquire a large number of counts necessary.[54-56] This scintigraphic blood pool technique allows accurate boundary detection of the LV and is useful in two ways.

1. End-diastolic volume (EDV) and end-systolic volume (ESV) can be estimated and LV ejection fraction (LVEF) derived using a simple formula:

$$LVEF = \frac{EDV - ESV}{EDV}$$

2. By observing relative motion of portions of the left ventricular wall during systole and diastole, segmental wall motion abnormality, if present, can be detected.

A real-time RCA procedure permits continuous monitoring and analysis of LV function during exercise.

Other radionuclide techniques are the first-pass methods and the nuclear stethoscope. First-pass methods enable separate visualization of right and left sides of the heart which is not possible with equilibrated blood pool imaging.

The nuclear stethoscope[57] is more sensitive than a scintillation camera and provides facility for beat to beat dynamic monitoring of cardiac cycle. Quantitative measurements including LVEF and diastolic filling rate are readily available with each cardiac cycle, although the instrument does not lend itself for studying regional wall motion. It is beyond the scope of this chapter to discuss in depth the relative merits and demerits of various radionuclide techniques.

CONCLUSION AND IMPLICATIONS FOR THE FUTURE

It has now become obvious that the days when a vascular surgeon requested a cardiac opinion concerning a patient's suitability to undergo anaesthesia and surgery and the cardiologist, after a bed-side clinical assessment using the stethoscope, the resting ECG and chest roentgenogram, would pronounce an opinion are over. It has been realized that the best results are obtained by a multidisciplinary approach and have come from units where there is team-work involving the skill and cooperation of a number of experts which include noninvasive technologists, peripheral vascular surgeons, cardiac surgeons, cardiologists, and experienced cardiac anaesthesiologists.

We can now detect and grade asymptomatic carotid, lower limb, and CAD noninvasively. This will benefit not only the individual patient because of a more cost effective and accurate diagnosis with minimum morbidity, but will also allow us to study the natural history and epidemiology of early atherosclerotic lesions.

The first era of vascular surgery was dominated by the development of surgical techniques. The second era saw the development of noninvasive investigations. We are now entering the third era of early detection of asymptomatic disease and better understanding of its natural history in relation to risk factors. The natural sequel of this, the development of effective prevention that can be applied when the disease is in its asymptomatic stage is no longer in the distant future.

REFERENCES

1. Julian DG: Coronary artery bypass surgery: The European prospective randomized study. Implications for management after infarction. Tex Heart Inst J 9:483, 1982
2. CASS Principal Investigators et al: Coronary artery surgery study (CASS): A randomized trial of coronary artery bypass surgery. Survival data. Circulation 68:939, 1983
3. Loop FD, Cosgrove DM, Lytle BW, et al: Life expectancy after coronary artery surgery. Am J Surg 141:665, 1981
4. Loop FD, Cosgrove DM, Ltyle BW, et al: An 11 year evolution of coronary arterial surgery (1967–1978). Ann Surg 190:444, 1979
5. Hall RJ: Coronary artery bypass: Facts and figures. Tex Heart Inst J 9:478, 1982
6. Cooley DA, Wakasch DC: Techniques in vascular surgery. Philadelphia, Saunders, 1979, p. 261
7. Jamieson WRE, Jancesz MT, Miyagishima RT, et al: Influence of ischaemic heart disease on early and late mortality after surgery for peripheral occlusive vascular disease. Circulation 66:92, 1982
8. Crawford ES, Bomberger RA, Glaeser DH, et al: Aorto-iliac occlusive disease: Factors influencing survival and function following reconstructive operation over a twenty-five year period. Surgery 90:1055, 1981
9. Burnham NR, Johnson G, Gurri JA: Mortality risks for survivors of vascular reconstructive procedures. Surgery 92:1072, 1982
10. Hertzer NR: Fatal myocardial infarction following lower extremity re-vascularization: 273 patients followed 6 to 11 postoperative years. Ann Surg 193:492, 1981
11. Bergan JJ, Veith FJ, Bernard VM, et al: Randomization of autogenous vein and polytetrafluoroethylene grafts in femoral-distal reconstruction. Surgery 92:921, 1982
12. DeBakey ME, Crawford ES, Morris GC, et al: Late results of vascular surgery in the treatment of arteriosclerosis. J Cardiovasc Surg 5:473, 1964
13. Minken SL, DeWeese JA, Southgate WA, et al: Aorto-iliac reconstruction for atherosclerotic occlusive disease. Surg Gynaecol Obstet 126:1056, 1968
14. Couch NP, Lane FC, Crane C: Management and mortality in resection of abdominal aortic aneurysms. Am J Surg 199:408, 1970
15. Lawrie GM, Morris GC: Factors influencing late survival after coronary bypass surgery. Ann Surg 187:665, 1978
16. Veith FJ, Gupta S, Samson R, et al: Progress in limb salvage by reconstructive arterial surgery combined with new or improved adjunctive procedures. Ann Surg 194:386, 1981
17. O'Donnell TF, Callow AD, Willet C, et al: The impact of coronary artery disease on carotid endarterectomy. Ann Surg 198:705, 1983
18. Hertzer NR, Bevan EG, Young JR, et al: Coronary artery disease in peripheral vascular patients. A classification of 1000 coronary angigrams and results of surgical management. Ann Surg 199:223, 1984
19. Cutler BS, Wheeler HB, Paraskos JA, et al: Assessment of operative risk with electrocardiographic exercise testing in patients with peripheral vascular disease. Am J Surg 137:484, 1979

20. Gage AA, Bhayana JN, Balu V, et al: Assessment of cardiac risk in surgical patients. Arch Surg 112:1488, 1977
21. McCabe CJ, Reidy NC, Abbott WM, et al: The value of electrocardiogram monitoring during treadmill testing for peripheral vascular disease. Surgery 89:183, 1981
22. Kovamees A, Bundin T: Continuous electrocardiographic recordings at examination of walking capacity in patients with intermittent claudication. J Cardiovasc Surg 509:12, 1976
23. Kanazawa M, Rose H, Vyden JK, et al: The importance of cardiac monitoring in tread-mill claudication testing. Prac Cardiol 7:48, 1981
24. Vecht RJ, Nicolaides AN, Brandao E, et al: Resting and treadmill electrocardiographic findings in patients with intermittent claudication. Int Angio 1:119, 1982
25. Carroll RM, Rose HB, Vyden J, et al: Cardiac arrhythmias associated with treadmill claudication testing. Surgery 83:284, 1978
26. Salmasi AM, Nicolaides AN, Vecht RJ, et al: Electrocardiographic chest wall mapping in the diagnosis of coronary artery disease. Br Med J 2:9, 1983
27. Goldman L, Caldera DL, Southwick FS, et al: Cardiac risk factors and complications in noncardiac surgery. Medicine 57:357, 1978
28. Salene DN, Homans DC, Isner JM: Management of cardiac disease in the general surgi-cal patient. Curr Prob Cardiol 5:22, 1980
29. Scher K, Tice DA: Operative risk in patients with previous coronary bypass. Arch Surg 111:807, 1976
30. McCollum CH, Garcia Rinalde R, Graham JM, et al: Myocardial infarction revascularization prior to subsequent major surgery in patients with coronary artery disease. Surgery 81:302, 1977
31. Edwards WH, Mulhein JL, Walker WE: Vascular reconstructive surgery following myo-cardial revascularization. Ann Surg 187:653, 1978
32. Wells PH, Kaplan JA: Optimal management of patients with ischaemic heart disease for noncardiac surgery by complementary anaesthesiologist and cardiologist interaction. Curr Cardiol St Louis, Mosby, 1981, pp. 1029–1037
33. Crawford ES, Morris GS, Howell JF, et al: Operative risk in patients with previous coronary artery bypass. Ann Thorac Surg 26:215, 1978
34. Ennix CL Jr, Lawrie GM, Morris GC Jr, et al: Improved results of carotid endarter-ectomy in patients with symptomatic coronary disease: An analysis of 1546 consecutive carotid operations. Stroke 10:122, 1979
35. Bernstein EF, Humber PB, Collins GM, et al: Life expectancy and late stroke following carotid endarterectomy. Ann Surg 198:80, 1983
36. Hertzer NR (1984) Personal communication
37. Kennedy HI, Caralis DG: Ambulatory electrocardiography: A clinical perspective. Ann Intern Med 87:729, 1977
38. Stern S, Tzivoni D: Early detection of silent ischaemic heart disease by 24 hour electro-cardiographic monitoring of active subjects. Br Heart J 36:481, 1974
39. Wolf E, Tzivoni D, Stern S: Comparison of exercise test and 24 hour ambulatory elec-trocardiographic monitoring in detection of active subjects. Br Heart J 36:90, 1974
40. Allen RD, Gettes LS, Phalan C, et al: Painless ST segment depression in patients with agina pectoris. Chest 69:467, 1976
41. Gillilan RE, Babitt HI, Warbasse JR: Clinical accuracy of ECG ischaemic ST segment changes by electro-magnetic tape and by radiotelemetry. Circulation 42:157, 1970
42. Reichek N: Uses and abuses of two-dimensional echocardiography. Int J Cardiol 1:221, 1982
43. Schnitger I, Gordon EP, Fitzgerald PJ, et al: Standardized intracardiac measurements of two-dimensional echocardiography. Am J Cardiol 2:934, 1983
44. Tortoledo FA, Quinones MA, Fernandez GC: Quantification of left ventricular volumes by two-dimensional echocardiography. A simplified and accurate approach. Circulation 67:579, 1983

45. Nicolaides AN, Salmasi SN, Salmasi AM, et al: Transaortic velography (TAV) in the assessment of left ventricular function of patients with coronary artery disease. Br J Surg 70:696, 1983
46. Light LH: Noninvasive ultrasonic technique of observing flow in the human aorta. Nature 224:1119, 1969
47. Cross G, Light LH: Noninvasive intrathoracic blood velocity measurement in the assessment of cardio-vascular function. Biomed Engin 9:464, 1974
48. Sequeira RF, Light LH, Cross G, et al: Br H J 38:443, 1976
49. Brotherhood J, Cross G, Hanson GC, et al: J Physiol 281:4, 1978
50. Botrinick EH, Taradach MR, Shames DM, et al: Thallium-201 myocardial perfusion scintigraphy for the clinical classification of normal, abnormal and equivocal electrocardiographic stress tests. Am J Cardiol 41:43, 1978
51. McCarthy DM, Blood DK, Sciacca RR, et al: Single dose myocardial perfusion imaging with thallium-201. Application in patients with nondiagnostic electrocardiographic stress tests. Am J Cardiol 43:899, 1979
52. Bodenheimer MW, Banka VS, Fooshee CM, et al: Comparative sensitivity of the exercise electrocardiogram, thallium imaging and stress radionuclide angiography to detect the presence and severity of coronary heart disease. Circulation 60:1270, 1979
53. Becker LC: Diagnosis of coronary artery disease with exercise radionuclide imaging. State of the art. Am J Cardiol 45:1301, 1980
54. Borer JS, Bacharach SL, Green MV, et al: Real-time radionuclide cine angiography in the noninvasive evaluation of global and regional left ventricular function at rest and during exercise in patients with coronary artery disease. N Engl J Med 296:839, 1977
55. Strauss HW, Zaret BL, Hurley PJ, et al: A scintiphotographic method for measuring left ventricular ejection fraction in man without cardiac catheterization. Am J Cardiol 28:575, 1973
56. Zaret BL, Strauss HW, Hurley PJ, et al: A noninvasive scintiphotographic method for detecting regional ventricular dysfunction in man. N Engl J Med 284:1165, 1971
57. Hoilund-Carlsen PF, Mrving J, Jensen G: Accuracy of left ventricular ejection fraction determined by the nuclear stethoscope. Int J Cardiol 2:237, 1982

Wolfgang Kox

6

Cardiovascular Monitoring in Patients Undergoing Major Vascular Surgery

It can be assumed that patients undergoing major vascular surgery such as repair of aortic aneurysm and aortic-iliac, aortic-bifemoral, femoro-distal, and axillo-femoral bypass operations have generalised arterial disease, including the coronary arteries, which explains the still remaining risk in this group of patients. To reduce the mortality of these patients, thorough cardiovascular assessment and monitoring is required even including, if necessary, invasive techniques such as indwelling arterial lines and the insertion of Swann-Ganz catheters. The objective is to monitor cardiac output, arterial pressure, and peripheral vascular resistance. This chapter describes these techniques and the information obtained from them.

ARTERIAL BLOOD PRESSURE MEASUREMENT

Intraarterial blood pressure measurement is one of the cornerstones of perioperative monitoring in vascular surgery. The intraarterial cannula (e.g., Abbocath G20) should be inserted at a site where the risk of thrombosis and contamination is minimal and the danger of accidental dislocation is avoidable. Before insertion of the cannula the collateral blood flow to the dependent parts of the chosen artery should be tested (e.g., Allan Test), and the insertion itself should be performed under sterile conditions and after the skin has been infiltrated with a local anaesthetic agent (Lignocaine 1%). Once the cannula is in situ a short, pressure-resistant piece of tubing is connected and the whole system is properly fixed to the patient's skin with sticky tape. The length of the tubing should not exceed 150 cm.[1] The tube is then locked to the pressure transducer (e.g., Statham). A continuous flushing system is introduced between the transducer and the cannula via an intraflow. The flushing fluid (heparinized saline) is kept under constant pressure (300 mmHg) by applying a pressure cuff to the saline bag.

DIAGNOSTIC TECHNIQUES AND ASSESSMENT
PROCEDURES IN VASCULAR SURGERY
© 1985 Grune & Stratton
ISBN 0-8089-1721-8 All rights reserved

The pressure transducer is preferably linked to an analogue and a calibrated digital monitor. The analogue pressure curves appear on the monitor screen continuously with the ECG and allow the detection of errors such as damping (due to air bubbles in the fluid system) as well as the diagnosis of major changes in amplitude and steepness of the slope of the arterial pressure curve. For absolute values, it is easier to rely on the digital output. Systolic, diastolic, and mean pressures can be read from the display on the monitor screen.

Indwelling arterial lines offer the advantage of taking arterial samples for blood gases, haemoglobin and haematocrit more frequently in the perioperative period, while avoiding potential risks and discomfort for the patient due to repeated arterial stabs.

SWANN-GANZ CATHETERIZATION

The Swann-Ganz catheter can be inserted percutaneously via one of the two internal jugular or one of the subclavian veins under absolutely sterile conditions. The introduction of the catheter via the cubital veins should be avoided because of the high risk of thrombophlebitis. The femoral veins are best avoided because they may be too close to the operating field; regardless, this route is inconvenient for nursing and subjects the patients to a higher risk of infection.

Before the catheter is implanted, the balloon at the catheter tip should be inflated and checked for tightness. The triple lumen catheter is filled with heparinized saline; the distal lumen of the catheter is connected to a pressure transducer via a piece of pressure tubing; the transducer is plugged into the second pressure channel of the monitor; and after calibration and equilibration of the transducer and monitor, the catheter is inserted into the venous system through an introducer sheath and the pressure curve is continuously observed. As the catheter reaches a central venous position, as indicated by the pressure curve, the balloon is inflated with approximately 1 mL of air and floated through the right atrium and the right ventricle into one of the branches of the pulmonary artery (PA). The typical trace of the pressure curve is shown in Figure 6-1. The balloon is deflated, the catheter is fixed to the skin, and the puncture site is covered with sterile 'Opsite'-foil. In case of difficulties during the insertion of the catheter, radiographic screening should be used to float the catheter into the right position. Whatever method is used for insertion, a chest roentgenogram should be taken to confirm the correct position of the catheter.

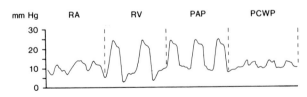

Fig. 6-1. Typical pressure curve when a Swann-Ganz catheter is inserted through the right atrium (RA), the right ventricle (RV) into the PA, and when wedged in the pulmonary artery (PCWP).

Directly measured variables are the central venous pressure (CVP) through the proximal lumen of the catheter, the pressure in the pulmonary artery (PAP), systolic, diastolic, and mean pressure, as well as the pulmonary capillary wedge pressure (PCWP) by inflating the balloon at the catheter tip (Fig. 6-2). Cardiac output can be measured with a thermodilution method by injecting 10 mL of cool saline of known temperature through a proximal lumen and measuring the change in temperature at the catheter tip when diluted in the circulating blood. The calculations are carried out by a connected computer (Edwards Laboratories) that can also display the patient's core temperature. The Swann-Ganz catheter can also provide information about ventricular filling, ventricular pressure, and contractility.

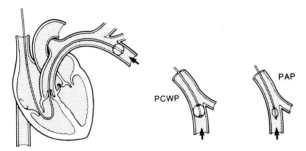

Fig. 6-2. Swann-Ganz catheter in situ with the balloon inflated (wedged) and deflated.

Filling

The filling can be assessed clinically by the CVP for the right ventricle and by the PCWP for the left ventricle. If the mitral valve is functioning normally the PCWP is identical to the end-diastolic filling pressure in the left ventricle.

Ventricular Pressure

A reasonable estimate of systolic ventricular pressure is given by the systolic arterial pressure. This pressure depends on the resistance against which the right or left ventricle has to pump the blood. The pulmonary vascular resistance (PVR) determines the resisting load for the right heart and can be calculated with the equation:

$$\text{PVR (dyn/sec/cm}^{-5}) = \frac{(\overline{\text{PAP}} - \text{PCWP}) \times 79.9}{\text{CO}}$$

$\overline{\text{PAP}}$ is the mean pressure in the pulmonary artery, and cardiac output (CO) can be replaced by cardiac index (CI) which is the CO divided by body surface area. The total peripheral resistance (TPR) is the resisting load for the left heart and is calculated as follows:

$$\text{TPR (dyn/sec/cm}^{-5}) = \frac{(\overline{\text{AP}} - \overline{\text{CVP}}) \times 79.9}{\text{CO}}$$

Where $\overline{AP}$ is the mean arterial pressure and again, CO can be replaced by CI and 79.9 is in both equations the conversion factor from mmHg × min/l to dyn/sec/cm^{-5}. Normal values for PVR lie between 150 and 250 dyn/sec/cm^{-5} and between 900 and 1500 dyn/sec/cm^{-5} for TPR. High peripheral or pulmonary resistance can be treated with vasodilators such as nitroprusside, nitroglycerine, isosorbide, or chlorpromazine.

Contractility

For a given volume and systolic pressure the heart can change its performance due to changes in its intrinsic property. These changes cannot be directly measured in an ejecting heart. For clinical purposes, indirect indices are used to give an idea of this function. During insertion of the Swann-Ganz catheter, the systolic and diastolic pressures of the right ventricle can be measured. It can be done repeatedly by pulling the catheter from its position in the PA back into the right ventricle. This should only be done by experienced physicians and only when additional information can be gained from this procedure. Differentiation of the ventricular rise in pressure gives an indication of the myocardial contractility of the right ventricle, provided the frequency response of the system is adequate. In a clinical situation it is easier to plot ventricle function curves, thereby getting an idea of the contractility of the heart.

The right and left ventricles perform as two pumps in series. To avoid a mismatch, the stroke volume of the two pumps has to be the same in the steady state. This is ensured by the Starling mechanism which governs the strength of contraction in relation to the end-diastolic length of the muscle fibres. The end-diastolic length is represented by the end-diastolic pressure in clinical terms. The end-diastolic pressure for the right ventricle is reflected by the CVP which can be measured through one of the proximal lumens of the Swann-Ganz catheter. The end-diastolic pressure of the left ventricle is assessed by the pulmonary artery wedge pressure and can be measured directly with the distal lumen of the catheter with the balloon inflated; this procedure results in a damped pressure trace on the monitor screen with respiratory fluctuations (Fig. 6-1). When the end-diastolic pressure is plotted on the abscissa of a graph and the ventricular stroke work is plotted on the ordinate, a ventricle function curve can be derived for each ventricle, where the right ventricular stroke work (RVSW) index is defined as:

$$RVSWI(gm/m^2) = SI \times (\overline{PA} - CVP) \times 0.0136$$

and the left ventricular stroke work (LVSW) as:

$$LVSWI(gm/m^2) = SI \times (\overline{AP} - PCWP) \times 0.0136$$

where SI is the stroke index which is the CO divided by heart rate and body surface area (mL/min/m^2) (see Fig. 6-3). The factor 0.0136 is the conversion factor from mmHg × cm^3 to gm.

The ventricle function curves are quite different for the right and the left ventri-

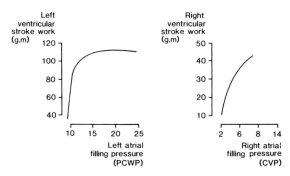

Fig. 6-3. Example for pressure stroke work relationship of the left and right ventricle. The main difference is the magnitude of the stroke work for the left and right ventricle.

cle in slope, steepness, and value. The CVP varies much less than PA pressure because the right side of the heart is more compliant. Thus, there is very little relationship between the end-diastolic pressure in the right ventricle and the LVSW, an indication of how important Swann-Ganz catheterization is for patients with expected heart failure.

A ventricle function curve can be plotted for each patient undergoing vascular surgery by taking measurements of the CVP and the PCWP as well as mean PA pressure and mean AP and repeating the measurements after two fluid challenges. If the pressure on the abscissa increases with administration of colloids (200 mL per challenge) but RVSW or LVSW stays the same or increases only marginally, ionotropic drugs should be given to increase the contractility of the muscle. If the pressure increases only slightly after the fluid challenge and the RVSW or LVSW is improved, more fluid would be indicated.

It can be concluded that the insertion of a Swann-Ganz catheter allows four very important cardiovascular variables to be monitored: (1) PCWP as an approximation to the left ventricular filling pressure; (2) the continuous measurement of mean PA pressure as an indication of clinical events such as hypoxaemia, pulmonary oedema, or pulmonary embolism; (3) the determination of systemic and pulmonary vascular resistances; (4) cardiac output.

For major vascular surgery, baseline measurements of all these variables should be performed the day before the operation, and optimal values established by giving either a fluid challenge or inotropic drugs. Once these optimal parameters are achieved, the patient is monitored permanently throughout the preoperative night and measurements are repeated the next morning after induction of anaesthesia. The ideal values are then attained before the start of the operation. Measurements are again taken during aortic clamping, at the end of the operation, and continued for at least 24 hours in intensive care. Should any intra- or postoperative cardiac "event" occur, a series of measurements should be performed and the appropriate treatment for amelioration should be chosen on the basis of full information concerning cardiovascular status.

These technical and practical points are detailed here and the results obtained at aortic clamping can be found in Chapter 18.

REFERENCE

1. Hughes VG, Prys-Roberts C: Intra-arterial pressure measurements: A review and analysis of methods relevant to anaesthesia and intensive care. Anaesthesia 26:511, 1971

FURTHER READING

Allardyce DB: Symposium on intensive care: Monitoring of the critically ill surgical patient. Can J Surg 21:75, 1978

Swann HJC; Ganz W, et al: Catheterization of the heart in man with use of a flow-directed balloon-tipped catheter. N Engl J Med 283:447, 1970

Swann HJC, Ganz W: Use of balloon-flotation catheters in critically ill patients. Surg Clin North Am 55:501, 1975

Gravenstein JS, Newbower RS, Ream AK, et al: An Integrated Approach to Monitoring. Boston, Butterworths, 1983.

John P. Woodcock

7

Principles of Doppler Ultrasound

In order to appreciate more fully the useful clinical information that can be gained by using Doppler ultrasound, it is important to understand the nature of the Doppler signal. The physical conditions in which the Doppler shift signal is detected puts certain constraints on the design of Doppler-shift flowmeters, which in turn limits the useful information that can be obtained. In this paper the principles of the detection of the Doppler shift and of the determination of flow direction will be discussed. Problems of signal to noise ratio, fixed echoes, and velocity ambiguities will also be discussed.

ULTRASONIC DOPPLER-SHIFT FLOWMETERS

Principle of Operation

The ultrasonic Doppler-shift flowmeter was first described in 1959.[1] An emitted high frequency sound wave, usually in the low megaHertz range, is incident on moving blood cells that scatter the incident radiation in all directions. This is the classical case of Rayleigh scattering where the wavelength is much larger than the target being irradiated. The scattered wave is received and a frequency difference is detected between the transmitted and received signals. This frequency shift is proportional to the velocity of the scatterers. The Doppler shift is based on two alterations in frequency between the emitter and receiver transducer, the first occurs as the ultrasound arrives at the scatterer, and the second as the ultrasound leaves. In the former case, the blood cells act as a moving receiver and it can be shown that the received frequency f_R is given by

$$f_R = (f_s + V_R/\lambda_s)$$

where f_s is the emitted frequency (source frequency), V_R the received velocity com-

DIAGNOSTIC TECHNIQUES AND ASSESSMENT
PROCEDURES IN VASCULAR SURGERY

© 1985 Grune & Stratton
ISBN 0-8089-1721-8 All rights reserved

ponent in the direction of the source, and λ_s the ultrasonic wavelength. This reduces to:

$$f_R - f_s = \frac{V_R}{C} f_s \tag{1}$$

where $(f_R - f_s)$ is the Doppler shift frequency and C the velocity of ultrasound in the blood.

The second change in Doppler shift occurs now, because the blood acts as a moving source for the receiving transducer. The moving source however, radiates ultrasound at an already Doppler shifted frequency f_R. The received frequency f'_R at the transducer is now given by:

$$f'_R = f_R + \frac{V_s}{C} f_R \tag{2}$$

Substituting the value of f_R from equation 1,

$$f_{R'} = f_s + \frac{V_R}{C} f_s + \frac{V_s}{C} \left(f_s + \frac{V_R}{C} \right) \tag{3}$$

Since $|V_R| = |V_s|$ $(= V)$ the target velocity, and because $V < C$ so that terms in $(V/C)^2$ can be neglected, equation 3 can be written as

$$f'_R = f_s + \frac{2V}{C} f_s \tag{4}$$

The Doppler shift frequency f_D is then given by:

$$f_D = \frac{2V}{C} f_s \tag{5}$$

The Doppler shift frequency, therefore, is a measure of the velocity of the blood. However, strictly speaking, a single frequency Doppler shift signal can only be produced if a plane target is moving at a constant velocity through a monochromatic ultrasonic field that extends over an infinitely wide beamwidth. This is obviously not the case when measuring blood flow, so it is necessary to see how this limits the practical application.

Consider the example of a finite width, monochromatic ultrasound beam, and a single target moving at a constant velocity. When the target enters the ultrasonic beam the incident ultrasound is frequency modulated (Doppler effect) but it is also amplitude modulated because of the finite size of the beam. Fine structure, due to diffraction effects in the ultrasound field from the transducer, modulates the amplitude of the back scattered signal. The resultant signal at the receiving transducer is both amplitude and frequency modulated. Fourier's theorem then says that if there is amplitude modulation of a single frequency, then the resultant Doppler signal at the receiver contains a spectrum of Doppler shift. The modulating function determines the shape of the frequency spectrum and the frequency spread is inversely proportional to the beam width.

Flowmeter Design

It has been shown in the previous section that there are very strict criteria for the correct use of the Doppler principle. However, flowmeters based on this principle work well in practice. There are two major types of flowmeter, namely, the continuous wave and the pulsed Doppler. In the continuous wave type there are usually two transducers, one emitting ultrasound continuously and the other acting as a receiver. The ultrasonic field occupies the continuous wave diffraction field of the transmitting transducer, but in practice it is only those targets moving within the beam common to both transducers that contribute to the Doppler output. The received signal is both amplitude and frequency modulated, as described in the previous section. Because the ultrasound is continuously emitted it is not known where the target is within the beam. If it is necessary to know the position of the target then the ultrasound must be pulsed. However, if the ultrasound is pulsed, in order to calculate this position, then certain limitations are imposed on the correct operation of the flowmeter. In the pulsed Doppler flowmeter, which was first described in 1969,[2] a single transducer acts as both emitter and receiver. During the interval between successive pulses, the transducer receives the scattered signal, and by means of a gated receiver, accepts signals from any point across the vessel lumen. The principle is illustrated in Figure 7-1. Since the speed of ultrasound in soft tissue is

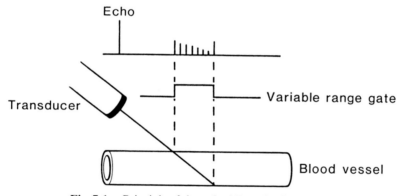

Fig. 7-1.   Principle of the pulsed Doppler flowmeter.

known, and since the elapsed time between emission and reception can be measured, then the distance of the target from the transducer can be calculated. There is a major disadvantage in pulsed systems, however, known as the velocity/range ambiguity, which arises in the following way. The pulse repetition frequency (PRF) is related to the maximum permissible range of the target R_M, and the velocity of ultrasound C in tissue by:

$$PRF < C/2R_M$$

In other words, the ultrasound pulse must be allowed to travel to the target and return to the transducer, before the next pulse is emitted. If the maximum Doppler shift frequency to be measured is f_{DM}, then sampling theory requires that:

$$PRF < 2f_{DM}$$

Since $f_{DM} = 2fV/C$, from the basic Doppler equation, then:

$$VR_M < C^2/8f$$

This means that the component of the blood velocity in the direction of the transducer multiplied by the maximum range is always less than a certain fixed value at the frequency used. This means that high velocities cannot be measured at long range without introducing an ambiguity. This ambiguity is usually referred to as "aliasing."

In a pulsed system the sample volume is determined by the pulse length and the diameter of the transducer. Suppose $\Delta\chi$ is the axial length of the sample volume, and suppose a target moves through the sample volume with an axial velocity v, then the transit time through the beam is given by:

$$\Delta t = \Delta\chi/v$$

From the previous discussion relating to amplitude modulation of the Doppler signal, the frequency spread Δf is inversely proportional to Δt, therefore:

$$\Delta f \propto v/\Delta\chi$$

For a given transmitted frequency, $\Delta v \propto \Delta f$, therefore

$$\frac{\Delta v}{v} \cdot \Delta\chi = \text{constant}$$

In other words the velocity and position of a target cannot be precisely calculated simultaneously. The introduction of a range measuring capability degrades the velocity resolution; and imposes a limit on the unambiguous measurement of velocity.

FLOW DIRECTION

Three major methods have been described to display flow direction, namely, single sideband detection, heterodyne detection, and phase quadrature detection.

If the ultrasonic carries frequency if and the measured Doppler shift frequency is f_D then for blood flow towards the probe the receiving transducer processes a signal of frequency $(f + f_D)$. For flow away from the probe the received frequency is $(f - f_D)$. In single sideband detection this received frequency is passed through two filters that have very steep filter characteristics. The characteristics are such that one filter passes $(f + f_D)$ and the other passes $(f - f_D)$. The outputs from these two filters can then be displayed.

In a heterodyne system[3] beats are produced between the received signal that contains the Doppler sidebands, and a local oscillator that operates at a frequency that is offset from that of the carrier. If f_H is the heterodyne or offset frequency then the total received signal is $(f + f_H) \pm f_D$. For flow towards the probe the demodulated received signal is $(f_H + f_D)$ and for flow away $(f_H - f_D)$. The disadvantage of this type of direction resolving system is that it is necessary to attenuate severely the carrier frequency component to prevent overloading.

In quadrature phase detection the returning signal $(f \pm f_D)$ is split into two parts, 90° out of phase. After synchronous detection, one channel leads the other in time and the flow direction is determined by which channel leads. This system has the disadvantage that if simultaneous forward and reverse flow exists it cannot be resolved. A more thorough review of the methods of flow direction processing has been produced.[3]

INSTRUMENTATION

The Doppler shift signal contains information about the way blood moves in a blood vessel, both in its velocity distribution across the lumen of the vessel and how this distribution varies with time over the cardiac cycle. These parameters them-selves are affected by the diameter and elastic properties of the blood vessel, and the impedance generated by the arterial system. It should, therefore, be possible to study physiological and pathological changes in the circulation by examining the Doppler spectrum. Because the continuous wave flowmeter obtains flow information from any blood vessel that intersects the ultrasonic beam from the transmitter, no depth information is available. If, however, the transmitter in the ultrasonic probe is pulsed, it is possible to determine from what part of the blood vessel the received Doppler signal is coming.

Doppler Imaging System

The simplest Doppler Imaging system consists of a continuous wave flowmeter linked to a position sensing arm and a display monitor. When a Doppler signal is detected a bright spot, corresponding to the probe position is stored on the monitor.

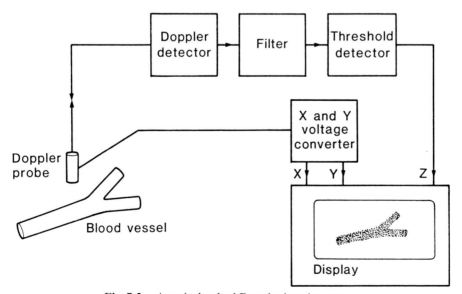

Fig. 7-2. A typical pulsed Doppler imaging system.

As the probe is moved over the skin overlying the blood vessel, an image of the projection of the blood vessel on the skin surface is generated on the screen. In the simple continuous wave systems only one projection can be obtained. In order to study the three dimensional flow image it is necessary to pulse the transmitted ultrasonic signal, and time-gate the received signal. Pulsed Doppler imaging systems require a position computer that combines the probe position signals and the signals corresponding to the position of the detected flow point in front of the transducer. A typical system is illustrated in Figure 7-2.

Duplex Scanners

Duplex scanners are a combination of a real-time B-scanner and a direction-resolving, pulsed, range-gated Doppler flowmeter. These instruments produce a real-time B-scan image of the area of interest and the sample volume of the flowmeter can be placed in the desired position within the scan plane. A typical system operates at 5 MHz and consists of three transducers mounted on a wheel which rotates continuously producing 30 frames per second.

The required image is stored, and one of the transducers acts as a gated pulsed Doppler transducer to sample the Doppler spectrum at a particular point within the blood vessel of interest. The position of the Doppler beam is indicated on the display by a white line and the position of the sample volume is shown as a white spot on this line. The position of the sample volume within the scan plane can be altered by means of an arm connected by a servomechanism to the transducer. A typical system is illustrated Figure 7-3.

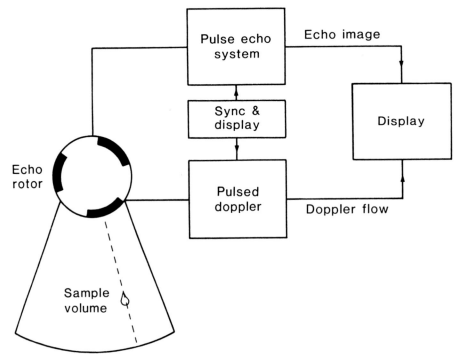

Fig. 7-3.   A typical Duplex scanner system.

Characterisation of the peripheral vascular bed is achieved by use of this type of equipment. The Doppler imaging systems and the Duplex scanners enable an image of the vessel lumen to be made and the Doppler spectrum from points within this image allow both localised and generalised information to be gained about the circulation.

Information Content of the Doppler Signal

As stated previously, the Doppler-shift spectrum contains information about the distribution of velocity across the vessel cross-section and the way it varies with time. This information is determined by the size of the blood vessels, their elastic properties, the impedance presented by the artery under investigation and the tissue bed fed by the artery. The vessel size can be determined by either the Doppler or the Duplex scanner but information concerning the impedance of the system can only be obtained by analysis of the variation of the Doppler spectrum over the cardiac cycle. A number of methods have been used including simple quantitative measurements of the maximum frequency envelope of the Doppler spectrum such as the Pulsatility Index, pattern recognition techniques such as Principle Components Analysis, and modelling techniques such as Laplace transform methods. Some of these methods are described in other chapters of this book and have been reviewed by Atkinson & Woodcock.[4]

REFERENCES

1. Satomura S: Study of the flow patterns in peripheral arteries by ultrasonics. J Acoust Soc Japan 15:151–158, 1959
2. Perronneau P, Leger F: Proc. 22nd Ann. Conf. on Engineering in Medicine & Biology, Chicago, p 10, (1969)
3. Coghlan BA, Taylor MG: Directional Doppler techniques for detection of blood velocities. Ultrasound Med Biol 2:171–179, 1976
4. Atkinson P, Woodcock JP: Doppler ultrasound and its use in clinical measurement. Academic Press, 1982

David S. Sumner
Dermot J. Moore
and Richard D. Miles

8

Ultrasonic Imaging

The dream of visualizing vascular morphology using noninvasive techniques has been brought closer to reality through the rapid advances in ultrasonic technology that have occurred over the past two decades. Ultrasonic imaging was first used successfully in the field of peripheral vascular diagnosis to assess the dimensions of abdominal aortic aneurysms.[1] The ability to outline the aneurysm wall accurately and consistently was quickly recognized as a major advantage not possessed by arteriograms which only delineate the lumen or lateral abdominal roentgenograms which depend on the vagaries of calcium deposition in the wall. The next area to receive attention was the extracranial carotid arterial system. Although the first attempts to image the carotid bifurcation were crude by today's standards, the results far surpassed those of the indirect noninvasive tests that were in use.[2] At present, ultrasonic imaging has become the preferred noninvasive method for diagnosing carotid arterial disease; not only does it accurately define the degree of stenosis but it also provides information concerning plaque morphology that cannot be attained in any other way.[3] Investigators, encouraged by the favorable results in the carotid system, have now begun to apply ultrasonic imaging to other areas where arteriography and routine noninvasive tests have proven deficient. Among the areas currently receiving attention are the diagnosis of renal and iliac arterial stenosis, intra- and postoperative assessment of vascular reconstructions, and the evaluation of deep venous thrombosis and valvular insufficiency.[4–7]

Two methods of ultrasonic imaging have been employed: Doppler flow-mapping and pulsed-echo methods. The most recent innovation, the Duplex scanner, combines pulsed-echo imaging and Doppler flow detection to provide both visual and physiologic information.

DOPPLER IMAGING

When an ultrasonic beam strikes a moving acoustic interface, such as a RBC, its frequency is altered according to the Doppler principle. The resulting frequency shift can be detected, amplified, and used to drive a speaker, to produce flow

DIAGNOSTIC TECHNIQUES AND ASSESSMENT
PROCEDURES IN VASCULAR SURGERY

© 1985 Grune & Stratton
ISBN 0-8089-1721-8 All rights reserved

recordings, or to unblank an oscilloscope screen. Early in the last decade, several groups of investigators independently and almost simultaneously conceived the idea of using the Doppler-shifted signal to map the flow stream—the underlying rationale being that the motion of blood could act as a contrast medium, analogous to the iodinated compounds used in conventional arteriography.[8–10]

Basically these instruments consist of an ultrasonic transducer, mounted on the end of a position-sensing arm, and a bistable storage oscilloscope (Fig. 8-1). As the transducer is moved over the surface of the skin, a spot appears on the oscilloscope screen when flow in an underlying blood vessel is detected. Since the location of the spot on the screen is determined by the position of the sensing arm, an image is gradually developed that resembles a conventional arteriographic picture—hence, the name "ultrasonic arteriography" (Fig. 8-2). The resulting image, which is essentially a projection of the arterial lumen in a plane paralleling that of the skin, is called a "plan view". Incorporation of direction-sensing circuitry permits the user to exclude flow in vessels carrying blood in the opposite direction from that in the vessel being studied. This avoids confusing the images of adjacent arteries and veins. In some instruments the colour of the dot appearing on the oscilloscope screen is modified to correspond to the frequency of the detected signal.[11] Since the frequency is directly related to the velocity of the blood, the color of the image helps define regions of stenosis where blood velocity is increased.

Two types of Doppler imaging devices are in use: those that use continuous-wave ultrasound and those that use pulsed-ultrasound. Pulsed-Doppler instruments, unlike those that use continuous-wave ultrasound, selectively detect blood flow at and only at a specific distance from the transducer. Discrete short bursts of ultrasound, each lasting for about 1.0 μsec, are emitted at a pulse repetition frequency (PRF) of about 16,000 times per second. The crystal used to transmit the sound remains quiescent for a short period and then is activated briefly to receive the

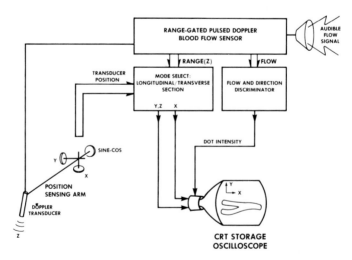

Fig. 8-1.   Block diagram of pulsed-Doppler imaging system. From Sumner DS, Russell JB, Miles RD: Pulsed-Doppler arteriography and computer assisted imaging of the carotid bifurcation, In Bergan JJ, Yao JST (eds): Cerebrovascular Insufficiency. Orlando, Fla, Grune & Stratton, 1983, pp 115–135.

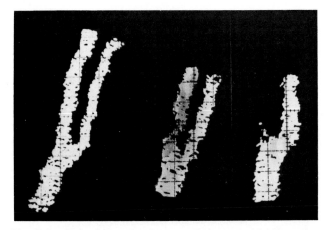

Fig. 8-2. Pulsed-Doppler images of the carotid bifurcation (plan views). Left, normal bifurcation; middle, stenosis of the internal carotid artery; right, total occlusion of the internal carotid artery. In each example, the internal carotid is on the left and the external on the right. From Sumner DS: Ultrasound, In Kempczinski RF, Yao JST (eds): Practical Noninvasive Vascular Diagnosis. Chicago, Year Book, 1982, pp 21–47.

backscattered signal, thus providing a "window" or "gate" for receiving the signal. Since the ultrasonic pulse, which travels at 1.56×10^5 cm/sec through the tissues, is reflected to a varying degree all along the way, only those signals that return when the gate is open are received. By adjusting the time between the transmission burst and activation of the gate, one can select the depth at which the flow signal will be detected. The volume of blood sampled depends on the geometry of the ultrasonic beam, the duration of the burst, and the length of time that the gate is open. When these parameters are properly adjusted, sample volumes may be restricted to a length of 1 to 2 mm.

Commercially available pulsed-Doppler imaging devices are equipped with multiple gates (6 to 30) that permit flow to be detected simultaneously at several different depths. When the transducer is oriented at right angles to the position sensing arm, spots will appear on the oscilloscope screen corresponding to each of the gates that are activated. A cross-sectional (depth) view will be obtained when the transducer is swept across the vessel perpendicular to its long axis, and a longitudinal (depth) view will be obtained when the transducer is used to trace the course of the vessel (Fig. 8-3). The plane of the longitudinal view is orthogonal (90°) to that of the usual plan view. In other words, if the plan view corresponds to an anterior-posterior (AP) arteriogram, the longitudinal view would correspond to a lateral arteriogram. When the transducer of a pulsed-Doppler imaging device is oriented in the same direction as the position sensing arm, all the spots coalesce into one on the oscilloscope screen, and the resulting image is of the plan type, identical to that developed with a continuous-wave device.

Pulsed-Doppler devices, having the ability to generate images in three planes, are therefore more versatile than the continuous-wave instruments. In addition, the ability to select the depth of flow recording, thereby eliminating unwanted signals,

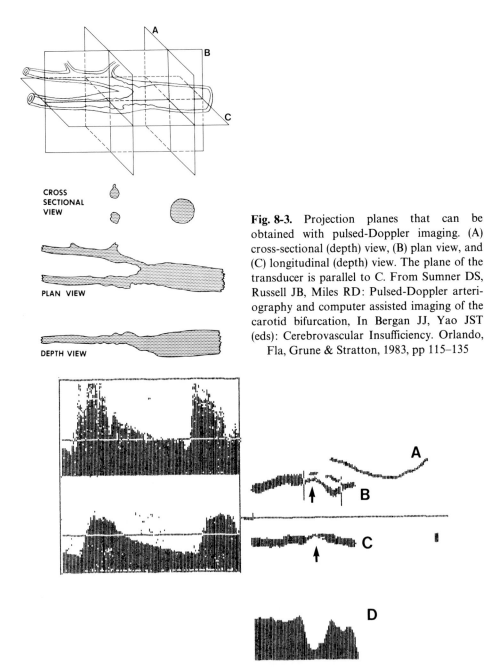

CROSS SECTIONAL VIEW

PLAN VIEW

DEPTH VIEW

Fig. 8-3. Projection planes that can be obtained with pulsed-Doppler imaging. (A) cross-sectional (depth) view, (B) plan view, and (C) longitudinal (depth) view. The plane of the transducer is parallel to C. From Sumner DS, Russell JB, Miles RD: Pulsed-Doppler arteriography and computer assisted imaging of the carotid bifurcation, In Bergan JJ, Yao JST (eds): Cerebrovascular Insufficiency. Orlando, Fla, Grune & Stratton, 1983, pp 115–135

A

B

C

D

Fig. 8-4. Thermal print of computerized pulsed-Doppler image showing a 60% stenosis of proximal internal carotid artery (arrows): (A) mandible, (B) plan (lateral) view, (C) longitudinal depth view (anterior-posterior projection), and (D) area histogram. Top spectrum is from distal internal carotid artery and bottom spectrum is from proximal internal carotid artery (see vertical lines on plan view). Both spectra show frequencies above 4000 Hz (horizontal line on spectra) and absence of systolic window.

makes the pulsed-Doppler arteriograph more discriminating than the non-depth sensitive continuous wave instruments. These advantages, however, are offset to some extent by the fact that pulsed-Dopplers are more difficult to use than continuous-wave instruments. Because reorientation of the probe to obtain cross-sectional and longitudinal depth views is cumbersome and time-consuming, most studies are performed in the plan mode, providing images similar to those obtained with the continuous wave instrument.

To overcome these difficulties, we have interfaced the pulsed-Doppler arterio-graph to a microcomputer, which is programmed to digitize the x-y position of the transducer and input flow signals from each of the range gates.[12] As the transducer probe is moved over the surface of the skin, both plan and depth views appear simultaneously on a video screen. Since the need to reposition the probe is elimi-nated, the process requires no more time and little more expertise than that required for conventional plan-view scanning. In addition, the computer has been prog-rammed to provide a simultaneous histogram depicting the cross-sectional area of the underlying vessel (Fig. 8-4).

Sources of Error

Calcification, which blocks the ultrasound beam, leads to confusing blank areas in the image, precluding the accurate estimation of stenosis. When the underlying vessels are tortuous or when flow is severely reduced, reversed, or stagnant, the image may defy interpretation. Arteries with a stenosis tight enough to restrict blood flow may appear occluded. Because the region of blood flow included in the sample volume is relatively large (even when a pulsed-Doppler instrument is used), it is impossible to define ulcers or irregularities of the vessel wall. Finally, unless scan-ning is done in multiple planes, asymmetrical stenoses may be misclassified.[12]

Many of these errors can be obviated by listening to the audible signal during the scanning process. For example, an astute technician hearing a normal Doppler signal distal to a blank area in the image would correctly ascribe the blank area to calcification rather than occlusion. To make the interpretation of flow signals more objective, most laboratories now routinely incorporate real-time spectral analysis into the scanning process. This identifies the source of the flow signals, avoids confu-sing one vessel for another, and allows selective interrogation of specific areas along the course of the vessel.

ECHO IMAGING

When short bursts of ultrasound are transmitted through the skin into the underlying tissues, some of the sonic energy is reflected from acoustic interfaces lying along the course of the sound beam. By timing the return of the echoes, one can determine the distance of the tissue boundaries from the transducer. Echo-imaging devices employ a B-mode display in which the amplitude of the echoes is indicated by the "brightness" of the dot appearing on a video screen. For static scanning, the transducer is mounted on a position-sensing arm, which, together with the range information derived from the time required for the echoes to return, serves to position the dots on the screen. As the transducer probe is swept over the skin surface, an image appears outlining all organs that have acoustic interfaces at their

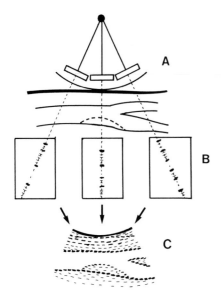

Fig. 8-5. Diagram illustrating real-time B-mode scanning. (A) Probe with transducer crystals in three positions. (B) Instantaneous echoes along course of sound beam. (C) Final image.

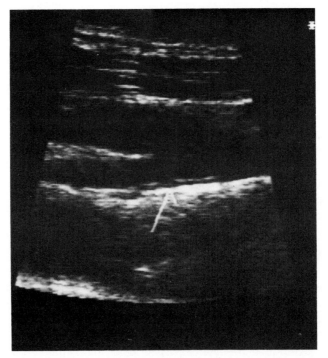

Fig. 8-6. Longitudinal real-time B-mode image of a normal carotid bifurcation. Arrow points to intimal "echogenic line," a normal finding.

boundaries. Static B-mode scanning is useful for measuring the dimensions of large arteries, such as the abdominal aorta, but the studies are too time consuming and cumbersome to be used in the routine investigation of peripheral vascular disease.

More recently, real-time B-mode instruments have become available. These employ a rotating or oscillating transducer or an oscillating beam-deflecting mirror encased in a water-filled probe. The ultrasonic beam sweeps through an arc producing a pie-shaped "sector scan" that is updated on a video screen 20 to 60 times per second (Fig. 8-5). Because all the insonated tissues are visualized continuously, these devices permit rapid surveillance of superficial arteries and veins, allow vascular wall motion to be perceived in real time, and guide the operator in positioning the probe to obtain an optimum image. Once a satisfactory image has been obtained, it can be frozen on the television screen for closer scrutiny or photographic recording (Fig. 8-6). All or selected positions of any study may be digitized and stored on floppy diskettes for future review.

To demonstrate luminal surface characteristics, the axial and lateral resolution should be less than 1.0 mm at the focal length of the transducer.[13] Excellent sensitivity and wide dynamic range (gray scale) are required for peripheral vascular work to distinguish plaques or thrombi of low echogenicity from blood. Transducers with a focal length of about 2 cm and a maximal focal zone extending to 4 cm are best for surveying the carotid and other superficial arteries and veins. For deeper structures, such as the abdominal aorta and renal arteries, greater focal lengths are preferred (Fig. 8-7).

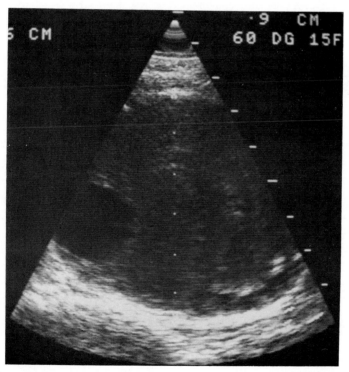

Fig. 8-7. Cross-sectional real-time B-mode image of a 5.6-cm abdominal aortic aneurysm. All of the lumen except for a small circular area to the left is filled with thrombus.

Sources of Error

Real-time B-mode scanners provide a two-dimensional image of a narrow slice (1–2 mm) of the insonated tissues. Since most objects in everyday experience are visualized by reflected or transmitted light, we are most familiar with projections or plan views, such as those produced by conventional arteriography. Consequently, it requires skill and concentration to become comfortable with images produced by B-mode scans. Interpretation is easiest when the plane of the scan is aligned with the long axis of the vessel and intersect the center of the vessel, thus producing a longitudinal section (Fig. 8-6). Cross-sectional images produced when the plane of the scan is orthogonal to the long axis of the vessel also present little difficulty (Fig. 8-8). Often, however, attempts to obtain these views are frustrated because the vessels bifurcate or curve out of the plane of the scan. For example, it may be impossible to image both the internal and external carotid arteries simultaneously, despite multiple attempts to find an appropriate plane.

When the artery is curved and the scan is tangentially placed, the image may suggest a stenosis even though none is present. Similarly, scans can totally miss, underestimate, or overestimate the severity of asymmetric plaques. Arteries with axi-symmetrical plaques may appear more stenotic (or even occluded) when the scan does not pass through the center of the vessel.[13]

Thrombus and soft-lipid-laden plaques, which have an acoustic impedance that differs little from blood, are often difficult to detect. Totally thrombosed vessels have been interpreted as being patent; in stenotic vessels, the degree of narrowing produced by such plaques is easily underestimated. Complicated plaques, especially those containing calcium, are highly echogenic. The shadow that they cause may

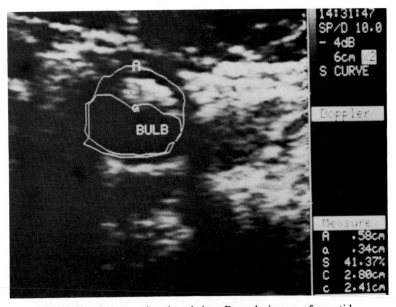

Fig. 8-8. Cross-sectional real-time B-mode image of carotid arterial bulb containing a brightly echogenic plaque. Planimeter function has been used to outline arterial wall and residual lumen. Calculated area stenosis was 41%.

obscure the opposite wall of the vessel or other parts of the atheroma. Soft plaques overlying a highly echogenic focus may be missed, causing the severity of the stenosis to be underestimated. Finally, depending upon the plane of the scan, the quality of the image, and the composition of the plaque, surface irregularities or ulcers can be missed when they are present and diagnosed when they are absent.

By scanning each vessel in multiple planes and by thinking three-dimensionally the skilled technician can reduce the number of these errors. It has, however, become the practice of many laboratories to supplement the image with an assessment of the flow pattern.

DUPLEX-IMAGING

Realization that real-time images are subject to errors of interpretation prompted the development of instruments that incorporate both real-time B-mode scanning and pulsed-Doppler flow-sensing capabilities.[14] The same crystal can be used for both echo-imaging and Doppler flow-sensing; or alternatively, a separate crystal dedicated to Doppler flow sensing may be placed in the probe adjacent to that used for echo imaging. Owing to interference between the signals, both studies cannot be accomplished simultaneously. In some instruments, a suitable frame of the real-time image is frozen on the video screen while flow in the imaged vessel is assessed. In others, the image is updated every few seconds to assure that the sample volume of the pulsed-Doppler remains in the proper position. Still other instruments utilize an M-mode display, allowing continuous monitoring of the position of the Doppler sample volume.

Once the image has been selected, the direction of the sound beam from the Doppler can be adjusted so that it intersects the flow stream at a defined angle, usually 45° or 60°. A line on the video screen indicates the direction of the sound beam. Some instruments provide another shorter line that can be placed in the direction of the flow stream to assist in the calculation of the angle of incidence (Fig. 8-9). By adjusting the range gate of the Doppler, one can place the sample volume in the center of the flow stream or at any point where one desires to examine the flow pattern. A dot, x, or other visual device that moves along the line defining the direction of the sound beam is used to indicate the location of the sample volume. Many instruments allow the length of the sample volume to be varied so that flow can be measured across the entire vessel lumen or restricted to only a small portion of the lumen (Fig. 8-9). The pulsed-Doppler signal can be interpreted audibly or it can be recorded in real-time. Although the signal can be processed with an analogue recorder, most instruments employ a fast-Fourier transform method to provide a frequency-spectrum analysis.

Duplex systems have many advantages. The image permits precise interrogation of the flow pattern at any desired spot along the artery (or vein) and at any specific point across its diameter. In this way, suspected lesions visualized on the scan can be assessed physiologically and their severity confirmed or denied by an additional modality, reducing the chance of missing a poorly echogenic thrombus or over-reading or under-reading the degree of stenosis. Since the angle at which the ultrasonic beam intersects the flow stream is critical to the accurate interpretation of the Doppler signal, the ability to select this angle is an important feature of Duplex

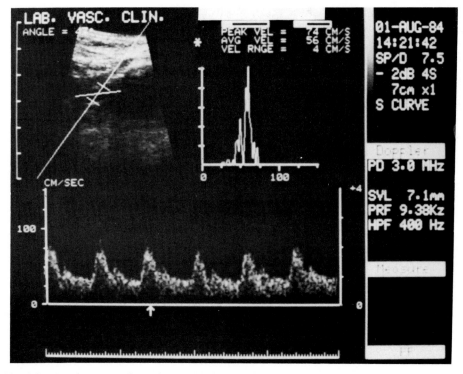

Fig. 8-9. Duplex scan of proximal internal carotid artery. The long line across sector scan indicates direction of pulsed-Doppler sound beam, which intersects the axis of the flow stream (shorter line) at a 47° angle. The two shortest lines indicate the length of the sample volume (7.1 mm). Spectrum shows peak velocity of 74 cm/sec (at arrow), with little spectral broadening.

systems. Lastly, the image may detect small plaques that do not produce flow disturbances and may supply information regarding the morphology and composition of the plaque, information that cannot be retrieved by the exclusive use of Doppler modalities. In turn, the audible Doppler signal facilitates the identification of the vessel being imaged, reducing the chance of confusing an artery for a vein or a high-resistance artery (such as the external carotid) for a lower-resistance artery (such as the internal carotid).

ACCURACY

The value of any diagnostic test ultimately depends on its accuracy in clinical applications. To reap the maximum benefit from a test, its limitations as well as its advantages must be carefully weighed, and the questions that it is supposed to answer must be rigidly defined. At the same time, it must be remembered that a test that gives superior results under one set of circumstances may give inferior results under another.

Extracranial Carotid Arterial Disease

The accuracy of ultrasonic imaging vis-à-vis conventional carotid arteriography has been carefully scrutinized by a large number of investigators. Their observations, therefore, provide a wealth of information that can be used not only to compare the accuracies of the various imaging devices but also to examine how accuracy varies according to diagnostic requirements.

Tables 8-1 through 8-4 summarize the parameters of accuracy from reports in which the data were sufficiently detailed to permit analysis. Accuracy is defined in terms of sensitivity (the ability to detect the presence of disease) and specificity (the ability to recognize the absence of disease). The utility of the test is described by the positive predictive value (the likelihood that a positive test result implies the presence of disease) and negative predictive value (the likelihood that a negative test result excludes the presence of disease).[47] For most of the parameters, the range of reported values was quite wide. In the case of the Duplex scanner (Table 8-4), accuracy has increased with refinements of the equipment; in other cases, the variation probably reflects gradations of experience or the vagaries of sampling. To simplify comparisons, mean values were calculated from the accumulated data.

For distinguishing between hemodynamically significant ($\geq 50\%$ diameter reduction) and non-hemodynamically significant lesions ($< 50\%$ diameter reduction)

Table 8-1

Accuracy of Pulsed Doppler Arteriography (UA) for Detecting Disease of the Internal Carotid Artery

References	Diagnostic Criteria	Sensitivity	Specificity	PPV	NPV
14–22	$<50\% \ v \geq 50\%$	87–96 (90)*	65–99 (87)	53–98 (80)	91–98 (94)
14, 17, 20–24	$0 \ v \geq 1\%$	70–96 (76)†	74–94 (80)	81–98 (88)	29–92 (64)
15, 17, 20–24	$\leq 99\% \ v \ 100\%$	61–100 (82)‡	95–100 (97)	64–100 (80)	96–100 (98)

Note. Data are range (mean) expressed as a percentage.
* 1393 studies.
† 1805 studies.
‡ 1411 studies.

Table 8-2

Accuracy of Continuous-Wave Doppler Imaging for Detecting Disease of the Internal Carotid Artery

References	Diagnostic Criteria	Sensitivity	Specificity	PPV	NPV
11, 25–31	$<50\% \ v \geq 50\%$	78–98 (91)*	77–99 (89)	62–99 (82)	88–99 (95)
11, 30, 32	$0 \ v \geq 1\%$	69–93 (75)†	53–94 (87)	81–96 (87)	44–82 (75)
11, 28, 30, 31	$\leq 99\% \ v \ 100\%$	58–88 (75)‡	96–99 (98)	78–88 (82)	93–99 (97)

Notes. Data are range (mean) expressed as a percentage.
* 1427 studies.
† 690 studies.
‡ 887 studies.

Table 8-3
Accuracy of B-Mode Real-Time Imaging for Detecting Disease of the
Internal Carotid Artery

References	Diagnostic Criteria	Sensitivity	Specificity	PPV	NPV
13, 23, 33–37	<50% v ≥50%	36–88 (84)*	67–98 (87)	42–92 (77)	77–93 (91)
23, 34	0 v ≥1%	84–100 (95)†	47–91 (75)	89–91 (89)	83–100 (87)
23, 34, 35	≤99% v 100%	27–67 (61)‡	99–100 (99)	80–100 (85)	88–98 (97)

Note. Data are range (mean) expressed as a percentage.
* 2529 studies.
† 168 studies.
‡ 1857 studies.

Table 8-4
Accuracy of Duplex Imaging for Detecting Disease of the
Internal Carotid Artery

References	Diagnostic Criteria	Sensitivity	Specificity	PPV	NPV
38–45	<50% v ≥50%	90–96 (93)*	82–98 (90)	82–97 (89)	87–96 (94)
38–40, 43, 45, 46	0 v ≥1%	93–100 (97)†	21–84 (64)	87–97 (95)	25–100 (74)
38–41, 43, 45, 46	≤99% v 100%	70–100 (88)‡	96–100 (98)	71–100 (88)	94–100 (98)

Note. Data are range (mean) expressed as a percentage.
* 1490 studies.
† 1214 studies.
‡ 1341 studies.

of the internal carotid arteries, all of the techniques had roughly the same mean specificity (87%–90%); but the sensitivity of B-mode imaging (84%) appeared to be somewhat inferior to that of the other modalities (90%–93%). Doppler imaging, of both varieties, was less sensitive (75%–76%) than B-mode (95%) or Duplex (97%) imaging for detecting any disease causing ≥1% diameter reduction. This finding merely reflects the superior resolving power of the echo technique compared with the Doppler flow-map. On the other hand, Doppler imaging was somewhat more specific (80%–87%) for identifying vessels without disease than the B-mode or Duplex devices (64%–75%). In other words, the echo techniques reveal (or appear to reveal) small lesions that are not perceptible on contrast arteriograms. Detecting total occlusions is best accomplished with the Duplex scan (sensitivity, 88%) and least well accomplished with the B-mode imager (sensitivity, 61%), testifying to the value of Doppler flow analysis for identifying weakly echogenic plaques and thrombi that occlude the carotid artery. The specificity of all methods was excellent (97%–99%) for demonstrating patency of stenotic but not occluded arteries.

Although sensitivity and specificity are useful for comparing the relative accuracies of diagnostic modalities, the positive (PPV) and negative (NPV) predictive values convey more information to the recipient of the test results. Because predictive values are greatly influenced by the prevalence of disease in the population studied and because disease prevalence varies from study to study, it is often inap-

propriate to compare raw predictive values.[47] To make predictive values comparable, they must all be normalized to the same disease prevalence. As shown in Table
8-5, the NPV of all the imaging methods was good (91%–96%) for identifying non-
hemodynamically significant lesions. In other words, if the study was read as
showing a less than 50% diameter reduction, there is only a 4%–9% chance that the
stenosis exceeds 50%. Similarly, an image from any of the devices showing a patent
vessel, regardless of the degree of stenosis, virtually rules out a complete occlusion
(NPV, 96%–99%). A normal B-mode or Duplex scan makes it unlikely that the
vessel is diseased (NPV, 89%–92%), but a normal Doppler scan is inconclusive for
the absence of disease (NPV, 64%–65%). Stated in another way, 35% of vessels with
negative Doppler scans can be expected to harbor arteriographically detectable
lesions.

The ability of the imaging devices to accurately predict the presence of disease
is, in general, inferior to their ability to rule out disease. A study suggesting a stenosis exceeding 50% diameter reduction has about a 20% chance of being incorrect
(PPV, 78%–82%). The presence of any disease, regardless of its severity, is predicted
with about 90% confidence by the Doppler and B-mode scans. Owing to its lower
specificity, the Duplex scan is a bit less accurate (PPV, 83%). For reasons that are
not apparent, pulsed-Doppler scans (PPV, 75%) seem less accurate for predicting
total occlusion than the other modalities. A B-mode scan that indicates a total
occlusion has the greatest chance (87%) of being correct. At any rate, the likelihood
that an apparent totally occluded vessel is in fact patent is high enough with any of
the devices (13%–25%) that confirmatory arteriography should be obtained.

In our laboratory, the accuracy of pulsed-Doppler arteriography has been
improved by computerizing the image and by routinely performing spectral
analysis.[12,48] When the two studies agreed, as they did in 89% of the carotid bifurcations, the sensitivity was 98% and the specificity was 94% for distinguishing
between hemodynamically and nonhemodynamically significant lesions. The PPV
was 84% and the NPV was 99%. The presence or absence of any disease was
detected with a sensitivity of 88%, a specificity of 93%, a PPV of 91%, and a NPV

Table 8-5
Predictive Values for Detecting Disease of the Internal Carotid Artery
(Normalized to Equivalent Disease Prevalences

Diagnostic Criteria	Prevalence (%)	Test	PPV (%)	NPV (%)
$<50\%$ v $\geq50\%$	35	Pulsed-Doppler	79	94
		C-W Doppler	82	95
		B-Mode	78	91
		Duplex	83	96
0 v $\geq1\%$	65	Pulsed-Doppler	88	64
		C-W Doppler	91	65
		B-Mode	88	89
		Duplex	83	92
$\leq99\%$ v 100%	10	Pulsed-Doppler	75	98
		C-W Doppler	81	97
		B-Mode	87	96
		Duplex	83	99

of 90%. Agreement between the image and spectrum occurred in 80% of the studies. If the overall results were called positive when either the spectrum or computerized image was positive and negative only when both were negative, the sensitivity was 96% for hemodynamically signficant lesions and 91% for any disease. Specificity, of course, suffered—falling to 83% and 74%, respectively.[48]

Ulcers cannot be detected with Doppler imaging. With their superior resolution, real-time B-mode images are capable of identifying ulcers, provided the plane of the scan is appropriate. Even so, according to Katz et al the sensitivity was only 33% for small craters (<2 mm) and 58% for larger craters (>2 mm).[49] Specificity was 84%; NPV was 62%; and PPV was 44%–85%, depending on the size of the ulcer. While these results are imperfect, they compare favorably with those of arteriography. Real-time imaging has been reported to detect intra-plaque hemorrhage with a sensitivity of 91% and a specificity of 65%.[3] This potentially very important information cannot be obtained arteriographically.

Other Areas

Norris et al have used the Duplex scanner to investigate renal artery stenosis.[4] Even in this relatively inaccessible area, they were able to distinguish between <60% and ≥60% stenosis with a sensitivity of 83% and a specificity of 97%. Using similar instrumentation, Jager et al have identified disease in all of the lower extremity arteries from the iliac to the popliteal with gratifying accuracy.[5] Particularly impressive were the data from the iliac and profunda femoris arteries, two areas that are notoriously difficult to examine by arteriography or by the usual noninvasive methods. In both arteries, the PPV for hemodynamically significant stenosis was 100%; and the NPV for excluding hemodynamically significant lesions was 92% and 98%, respectively.

The accuracy of imaging in other areas has received more attention and will be discussed later in this book.

CLINICAL APPLICATION—PRINCIPLES

Of all the applications of ultrasonic imaging none has excited more interest or has been more thoroughly studied than its use in the diagnosis of suspected disease of the extracranial carotid arteries. Imaging methods avoid many of the errors inherent in indirect noninvasive testing, which include inability to detect non-stenotic plaques and relative insensitivity to diameter stenosis in the 50%–75% range.[2] But, at present, the imaging methods are not infallible, and their rational application must be determined by the demands of the clinical situation. Several guidelines can be formulated.

Hemodynamically Significant Disease

All of the imaging modalities are capable of ruling out hemodynamically significant disease. Patients with asymptomatic bruits and those will ill-defined non-hemispheric symptoms can therefore be spared arteriography when the results are negative. A positive test result, however, requires arteriographic confirmation if surgical intervention is to be restricted to arteries with hemodynamically significant lesions.

Non-Stenotic Lesions

Doppler imaging techniques do not reliably rule out low-grade lesions. A negative B-mode or Duplex study does tend to rule out disease, but not with an accuracy sufficient to obviate the need for arteriography if the patient's symptoms are compatible with an embolic focus. Likewise, a positive result with any of the methods—though highly suggestive of disease—should be confirmed with arteriography. On the other hand, a positive image—especially a B-mode image that shows an ulcer or a heterogeneous plaque—should be taken seriously and acted upon if the clinical situation dictates, even when a less significant lesion is visualized arteriographically.[3,35,50]

Total Occlusion

Ultrasonic images that demonstrate a patent artery are apt to be correct. Thus, arteriograms that appear occluded when the image indicates patency should be viewed skeptically; in some cases, surgical exploration may be indicated to establish the diagnosis and to forestall progression of a highly stenotic lesion to total occlusion.[51] Ultrasonic images cannot be relied on to diagnose total occlusion. All apparent occlusions should be verified arteriographically.[52]

Based on these considerations, ultasonic imaging is a particularly good method for screening patients with asymptomatic bruits or ill-defined symptoms or for evaluating patients scheduled to undergo cardiovascular or peripheral vascular surgery. Even in patients with hemispheric symptoms (transient ischemic attack, stroke, amaurosis fugax), the images can supply valuable supplementary information, particularly when arteriographic findings do not coincide with clinical impressions. In the rare patient on whom arteriography cannot be performed—either because of severe allergy to contrast or lack of vascular access—imaging can function as the only diagnostic method prior to surgery.[53,54] Finally, imaging is ideally suited for population surveys, for following patients after surgery, and for detecting advancing lesions in patients on whom no surgery has been performed.[55,56] For these purposes, arteriography is too invasive and indirect noninvasive testing is far too inaccurate.

Other chapters will further develop the diagnostic approach to cerebrovascular disease and will discuss the application of ultrasonic imaging to the diagnosis of aneurysms, to the detection of intraoperative mishaps, and to the evaluation of deep venous thrombosis. For each area, specific guidelines must be formulated in order to capitalize on the strengths and to minimize the weaknesses of ultrasonic imaging.

CONCLUSION

It is hardly an exaggeration to state that ultrasonic imaging is in the process of revolutionizing the diagnostic approach to peripheral vascular disease. Imaging techniques have already had a major impact on the diagnosis of cerebrovascular disease, having replaced indirect tests in many laboratories. Promising new applications are being reported in the areas of renal, visceral, and peripheral arterial disease—even in the area of venous thrombosis and valvular insufficiency. The ability to define plaque morphology, measure stenoses accurately, and investigate local flow disturbances makes ultrasonic imaging ideally suited for population surveys and follow-up studies. As a result, contributions to the understanding of the natural history of vascular disease are beginning to appear in the literature, providing knowledge that may alter prevailing therapeutic concepts. All this has been made possible by the continuing interaction between clinical investigators and their engineering counterparts, who are almost daily improving the quality of the image, probe design, Doppler capabilities, and signal processing. Much remains to be accomplished, but the future looks bright.

REFERENCES

1. Segal BL, Likoff W, Asperger F, et al: Ultrasound diagnosis of an abdominal aortic aneurysm. Am J Cardiol 17:101, 1966
2. Sumner DS: Noninvasive methods for preoperative assessment of carotid occlusive disease. Part 1. Statistical interpretation of test results. Vasc Diag Therapy 2:41, 1981
3. Reilly LM, Lusby RJ, Hughes L, et al: Carotid plaque histology using real-time ultrasonography. Clinical and therapeutic implications. Am J Surg 146:188, 1983
4. Norris CS, Pfeiffer JS, Rittgers SE, et al: Noninvasive evaluation of renal artery stenosis and renovascular resistance. Experimental and clinical studies. J Vasc Surg 1:192, 1984
5. Jager KA, Phillips DJ, Martin RL, et al: Noninvasive mapping of lower limb arterial lesions. Ultrasound Med Biol 1985 (in press)
6. Sigel B, Coelho JCU, Flanigan DP: Ultrasonic imaging during vascular surgery. Arch Surg 117:764, 1982
7. Sullivan ED, Peter DJ, Cranley JJ: Real-time B-mode venous ultrasound. J Vasc Surg 1:465, 1984
8. Mozersky DJ, Hokanson DE, Baker DW, et al: Ultrasonic arteriography. Arch Surg 103:663, 1971
9. Fish PJ: Visualizing blood vessels by ultrasound. In Roberts VC (ed): Blood Flow Measurement. London, Sector Publishing Ltd, 1972, pp 29–32
10. Reid JM, Spencer MP: Ultrasonic Doppler technique for imaging blood vessels. Science 176:1235, 1972
11. White DN, Curry GR: A comparison of 424 carotid bifurcations examined by angiography and the Doppler echoflow. In White D, Lyons EA (eds): Ultrasound in Medicine. Vol 4, New York, Plenum, 1978, pp 363–376
12. Miles RD, Russell JB, Modi JR, et al: Computerized multiplanar imaging and lumen area plotting for noninvasive diagnosis of carotid artery disease. Surgery 93:676, 1983
13. Comerota AJ, Cranley JJ, Cook SE: Real-time B-mode carotid imaging in diagnosis of cerebrovascular disease. Surgery 89:718, 1981
14. Blackshear WM Jr, Phillips DJ, Thiele BL, et al: Detection of carotid occlusive disease by ultrasonic imaging and pulsed Doppler spectrum analysis. Surgery 86:698, 1979
15. Barnes RW, Bone GE, Reinertson J, et al: Noninvasive ultrasonic angiography: Prospective validation by contrast arteriography. Surgery 80:328, 1976
16. Wolf EA Jr: Discussion of Sumner DS, Russell JB, Ramsey DE, et al: Noninvasive diagnosis of extracranial carotid arterial disease. Arch Surg 114:1222, 1979
17. Cardullo PA, Cutler BS, Wheeler HB, et al: Noninvasive detection of carotid disease: An evaluation of oculoplethysmography, carotid phonoangiography, and pulsed Doppler ultrasonic arteriography. Bruit 5:26, 1981

18. Hobson RW II, Berry SM, Jamil Z, et al: Oculoplethysmography and pulsed Doppler ultrasonic imaging in the diagnosis of carotid occlusive disease. Surg Gynecol Obstet 152:433, 1981

19. Bodily KC, Modene B, Chikos PM, et al: Ultrasonic arteriography: Implications in patient management. West J Med 135:183, 1981

20. Sumner DS, Russell JB, Miles RD: Are noninvasive tests sufficiently accurate to identify patients in need of carotid arteriography? Surgery 91:700, 1982

21. Doorly TPG, Atkinson PI, Kingston V, et al: Carotid ultrasonic arteriography combined with real-time spectral analysis: A comparison with angiography. J Cardiovasc Surg 23:243, 1982

22. Wasserman DH, Hobson, RW II, Lynch TG, et al: Ultrasonic imaging and oculoplethysmography in diagnosis of carotid occlusive disease. Arch Surg 118:1161, 1983

23. Hobson RW II, Berry SM, Katocs AS Jr, et al: Comparison of pulsed-Doppler and real-time B-mode echo arteriography for noninvasive imaging of the extracranial carotid arteries. Surgery 87:286, 1980

24. Warlow CP, Fish PJ: Pulsed Doppler imaging of the carotid artery. J Neurol Sci 45:135, 1980

25. Spencer MP, Brockenbrough EC, Davis DL, et al: Cerebrovascular evaluation using Doppler C-W ultrasound. In White D, Brown RE (eds): Ultrasound in Medicine. Vol. 3B. New York, Plenum, 1977, pp 1291–1310

26. Blackwell E, Merory J, Toole JF, et al: Doppler ultrasound scanning of the carotid bifurcation. Arch Neurol 34:145, 1977

27. Shoumaker RD, Bloch S: Cerebrovascular evaluation: Assessment of Doppler scanning of carotid arteries, opthalmic Doppler flow, and cervical bruits. Stroke 9:563, 1978

28. Lynch TG, Wright CB, Miller EV, et al: Comparison of continuous-wave Doppler imaging, oculopneumoplethysmography, and the cerebrovascular Doppler examination. Circulation 66(Supp 1):106, 1982

29. O'Leary DH, Clouse ME, Persson, AB, et al: Noninvasive testing for carotid artery stenosis. II. Clinical application of accuracy assessments. AJR 138:109, 1982

30. Turnispeed WD, Sackett JF, Strother CM, et al: A comparison of standard cerebral arteriography with noninvasive Doppler imaging and intravenous angiography. Arch Surg 117:419, 1982

31. D'Alton JB, Norris JW: Carotid Doppler evaluation in cerebrovascular disease. Can Med Assoc J 129:1184, 1983

32. Weaver RG Jr, Howard G, McKinney WM, et al: Comparison of Doppler ultrasonography with arteriography of the carotid bifurcation. Stroke 11:402, 1980

33. Humber PR, Leopold GR, Wickbom IG, et al: Ultrasonic imaging of the carotid arterial system. Am J Surg 140:199, 1980

34. Wolverson MK, Heiberg E, Sundaram M, et al: Carotid atherosclerosis: High resolution real-time sonography correlated with angiography. AJR 140:355, 1983

35. Comerota AJ, Cranley JJ, Katz ML, et al: Real-time B-mode carotid imaging. A three-year multicenter experience. J Vasc Surg 1:84, 1984

36. Herring MB, Russ M, Benge C, et al: A comparison of Doppler flow measurement, ultrasonic and arteriographic imaging in the evaluation of stenoses of the carotid artery. Surg Gynecol Obstet 159:67, 1984

37. Farber R, Bromer M, Anderson D, et al: B-mode real-time ultrasonic carotid imaging: Impact on decision-making and prediction of surgical findings. Neurology 34:541, 1984

38. Fell G, Phillips DJ, Chikos PM, et al: Ultrasonic Duplex scanning for disease of the carotid artery. Circulation 64:1191, 1981

39. Breslau PJ, Knox RA, Beach KW, et al: Ultrasonic Duplex scanning with spectral analysis in extracranial carotid artery disease. Comparison with contrast arteriography. Vasc Diag Therapy 3:17, 1982

40. Roederer GO, Langlois YE, Chan AW, et al: Ultrasonic Duplex scanning of extracranial

carotid arteries: Improved accuracy using new features from the common carotid artery. J Cardiovasc Ultrasonography 1:373, 1982

41. Daigle RJ, Gardner M, Smazal SF, et al: Accuracy of Duplex ultrasound scanning in the evaluation of carotid artery disease. Bruit 7:17, 1983

42. Wetzner SM, Kiser LC, Bezrek JS: Duplex ultrasound imaging: Vascular applications. Radiology 150:507, 1984

43. Eikelboom BC, Ackerstaff RGA, Ludwig JW, et al: Digital video subtraction angiography and duplex scanning in assessment of carotid artery disease: Comparison with conventional angiography. Surgery 94:821, 1983

44. Matsumoto GH, Rumwell CB: Screening of carotid arteries by noninvasive Duplex scanning. Am J Surg 145:609, 1983

45. Cardullo PA, Cutler BS, Wheeler HB, et al: Accuracy of Duplex scanning in the detection of carotid artery disease. Bruit 8:181, 1984

46. Glover JL, Bendick PJ, Jackson VP, et al: Duplex ultrasonography, digital subtraction angiography, and conventional angiography in assessing carotid atherosclerosis. Arch Surg 119:664, 1984

47. Sumner DS: Evaluation of noninvasive testing procedures, data analysis and interpretation. In Bernstein EF (ed): Noninvasive Diagnostic Techniques in Vascular Disease. 3 ed, St. Louis, Mosby, 1985, (in press)

48. Sumner DS, Moore DJ, Miles RD: Doppler ultrasonic arteriography and flow velocity analysis in carotid disease. In Bernstein EF (ed): Noninvasive Diagnostic Techniques in Vascular Disease. 3 ed, St. Louis, Mosby, 1985, (in press)

49. Katz ML, Johnson M, Pomajzl MJ, et al: The sensitivity of real-time B-mode carotid imaging in the detection of ulcerated plaques. Bruit 8:13, 1983

50 Johnson JM, Ansel AL, Morgan S: Ultrasonographic screening for evaluation and follow-up of carotid artery ulceration. A new basis for assessing risk. Am J Surg 144:614, 1982

51. Poole MA, Boone SC: Distinguishing subtotal from total carotid occlusion. Complementary roles of angiography and Doppler study. Vasc Diag Ther 4:19, 1983

52. O'Leary DH, Gibbons GW, Pinel DF: Limitations of noninvasive testing in assessing the "occluded" carotid artery. AJNR 4:759, 1983

53. Blakshear W Jr, Connar RG: Carotid endarterectomy without angiography. J Cardiovasc Surg 23:477, 1982

54. Ricotta, JJ, Holen J, Schenk E, et al: Is routine angiography necessary prior to carotid endarterectomy? J Vasc Surg 1:96, 1984

55. Zierler RE, Bandyk DF, Thiele BL, et al: Carotid artery stenosis following endarterectomy. Arch Surg 117:1408, 1982

56. Roederer GO, Langlois YE, Jager KA, et al: The natural history of carotid arterial disease in asymptomatic patients with cervical bruits. Stroke 15:605, 1984

J. W. Ludwig, B. C. Eikelboom
C. C. van Schaik, A. J. Taams
and C. Teeuwen

9

Digital Subtraction Angiography (DSA)

Besides the non-invasive techniques, angiography remains essential. The disadvantages of angiography are the complexity of the procedure and the possibility of complications. Digital subtraction angiography (DSA) is a considerable improvement in the examination of vessels. In DSA, subtraction combined with enhancement of the signals allows the use of intravenous injection to obtain good images of the arteries. However, when the contrast material is supplied intravenously, a rather large amount of contrast material is necessary to obtain images of good quality. Quantities of 30–40 cc of contrast material are required. The advantage of the intravenous injection of contrast material rather than the use of a catheter to deliver the contrast material in loco is that it is almost non-invasive thus circumventing the complications caused by catheter manipulation in the arterial system. This makes it possible to apply this method on an out-patient basis.

To obtain good images with the intravenous DSA several conditions must be fulfilled. The most important is good cooperation of the patient to prevent motion artefacts in the subtraction technique and a second condition is a good circulation to optimize the iodine concentration in the arteries that are to be examined.

DSA can also be applied with intra-arterial selective injection of the contrast material. In this case, the strong enhancement with DSA allows the use of a small quantity of contrast material while still obtaining images of the vessels with good contrast definition. For instance 2 to 3 cc of contrast material diluted with saline solution to 8–10 ml suffices for the examination of the carotid arteries. Through the enhancement of the signal with DSA good images can still be obtained even with less selective injection of the contrast material.

Cerebrovascular Disease

For reasons mentioned above we prefer intravenous DSA as long as it provides sufficient information. This means that one needs not only accurate information on the carotid bifurcations in two different planes, but also visualisation of aortic arch vessels and intracranial circulation. The resolution of intravenous DSA is good enough to obtain this goal, even for the carotid syphons. The major problem is the limited amount of contrast that can be given. Visualisation of all these areas in two

DIAGNOSTIC TECHNIQUES AND ASSESSMENT
PROCEDURES IN VASCULAR SURGERY © 1985 Grune & Stratton
ISBN 0-8089-1721-8 All rights reserved

different planes requires too many injections of contrast material. This has led many users of DSA to its intra-arterial application. In our experience this is not necessary if DSA is preceded by a good non-invasive evaluation. Duplex scanning combines B-mode imaging with spectrum analysis of a pulsed Doppler signal and allows accurate evaluation of all extracranial vessels. This information is given to the radiologist which allows him to make optimal use of the limited amount of contrast. By adopting this policy we obtain sufficient information with intravenous DSA in 91% of our patients for carotid surgery. Intra-arterial DSA is only necessary in complex multivessel disease, if there is disagreement between Duplex and intravenous DSA and in poor quality intravenous DSA.

Abdominal Aorta

Examination of the abdominal aorta with intravenous DSA gives excellent results in cooperative patients with a good circulation. To study the aorta in patients with dysbasia or in cases of suspicion of an aneurysm the intravenous application of contrast material provides sufficient information in almost all cases. The origin of renal arteries can be determined in respect to the aneurysm almost always. With intravenous DSA as in conventional angiography only the lumen can be visualized and not the exact diameter of an aneurysm if an attached thrombus exists. In a series of 65 patients, 92% of the cases, the angiographic information in combination with non-invasive examinations such as ultra sound, or CT, suffices for surgical treatment.

Renal Arteries

In patients with hypertension an examination of renal arteries can be of great value. With intravenous DSA reliable information about stenosis of renal arteries can be achieved. Correlation between diagnosis with intravenous DSA and intraarterial application of contrast material in studies done with the DVI-II machine (Philips corporation) is now an average of about 95%, approximately the same as other authors describe. After treatment by angioplasty or renal artery surgery, a check with intravenous DSA can easily be performed.

Iliac Arteries

The examination of the iliac arteries can be done with intravenous DSA. To obtain good images of these arteries interfering bowel movement artefacts must be prevented. For this we inject a drug. The best results we obtain with intervenous application of Scopolamine bromide 40 mgr (Buscopan®, Boehringer Ing.) and if a contra indication for this exists we use Glucagon intravenously 1 mg. In cooperative patients with a good circulation we can do a good study of the iliac arteries on an out-patient basis.

DSA After Intervention

The results of surgery or interventional radiology can be checked with intravenous DSA. The almost harmless procedure with a small inconvenience for the patient allows these studies. The easy imaging of vessels can be helpful to evaluate the surgical or radiological intervention.

Peripheral Arteries

In patients with lower limb ischemia, there is a place for intravenous DSA, intraarterial DSA and conventional arteriography, depending on the extent and location of the disease. Intravenous DSA provides sufficient information on the femoro-popliteal segment. If the disease is limited to this segment as in claudication, surgery can often be performed on intravenous DSA only. However, patients with rest pain or gangrene require more detailed information on the tibial and peroneal arteries. This can not be obtained by intravenous DSA and a choice has to be made between intraarterial DSA and conventional arteriography by femoral puncture. If a tibial bypass is considered, conventional arteriography is superior to intraarterial DSA in assessment of the quality of these vessels, due to its better spatial resolution. However, intraarterial DSA is undoubtedly the best technique for visualisation of pedal and toe vessels. This applies also to the examination of the hand and digits in Raynaud's disease. Arm and forearm arteries can be assessed by intravenous DSA.

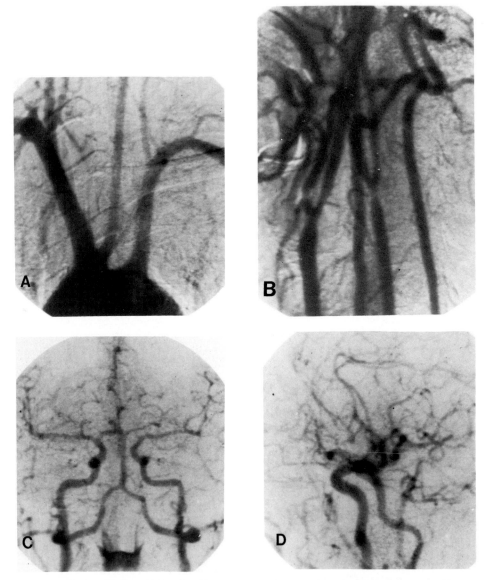

Fig. 9-1. This is a 54 year old female with a history of drop attacks and with bruits over the left and right carotid bifurcations. (A) Intravenous DSA. Truncus bicaroticus. No lesions are seen in the left and right subclavian arteries or proximal parts of the common carotid arteries. There is filling of both vertebral arteries with no lesions visible. (B) Intravenous DSA carotid bifurcations. Right: distal part common carotid artery stenosis 50–60%; internal carotid artery stenosis 70%; external carotid artery 40%. Left: common carotid artery stenosis 80%. (C) Intravenous DSA. A.P.-projection of syphons, vertebral arteries, basilar artery and intracranial arteries. No lesions visible. (D) Intravenous DSA. No lesions are visible on the lateral projection.

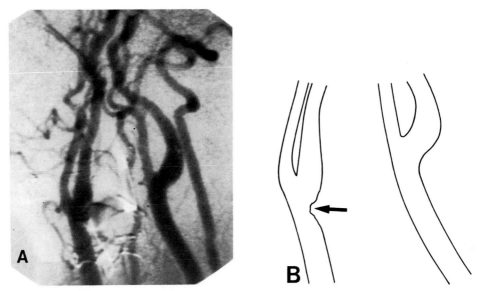

Fig. 9-2. (A) In this 60 year old male, transient ischaemic attacks had occurred involving hemiparesis of the left hand side. Intravenous DSA was performed for the aortic arch with branches, syphons, basilar artery, intracranial arteries and no lesions were found. The carotid bifurcations are shown in the figure. Left: no lesions. Right: common carotid artery—no lesions; external carotid artery—no lesions; internal carotid artery—irregularity with stenosis of maximum 20%. (B) The arrow indicates the diseased portion.

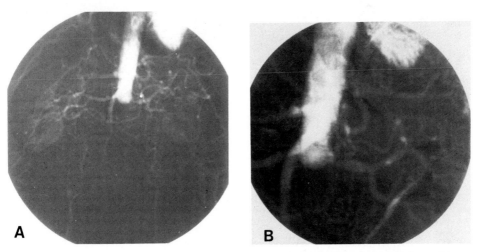

Fig. 9-3. This 59 year old male patient complained of bilateral calf and buttock claudication and impotence. Very poor pulsations in both groins were found on clinical examination. (A) Intravenous DSA. Occlusion of abdominal aorta at the origin of renal arteries. (B) Magnification of occlusion of aorta. Left renal artery stenosis of approximately 80%.

85

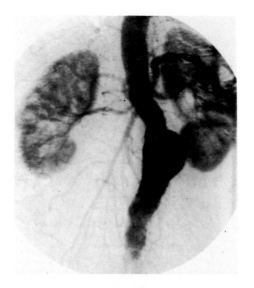

Fig. 9-4. Here is a 67 year old male patient with suspicion of aneurysm. Intravenous DSA abdominal aorta: this shows an abdominal aortic aneurysm with the siting of the renal arteries.

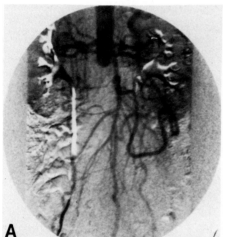

A

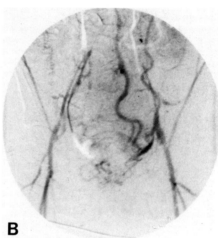

B

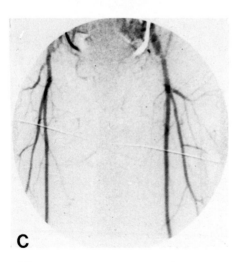

C

Fig. 9-5. This 57 year old male patient had claudication of both legs. There were reasonable pulsations in the femoral arteries. Comparison with former angiographic pictures showed a progression of occlusion more proximal in the aorta. (A) Total occlusion of the aorta below the renal arteries. Filling of the anastomosis of Riolan. (B) Fast filling via the superior rectal artery and deep ileo. (C) No abnormalities of the common-, superficial- and deep femoral arteries.

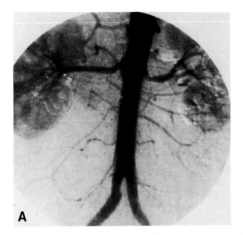

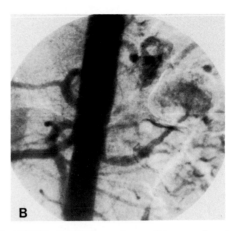

Fig. 9-6. This is a 43 year old hypertensive male (BP. 180/120). On I.V.P. no abnormalities were found with equal nephrogenic phase for both kidneys. (A) Intravenous DSA abdominal aorta. Stenosis of left renal artery. Right renal artery is normal. (B) Magnification of left renal artery. Stenosis of left renal artery approximately 75%. This was confirmed by intraarterial injection of contrast material at the time of the angioplasty procedure.

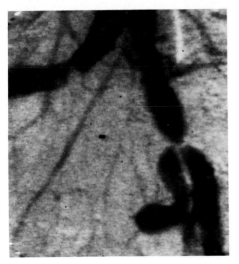

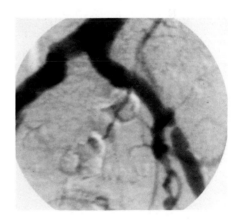

Fig. 9-7. This 60 year old male patient with severe bilateral claudication had weak pulses in both groins. Intravenous DSA: Severe stenoses in left and right iliac artery.

Fig. 9-8. This 54 year old male patient complained of claudication in the left leg. Intravenous DSA: Subtotal stenosis in left external iliac artery.

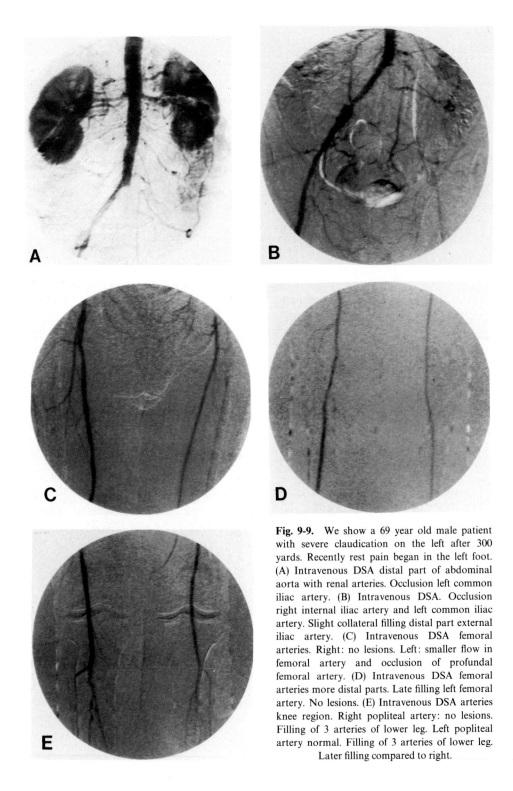

Fig. 9-9. We show a 69 year old male patient with severe claudication on the left after 300 yards. Recently rest pain began in the left foot. (A) Intravenous DSA distal part of abdominal aorta with renal arteries. Occlusion left common iliac artery. (B) Intravenous DSA. Occlusion right internal iliac artery and left common iliac artery. Slight collateral filling distal part external iliac artery. (C) Intravenous DSA femoral arteries. Right: no lesions. Left: smaller flow in femoral artery and occlusion of profundal femoral artery. (D) Intravenous DSA femoral arteries more distal parts. Late filling left femoral artery. No lesions. (E) Intravenous DSA arteries knee region. Right popliteal artery: no lesions. Filling of 3 arteries of lower leg. Left popliteal artery normal. Filling of 3 arteries of lower leg. Later filling compared to right.

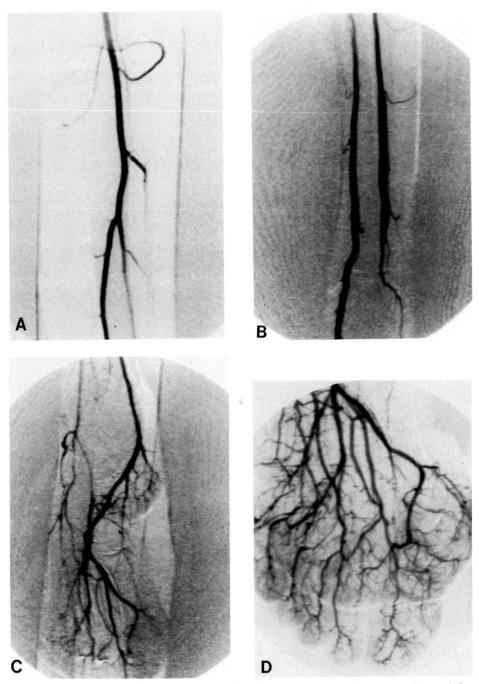

Fig. 9-10. This 75 year old male patient complained of rest pain in both feet. Examination before injection of Tolazoline showed a remarkable spasm of the distal parts of the arteries in the lower leg. (A) Intraarterial DSA knee region and proximal part of the lower leg. 40 mg. Tolazoline (Priscol) was inject- ed intraarterially. No lesions were seen. (B) Intraarterial DSA of the distal part of the lower leg and ankle. No lesions were seen. (C) Intraarterial DSA ankle and foot. Also in this region no lesions. (D) Intraarterial DSA foot. Magnification × 2. Shows an excellent outline of the digital nerves.

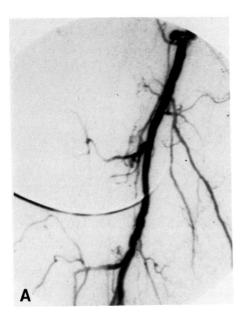

A

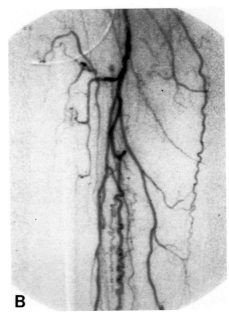

B

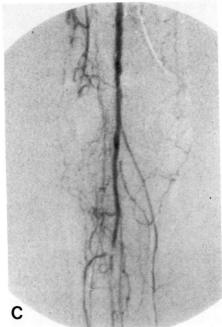

C

Fig. 9-11. This 63 year old male patient had rest pain of the right leg and foot. The patient suffered from diabetes mellitus, hypertension and alcohol abuse. (A) Intraarterial DSA. Puncture in right femoral artery. Infection by hand, with 5 cc contrast and 5 cc saline solution. In the proximal region the right femoral artery wall shows irregularities. (B) Intraarterial DSA distal right superficial femoral artery. Occlusion of the right artery and collateral circulation to popliteal artery. (C) Intraarterial DSA. Here in the knee region there is occlusion of the distal part of the popliteal artery. Collateral circulation is seen especially to the anterior tibial artery. (*Fig. 9-11 continues.*)

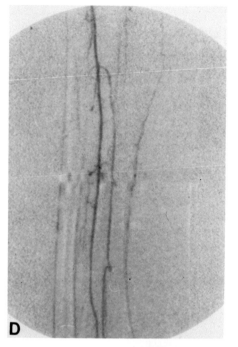

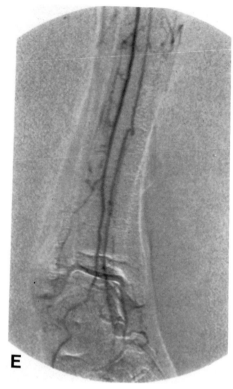

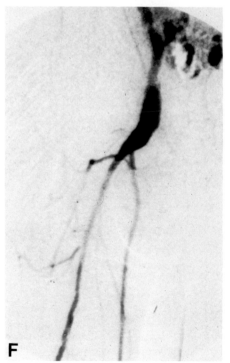

(D) Intraarterial DSA of the proximal part of the lower leg. Occlusion of peroneal artery and posterior tibial artery. Normal patency and no stenosis visible of anterior tibial artery. (E) Intraarterial DSA distal part lower leg and ankle region. Good patency of the anterior tibial artery and collateral circulation from peroneal artery to the foot. (F) Postoperative intravenous DSA right leg of same patient. Intravenous DSA proximal part of femoral artery showing profund endarterectomy and the proximal part of a femoral-popliteal bypass and jumpgraft onto the anterior tibial artery. (*Fig. 9-11 continues.*)

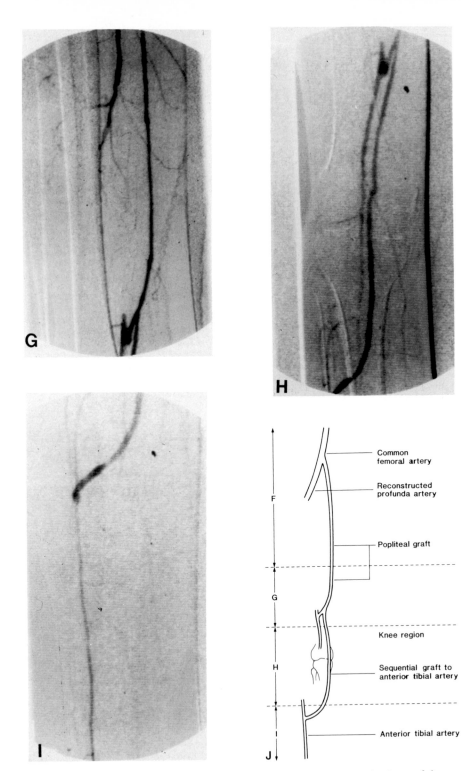

(G) Intravenous DSA of the distal part of the femoral popliteal bypass and proximal part of the sequentialgraft to the anterior tibial artery. (H) Intravenous DSA knee region with sequentialgraft and distal part of sequentialgraft. (I) Intravenous DSA. Sequentialgraft to anterior tibial artery. (J) Schematic drawing.

Fig. 9-12. This shows a 38 year old woman with attack of varospasm of both hands and gangrene of the second right digit. In order to investigate the problem, intraarterial digital subtraction angiography was performed after slow injection of 40 mg. Tolazoline through the catheter with the tip in the right brachial artery. Intraarterial DSA: good filling of the arteries and capillary bed of the 4th and 5th finger; loss of the medial digital artery in the distal part of the 2nd finger; good filling of the medial and lateral digital artery and no capillary filling of the distal part of the 3rd and 2nd finger.

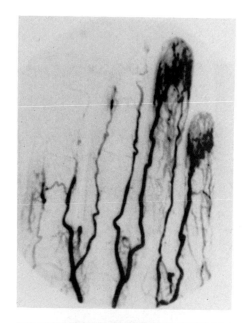

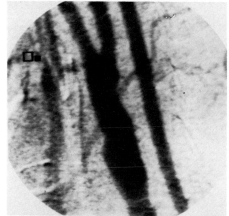

Fig. 9-13. This is a 58 year old male patient who had surgery to the left common carotid artery. Intravenous DSA left carotid artery. Endarterectomy. Irregular wall of distal part of common carotid artery. No stenosis. Good filling of left internal and external carotid artery.

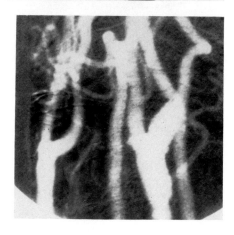

Fig. 9-14. This is a 54 year old female patient. Endarterectomy of the left common and internal carotid artery had been performed. Intravenous DSA 1 year after surgery. Kinking at the distal endpoint of the endarterectomy.

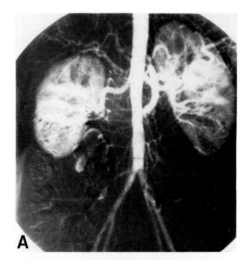

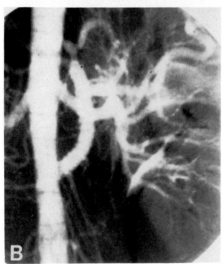

Fig. 9-15. This is a postoperative study of a 46 year old female patient. Implantation of a prosthesis between aorta and coeliac artery for abdominal angina had been performed. (A) Intravenous DSA abdominal aorta. Good filling of prosthesis between aorta and coeliac artery. (B) Original magnification. Clear view of prosthesis with anastomoses.

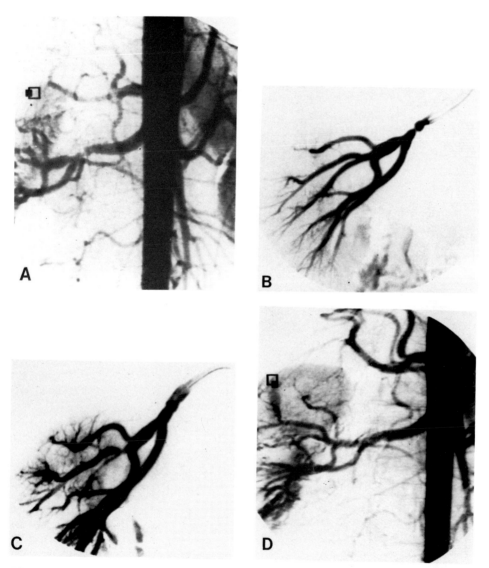

Fig. 9-16. This shows a 35 year old hypertensive female. BP. 220/120 without treatment. (A) Intravenous DSA abdominal aorta. Right renal artery: proximal part no abnormalities; more distal just before branching a stenosis at a rough estimation of 75%. Left renal artery normal. (B) Intravenous DSA. Stenosis in right renal artery of 80% probably caused by fibromuscular dysplasia. (C) Angioplasty procedure. After dilatation still an irregular wall. Stenosis disappeared. (D) Intravenous DSA check. Still irregular wall of renal artery. No severe stenosis. BP. now 140/75.

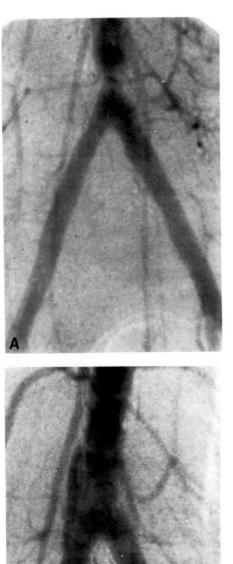

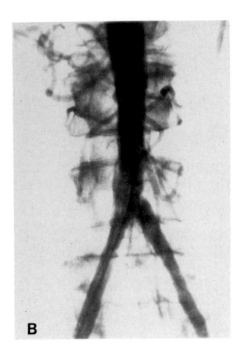

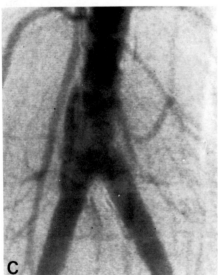

Fig. 9-17. This 52 year old male had the Leriche syndrome. On examination a murmur just below the umbilica was heard. (A) Intravenous DSA abdominal aorta and proximal part of iliac arteries. Stenosis of 90% in distal part of the aorta. The femoral arteries showed no lesions. (B) Angioplasty procedure. Conventional angiography after the dilatation. (C) Intravenous DSA check one day after angioplasty. Same information as in B.

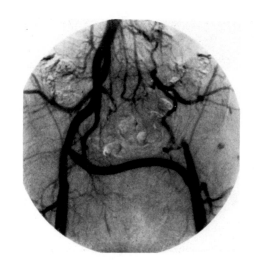

Fig. 9-18. This 74 year old male patient had surgery and a femoro-femoral crossover graft was performed. Intravenous DSA shows the graft crossing from right to left in an S shaped configuration.

PART II

Cerebral Revascularisation

Roger N. Baird, M. I. Aldoori,
Susan E. A. Cole, and W. D. Jeans

10

Preoperative Assessments—Cerebral Revascularisation

Selection of patients for carotid endarterectomy depends on the surgeon being satisfied that there is an increased risk of stroke that can be modified by correction of localised atheroma at the origin of the internal carotid artery. Arteriography is the definitive preoperative investigation, which ideally produces an unrivalled view of the carotid bifurcation in three projections, together with the carotid syphon, cerebral and vertebral circulations. But the investigation is invasive, carries risks, and involves an overnight stay in the hospital. Because of this, preliminary screening is required for those with clinical features that suggest carotid disease. In the past five years, direct noninvasive imaging of the carotid bifurcation has become widely available, using Duplex ultrasound scanners combining real-time imaging (Fig. 10-1) and Doppler to evaluate flow. These direct techniques provide more selective information than earlier indirect methods e.g., oculoplethysmography, temporal artery occlusion test. An exciting potential alternative to Duplex scanning is Digital Subtraction Angiography (DSA). DSA is accurate and safer than conventional arteriography. Problems with small field size, lack of fine detail, motion artefact and overlap of the carotid and vertebral vessels will be overcome as DSA undergoes further refinement and improvement.

This chapter considers the investigation of 1288 patients who underwent direct ultrasound imaging of the carotid arteries in the neck for suspected carotid stenosis and ulceration from 1979 to 1984. Based on the ultrasound results and clinical features 414 patients underwent carotid arteriography and 78 carotid endarterectomies were done.

CAROTID ARTERY DISEASE

Pathophysiology

Atheroma at the origin of the internal carotid artery in the neck causes symptoms by two pathological mechanisms—emboli to the cerebral hemispheres and cerebral hypoperfusion. Emboli arise from irregular athcromatous ulcers, consisting

DIAGNOSTIC TECHNIQUES AND ASSESSMENT
PROCEDURES IN VASCULAR SURGERY

© 1985 Grune & Stratton
ISBN 0-8089-1721-8 All rights reserved

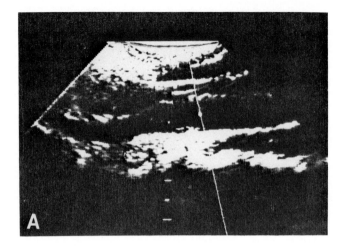

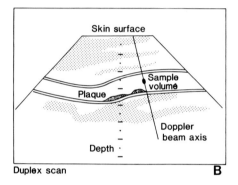

Fig. 10-1. (A, B) A.T.L. Duplex scan illustrating carotid stenosis.

of fibrin/platelet thrombi and fragments of cholesterol. They lodge in retinal arteries where they can be observed with an ophthalmoscope, and in the cerebral hemispheres, resulting in radiolucent areas visible on computed tomography (CT) brain scans. Hypoperfusion from carotid stenosis is compensated for by cerebral perfusion via the circle of Willis unless other feeding vessels are atheromatous. In a series of 135 carotid arteriograms reported below, the nonsymptomatic carotid artery was frequently diseased, as were the vertebral arteries (18%) and the carotid syphon (14%). Kinks and coils of the internal carotid artery were noted in 13% and were of uncertain pathophysiological effect.

Clinical Features

The diagnosis of cerebral ischaemia depends on a history of focal transient ischaemic attacks (TIAs), manifest as weakness, numbness, or parasthesia of the face, arm, and leg, usually of a few minutes duration and followed by complete recovery. The patient and his relatives are naturally anxious lest a further episode occur or permanent stroke develop. An alternative presentation is of amaurosis fugax—a temporary curtain-like loss of vision—again with full recovery. Between attacks, there is no visual or neurological defect on examination. In more advanced cases, there are persistent, progressive changes requiring urgent appraisal. Permanent neurological damage can occasionally be prevented by timely intervention.

Carotid Murmurs

Murmurs on auscultation of the carotid arteries in the neck result from vortical eddies within turbulent arterial flow.[1] They are mainly caused by local atheromatous encroachment of the arterial lumen at the carotid bifurcation. Alternatively, they are propagated from the heart, or caused by greatly augmented flow in a normal carotid system to compensate for occlusions of other cerebral vessels.

Murmurs are present less than half of the patients presenting with symptoms of cerebral ischaemia. In a recent study[2] of 135 patients with classic TIAs or amaurosis fugax, a cervical murmur over the appropriate carotid artery was present in 62 (45%). Murmurs are detectable in a minority of carotid stenoses. In an arteriographic review described below of 262 carotid bifurcations, a murmur was present in 51 (44%) of 117 stenoses or ulcers of the internal carotid artery. These findings are similar to other published results (Table 10-1).

Table 10-1
Murmurs in Carotid Stenosis

Author	Incidence	
Peart & Rob[3]	59/103	57%
Humphrey & Marshall[4]	14/30	47%
Murie, Sheldon, & Quinn[5]	35/55	69%

ULTRASOUND IMAGING

Historical Review

The first ultrasound images of the carotid arteries were obtained in 1969 by Olinger using a pulsed echo system.[6] An important limitation was its failure to discriminate patency from occlusion in the internal carotid artery. To overcome this problem, the scanner was linked with a Doppler probe to detect blood flow-velocity signals within the imaged vessel. The first such Duplex scanner was described by Strandness' group in Seattle in 1974[7] and became commercially available six years later. Since then, there have been improvements in image quality, signal processing, and computing[2,8,9] and today highly competitive systems are available from several manufacturers.

Systems have also been devised in which an image of blood flowing within an artery (a flow map) is obtained from the return signals of a range gated pulsed Doppler instrument by Fish[10] and Hokanson.[11] These systems are effective in identifying carotid artery disease[12] but the images take longer to build up than with Duplex scanning and fine detail is less well shown.

Accuracy

The accuracy of Duplex scanning was assessed in a study of the origins of 78 internal carotid arteries in which ultrasound scans and arteriograms were compared (Table 10-2). The results were that Duplex scans had a sensitivity of 93% and specificity of 94% compared with arteriograms in detecting stenoses at the origin of the internal carotid artery.[2] Similar results have been reported by Strandness' group.[8] Carotid ultrasound scanning is a painless safe outpatient procedure that takes about 20 minutes. Training in scanning techniques and operation of the equipment are required for accurate, reproducible results to be obtained.

Table 10-2
Comparison of Ultrasonic and Angiographic Results of
78 Internal Carotid Artery Origins

Arteriograms	normal	25%	25–50%	50–90%	occluded
normal	15	1	–	–	–
less than 25%	4	19	3	–	–
25–50%	–	–	16	1	–
50–99%	–	–	–	13	1
occluded	–	–	1	–	4

From Lusby RJ, Machleder HI, Jeans WD, et al: Vessel wall and blood flow dynamics in arterial disease. Phil Trans R Soc Lond B. 294:231, 1981. With permission.

Referrals

Requests for carotid scans came from a wide variety of sources (Table 10-3). The finding of a high grade stenosis of greater than 50% diameter reduction usually resulted in an arteriogram with a view to an endarterectomy, unless consideration of operation was deferred because of advanced age, infirmity, reduced life expectancy, or other adverse factor. From 1979–1982, 61 patients with focal neurological symptoms and minor carotid disease (<50% stenosis) on ultrasound were managed medically including antiplatelet agents. They were reviewed and rescanned some

Table 10-3
Referrals for 1288 Carotid Scans

Medical		Surgical	
Neurology	219 (17%)	Vascular	123 (9.5%)
Cardiology	72 (5.5%)	Ophthalmology	295 (23%)
Other medical	344 (26%)	Other surgical	245 (19%)
(general, radiotherapy general practice)		(general, cardiac neuro, ENT)	

two years later in 1984. There were no strokes and no progression of carotid disease in 54 repeat scans. One patient was well at telephone review and was not scanned, two were lost to follow up and four died (malignant disease—2, myocardial infarct—2).

A study was made of the prevalance of carotid artery disease in 104 patients prior to coronary artery bypass and heart valve replacement. Greater than 50% carotid stenoses were identified in 11 internal carotid arteries in 6 of 56 patients (11%) prior to coronary artery bypass. One high grade carotid stenosis was found in 48 patients (2%) prior to mitral and aortic valve replacement. These results show the expected high frequency of multifocal atheroma in patients undergoing coronary artery operations. Carotid endarterectomy was undertaken without perioperative stroke or mortality in five patients undergoing coronary artery bypass and one valve replacement.

New Technology

Rapid advances in ultrasound technology have occurred in the last five years. The earliest scanners had fairly basic zero-crossing Doppler signal processing to which a spectral analyser was later added. The latest systems have onboard computing to measure volume blood flow. In order to do this, the vessel diameter is measured using electronic calipers (Fig. 10-2) and the angle at which the ultrasound

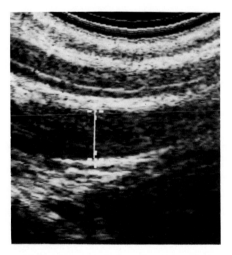

Fig. 10-2. Measurement of the diameter of the common carotid artery by a Technicare scanner. The crosses of the electronic calipers are aligned with the vessel wall.

beam cuts the longitudinal vessel axis is measured (Fig. 10-3). Preliminary results suggest that volume flow measurements made in this way are accurate and reproducible and are an exciting addition to the repertoire of noninvasive measurements of the carotid arteries and elsewhere.

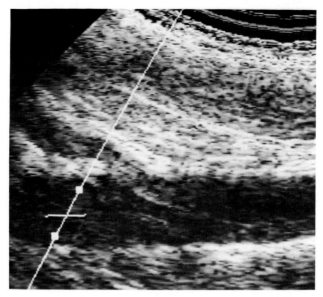

Fig. 10-3.   Measurement of beam vessel angle. The limits of
the range—gated, pulsed Doppler signal are shown.

CAROTID ARTERIOGRAPHY

A prospective study was undertaken of carotid arteriograms in 135 consecutive
patients presenting with cerebral, ocular, or cervical manifestations of the prestroke
syndrome during the three year period 1980–1982. During this time, 597 Duplex
ultrasound scans, 41 carotid endarterectomies, and 6 superficial temporal artery to
middle cerebral artery bypasses were done.

Technique

The brachio-cephalic arteries were catheterised by the transfemoral route.
Views of the carotid artery were obtained with the head turned towards (soft tissue
oblique) and away (bone oblique) from the side being injected. A horizontal beam
lateral film was also obtained (Fig. 10-4). The study included films of the origins of
the carotid and vertebral arteries, the carotid syphon, and cerebral vessels.

Complications

There was one death (0.7%). Four strokes (3%) occurred with a permanent
deficit. Six patients (4%) were rendered temporarily dysphasic or hemiparetic followed by full recovery, and there were 19 groin haematomas.

Results

Atheroma was defined as a smooth or irregular change in the margin of the
column of contrast medium. Occlusion was the failure to demonstrate the outline of
the internal carotid artery. Stenosis was defined as a percentage narrowing com-

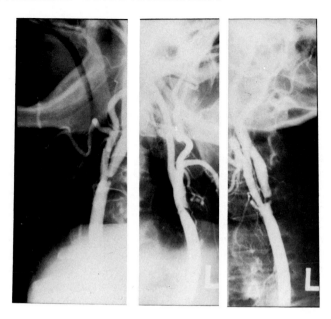

Fig. 10-4. Arteriogram showing carotid stenosis in lateral
and two oblique views.

pared with the distal internal carotid artery. But the carotid bulb is normally dilated
and highly distensible so that considerable atheroma has to be laid down before a
measurable stenosis occurs. An ulcer was identified if there was a crater with edges
on either side. No attempt was made to distinguish different categories of ulcers.[13]

The results in 262 internal carotid arteries of 135 patients are given in Table
10-4. Eight vessels were not shown, mainly the nonrelevant side in a difficult or
prolonged catheterisation. The origins of 117 internal carotid arteries were stenosed
and/or ulcerated, 17 were occluded, and 124 were normal or minimally diseased. In
only 16 patients were both internal carotid arteries normal.

The usefulness of three projections in demonstrating 117 stenoses and/or ulcers
was examined. In 41, the lesion was only seen on a single radiographic view: the
lateral in 17, bone oblique in 12, and soft tissue oblique in 12. Failure to visualise
disease was usually because of overlap of the external carotid artery or its branches.
The configuration of the carotid bifurcation was so variable that no less than three
views are required to display reliably the origin of the internal carotid artery.

Table 10-4
Angiographic Appearances
of 262 Internal Carotid
Artery Origins.

Normal	64
Atheroma	64
Stenosis & Ulcer	117
Occlusion	17

Conclusions

How then should the patient with cerebral ischaemia be investigated with surgical revascularisation in mind? As mentioned above, the diagnosis rests on a history of a focal TIA. Clinical examination between attacks is normal. A cardiac source of emboli is excluded. An arterial murmur localised at the relevant carotid bifurcation is useful but it is only heard in about half of carotid stenoses. In these circumstances, Duplex ultrasound scanning of the carotid bifurcations in the neck is a safe, accurate, painless, rapid, and convenient out-patient method of identifying atheroma at the origin of the internal carotid artery in the neck. The next step is carotid arteriography, which is done as a preoperative investigation before carotid endarterectomy. With few exceptions, patients undergoing arteriography should have carotid stenosis of ulceration on ultrasound, and be amenable to and fit for operation. The exceptions are progressive, persistent focal TIAs, reversible ischaemia lasting more than 24 hours, and stroke in evolution. These require immediate hospitalisation, anticoagulation with heparin, and consideration of an arteriogram if their cerebral state permits. Recognition of reversible ischaemia can be very difficult in these circumstances. Carotid endarterectomy cannot reverse neurological defects following cerebral infarction and, in the acute phase, usually leads to worsening of the stroke and death. CT scans are unhelpful in the hours following the onset of a hemiparesis. Diminished density of the cerebral substance and enhancement with contrast medium are usually not seen during the first 24 hours after an infarct has occurred.[14] Patients with completed strokes are candidates for operation only if there is a mild residual deficit and six weeks have passed to allow the infarct to stabilise.

Duplex scanning has reliably identified atheromatous ulcers, stenoses, and occlusions in patients with symptomatic cerebral ischaemia. This has led to its use as a screening technique. The selection process for each carotid endarterectomy currently involves, on average, 20 Duplex scans leading to 3 carotid arteriograms. Following endarterectomy, serial scans show that technical failures occur, leading to internal carotid artery occlusions. Months later, carotid restenosis can develop. Fortunately, most are asymptomatic and reoperation is rarely necessary or desirable.

REFERENCES

1. Baird RN: Carotid Murmurs. Br J Surg 70:83, 1983
2. Lusby RJ, Machleder HI, Jeans WD, et al: Vessel wall and blood flow dynamics in arterial disease. Phil Trans R Soc Lond B 294:231, 1981
3. Peart WS, Rob C: Arterial auscultation. Lancet 2:219, 1960
4. Humphrey PRD, Marshall J: Transient ischaemic attacks and strokes with recovery: Prognosis and investigation. Stroke 12:765, 1981
5. Murie JA, Sheldon CD, Quin RO: Carotid artery bruit: Association with internal carotid stenosis and intraluminal turbulence. Br J Surg 71:50, 1984.
6. Olinger CP: Ultrasonic carotid echoarteriography. Am J Roentgen Rad Ther Nucl Med 106:282, 1969
7. Barber FE, Baker DW, Strandness DE (Jr.), et al: Duplex scanner II: For simultaneous imaging of artery tissues and flow. In Ultrasonic Symptomsium Proceedings, IEEE Cat. 74:CHO 896. International Society of Ultrasonologists.

8. Fell G, Phillips DJ, Chikos PM, et al: Ultrasonic Duplex scanning for disease of the carotid artery. Circulation 64:1191, 1981
9. Breslau PJ, Knox RA, Greep JM, et al: The influence of ultrasonic Duplex scanning on the management of carotid artery disease. Br J Surg 70:264, 1983
10. Fish PJ: Visualising blood vessels by ultrasound. In: Blood Flow Measurement. Roberts VC (Ed.). Sector, London: 29, 1972
11. Mozersky DJ, Hokanson DE, Baker DW, et al: Ultrasonic Arteriography. Arch Surg 103:663, 1971
12. Lusby RJ, Woodcock JP, Skidmore R, et al: Carotid artery disease: A prospective evaluation of pulsed Doppler imaging. Ultrasound Med Bio 7:365, 1981
13. Moore WS, Boran C, Malone JM, et al: Natural history of non-stenotic, asymptomatic ulcerative lesions of the carotid artery. Arch Surg 113:1352, 1978
14. Norris JW; Hachinski VC: Misdiagnosis of stroke. Lancet 1:328, 1982

Robert Courbier, J. M Jausseran M. Reggi,
P. Bergeron, M. Formichi, and M. Ferdani

11

Peroperative Carotid Arteriography

In our team, carotid surgery is routinely controlled by peroperative arteriography in the same way as a peripheral reconstruction. There are two advantages to that; a residual lesion can be operated on in the same time before the occlusive stage—we can assess the integrity of the artery, and in case of restenosis, be sure that this stenosis did not exist after the operation and developed secondarily.

The purpose of this work is to study peroperative arteriographic aspects to find the favorable evolutive ones and detect those that represent permanent and threatening lesions.

CLINICAL MATERIAL

Surgical Management

Surgical management consisted in a classical thrombo-endarterectomy (TED) of the carotid bifurcation. A systemic administration of 500 IU of sodium heparin was always performed. A temporary carotid shunt was used when stump pressure was below 50 mm Hg (22% of cases). Since September 1983 a tapered stent (USCI) has routinely been inserted in the internal carotid artery to stitch the endarterectomy. Inspection of the repaired artery showed a normal external arterial diameter and normal arterial beats. Only the upper point of the stitch could show a stenosis. In some cases after X-ray control an immediate reoperation was performed to complete the TED or to increase the diameter by a venous patch or to insert saphenous vein bypass.

Per Operative X-Ray Control

After having located the area to be injected on a T.V. screen, peroperative carotid angiography consisted in 5 ml of Diatrizoate injected manually. The concentration was 60%. The dye progression is followed and at the time of optimum injec-

DIAGNOSTIC TECHNIQUES AND ASSESSMENT
PROCEDURES IN VASCULAR SURGERY

© 1985 Grune & Stratton
ISBN 0-8089-1721-8 All rights reserved

tion, the image is fixed on the screen. A 10 × 10 cm picture of the screen is taken. A reoperation of the TED can immediately be decided. We note that an intracerebral defect due to embolism cannot be detected by these techniques.

Postoperative Angiography

Postoperative angiography was performed by percutaneous puncture of the common carotid artery (patient under general anesthesia) or more recently by digital substraction angiography (DSA). Clinical records and X-ray detected lesions were correlated. All the patients with neurologic deficit were controlled. All the films were studied by three observers to describe the lesions. The internal carotid artery diameter was measured at the level of the stenosed portion and of the widest portion above the TED to assess the degree of stenosis.

Patients

In our experience, 1030 patients were operated on until February 1984. Until 1979 peroperative arteriography was exceptional, it became later more and more frequent and since 1980 it has been performed routinely. Therefore we studied three groups of patients to get a comparative value.

Group A. 65 patients (72 TED) had a peroperative arteriography and were secondarily controlled by another arteriography.

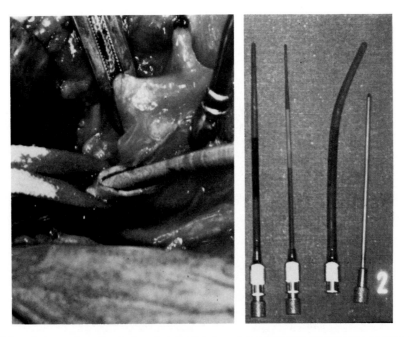

Fig. 11-1. A tapered probe is inserted in the superior part of the internal carotid artery before begining the suture.

Group B. A control series of 182 patients (206 TED), operated on before 1979, had no peroperative control.

Group C. One hundred most recent patients operated on consecutively (until February 1984) had a peroperative arteriography and benefited from the TED technical improvements using a probe* for the suture (Fig. 11-1)

RESULTS

Group A

Sixty-five patients (51 males and 14 females) underwent 72 TED of the internal carotid artery (7 bilateral). The mean age of 66.1 years was similar for females and males (extremes for 49 to 78 years). Operative indications were the following: 32 asymptomatic, 39 TIA, 1 stroke. All patients had a late arteriographic control at 22.9 months as an average (maximum 71 months).

Clinical Results

Operative mortality was zero. Three immediate reinterventions were performed (1 stenosis, 1 flap, 1 stenosing irregularity).

Secondarily four restenoses occurred of which three were operated on (3 months and 12 months later). There were two recurring TIA and two asymptomatic patients.

Anatomical Result

On the common carotid artery the 55 cases without shelf remained normal. In 17 cases with shelves, 14 normalizations (Fig. 11-2) and 3 residual stenoses occurred (Fig. 11-3).

At the external carotid artery level the control was normal in 47 cases with only one late stenosis and among 25 cases with initial stenosis, 15 became normal (Fig. 11-4), 8 did not change, and 2 showed thrombosis.

At the internal carotid level, in the 39 cases with an originally normal artery, a recurrent stenosis occurred in 2 cases; one spasm disappeared secondarily. Extensive irregularities (17) became normal (Fig. 11-5) (14) and left a stenosis in three cases. The apical arteriotomy suture (9) seen on the peroperative radiography became normal eight times (Fig. 11-4) and persisted in one case. Two flaps gave one normalization and one stenosis. Thirteen non reoperated stenoses gave eight normalizations, two secondary stenoses (Fig. 11-6) and three occlusions. In three cases where reconstructive surgery was performed immediately, results were perfect.

We can sum up the residual lesions of the internal carotid artery by stating the stenosis degree: 8 times less than 30% with 7 normalizations and 1 occlusion; 1 between 30% and 50% with one occlusion; 7 times over 50% with 1 normalization, 1 improvement, 1 unchanged, 1 occlusion; and 3 with secondary operation.

---

*Probe made specially by USCI.

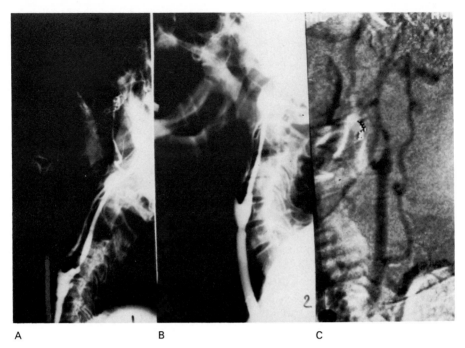

A   B   C

Fig. 11-2. (A) Before the TED.
          (B) Peroperative control (residual shelf on CCA).
          (C) Ten months later the shelf disappeared. A stenosis developed on the ICA.

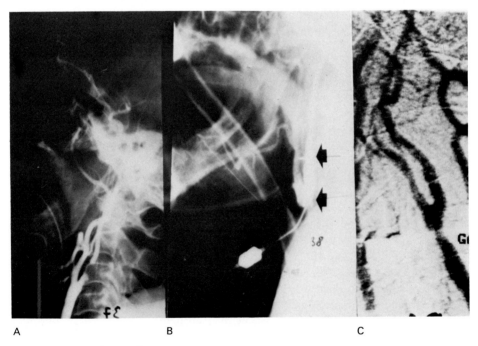

A   B   C

Fig. 11-3. (A) Before TED.
          (B) Peroperative control (the injection is made too high and the shelf is not obvious).
          (C) Sixteen months later, stenosis of CCA

114

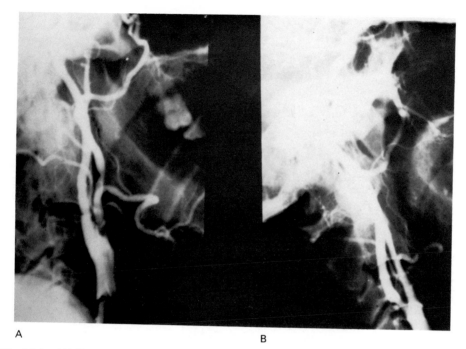

A   B

Fig. 11.4. (A) Peroperative control (debris in the ECA. The apical arteriotomy suture is causing a stenosis.)

           (B) Twenty months later, normalization of the ECA. Stenosis at the origin of the ICA. The apical arteriotomy suture appears normal.

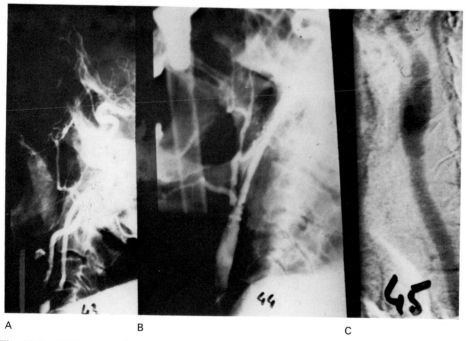

A   B   C

Fig. 11-5. (A) Preoperative X-ray.

           (B) Peroperative X-ray (irregularities on the ICA).

           (C) Three months later; Normalization of the ICA.

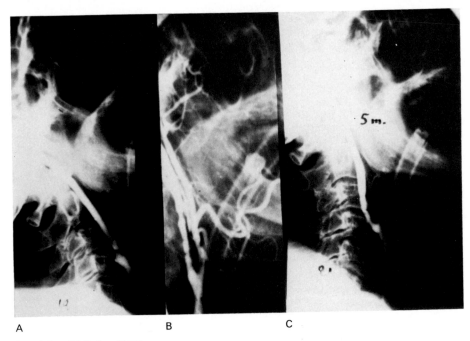

A   B   C

Fig. 11-6. (A) Before TED.
(B) Peroperative X-ray. Irregularities of the ICA. Partial reconstruction of the ECA.
(C) Five months later. Stenosis of the ICA. Occlusion of ECA.

Group B

One hundred and eighty two patients operated on before 1979 without peroperative angiography underwent 206 TED (69 asymptomatic, 121 TIA, 14 impending strokes, 2 strokes).

Operative mortality was six or 2.9% (3 neurologic and 3 cardiac origins). Transient neurologic deficit with complete recovery was 13 or 6.31% (4 hemiplegia, 5 hemiparesis, 4 partial paralysis). Permanent deficit was 4 (1.94%).

Group C

In comparison, 100 last consecutive TED (58 asymptomatic, 40 TIA, 1 impending stroke, 1 completed stroke) had technical modifications and X-ray control. Four patients had an immediate correction. Two were reoperated on in the following days. Operative mortality was 1 or 1% (hemiplegia on the 15th day). Transient deficit was 1 or 1%. Completed stroke was 1 or 1%. There were 3 restenosis operated on in the 12 months following the operation.

DISCUSSION

Carotid surgery has become very common. Even if the number of postoperative strokes represents a low incidence, a poor technical result in carotid reconstruction can explain secondary microembolization or internal carotid occlusion. Recurrent carotid artery stenosis may be due to incomplete reconstruction with technical problems.

As soon as 1967, Blaisdell performed peroperative arteriographies and observed 26% of patients who needed an immediate revision.[2-3] The immediate reoperation rate differs according to the authors (Table 11-1).

Table 11-1
Immediate Reoperation Rate

Author	Year	Reference	Rate
Blaisdell	1967	(2–3)	26%
Gaspar	1974	(5)	8.07%
Andersen	1978	(1)	5.3%
Courbier	1979	(4)	4.4%
Larson	1982	(7)	8.09%
Scott	1982	(10)	12%

Gaspar[5] realized that after having rectified the former technical mistakes, the percentage of reoperations did not change with experience of the team (1974, 8.07%–1982, 8.09%). For us this peroperative X-ray control is routinely used to avoid technical mistakes and to be allowed to study the evolution of the operated internal carotid arteries more objectively.

In practice, these peroperative angiographies did not lead to complications provided there was not too much dye injected (5 ml) and provided the patient had been heparinized until the surgeon was sure that immediate reoperation was not necessary. The possible subintimal injection of dye or dislodgement of atheroma or cumulative doses of irradiation to patients and physicians[1] is not a real argument. In the same way the operating time is always extended to a few minutes when there is the necessary organization in the operating room.

Interpretation of angiography is easy for the surgeon. Noninvasive techniques[10] need a supplementary specialist in the operating room at the right time.

Influence of Peroperative Angiography on Immediate Results

As we have used this technique routinely only since 1980 we can compare two groups of patients operated on with or without peroperative angiography. We compared a first Group B of 182 patients (206 operations) with a second Group C of the last 100 patients operated on consecutively (Table 11-2).

Table 11-2
Comparison of Groups B and C

	Group B	Group C
	206 operations	100 operations
Operative mortality	6* (2.91%)	1† (1%)
Completely regressive stroke	13 (6.31%)	1%
Completed stroke	4 (1.94%)	1%

* 3 were neurologic and 3 were cardiac origins
† neurologic origin

The decrease of the number of myocardial infarctions can be related to the improvement of intensive care techniques (Trinitrine, perfusion, monitoring, . . .). On the other hand, the evolution of strokes is significant. The use of higher doses of heparin (10.000 IU) each time a shunt is inserted may play a part.

Even if the artery looks normal "from the outside" and beats normally, after a TED the peroperative arteriography does not always confirm this reassuring aspect.

Identification of Lesions on the Peroperative Arteriogram

At the common carotid artery level, an atheromatous shelf that is located between the normal arterial wall and the endarterectomized portion is more or less prominant according to the importance of atheromatous overloading. In 14 cases, this image progressively disappeared and became normal at control. Three flaps turned into relative stenosis, less than 30%.

Yet, if this lesion cannot be avoided in some patients because the atheroma goes down to the aortic arch (Hertzer[6]) it is important to note that normalization is only possible with the formation of a fibrin deposit that "fills the shelf in" but it leaves for a few months the possibility of embolism. Larson[7] reported one case of stroke.

At the external carotid artery level when the plaque does not end smoothly towards the distal artery the number of residual lesions increases. Fifteen low grade peroperative stenoses disappeared at control, 8 increased and 2 led to occlusions. Only one artery that was normal at control developed a secondary stenosis. We prefer to cut the atheroma at the ostium level. An endarterectomy[7] that was blind-ended by pulling fragments down only gave an immediate patency with secondary occlusion. The technique of external carotid artery endarterectomy remains difficult to improve.[7]

At the internal carotid artery level lesions are very different. Spasm occurred when the arteriotomy is located on the very upper part of the dissected area. We observed the same finding on external iliac arteries after extensive dissection.

Extensive irregularities correspond to incomplete endarterectomy leaving circular muscular fibers of the media, or more often to the suture of the endarterectomized wall. For if the remaining wall is very thin, the pulling of the needle after the thread has passed through takes more or less tissue and we cannot be aware of it for there is no tensile strength in the posterior wall following the pulling (Fig. 11-7).

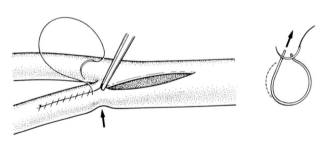

Fig. 11-7. A more or less amount of tissue is taken by each point.

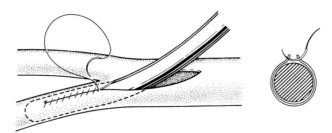

Fig. 11-8. (A) Probe inserted in the artery lumen avoids any
stenosis.
(B) The first point is checked, pulling the probe.
(C) The probe is reinserted in the artery to keep
the same diameter.

In 14 cases, the artery appearance became normal later. In three cases there was a
permanent stenosis. When a probe is used it keeps the artery lumen during the
arteriotomy stitching to the same diameter and avoids these irregularities. (Fig. 11-8)

Stenoses are due to different mechanisms. The site of the apical arteriotomy
suture is perceptible (9 times) but it disappears later (8 times). This can be observed
particularly when the arteriotomy goes beyond the upper limit of the plaque. The
overshoot is thus performed on a healthy portion of the internal carotid artery and
so reduces the artery circumference. A slight inversion of the endarterectomized wall
can be found most of the time when the artery is very atheromatous and rigid and
when the endarterectomy leaves a particularly thin wall. In the same way a supplementary hemostatic stitch on the arteriotomy after removal of the clamp leaves a
mark. Secondarily, the flexibility of the wall compensates the lesion.

A limited flap can be individualized. In one case it secondarily clung to the wall
and it gave a stenosis in another case. When this dissection is larger a thrombosis
occurs. In all these cases insertion of tacking suture secures the arterial intima.

Finally the most frequent stenoses are due to debris or to a technical fault in
the suture. Among 13 cases without immediate reoperations there were 8 normalizations, 2 secondary stenosis, and 3 occlusions. In 3 cases with immediate reoperation we had 3 normal late aspects. In all cases where the reduction of diameter is
inferior to 30%, late prognosis is good.

The disappearing of defects was described by Schutz[9] Hertzer,[6] and Zieler.[12] It
is linked to fibrin formation on the recently endarterectomized wall. We found the
same results in peripheral arterial surgery (Dos Santos False positives 4).

Finally the modifications found after operation by noninvasive techniques or
angiographies can only be acknowledged when the exact appearance immediately
after endarterectomy is known.[11]

When Should Immediate Reoperation be Undertaken?

The risk of repeated carotid clamping in high risk patients or with coronary
diseases made us hesitate to restore a "nonsatisfactory image" and thus accept an
incomplete TED. Are there peremptory criteria to reoperate these patients?

At the common carotid artery level visual control of the endarterectomized wall
seems sufficient and we never had to perform a larger endarterectomy downwards

after a X-ray control. Therefore an extensive thromboendarterectomy is not necessary on the common carotid artery. The recurrence of stenosis does not occur at this level.

On the external carotid artery a stenosis more than 50% needs immediate reoperation. After clamping the artery origin, a short arteriotomy is performed for thrombectomy. But a secondary thrombosis can more easily occur on these endarterectomized arteries because the atheromatous plaque is less limited than on the internal carotid artery.

At the internal carotid artery level a stenosis less than 30%, whatever may be its origin, is most likely to disappear secondarily.[7] On the contrary, if there is a higher grade stenosis, reoperation becomes necessary most after with a venous patch. When the wall is of poor quality we prefer a venous bypass that eliminates the endarterectomized area, which in our former experience was the origin of thrombosis.

Finally, immediate thrombosis must lead to saphenous vein bypass to find a healty artery higher on the internal carotid artery. The indications of reconstructive surgery of a TED must be cautious; the risk of a second carotid clamping must be taken if we are sure that the first operation can anatomically and hemodynamically be improved. At present, the risk of a prolonged clamping seems to be reasonable because of cerebral protection due to heparinization and to the shunt technique.

The technical difficulties to get good peroperative angiography are completely solved so that if the angiograph shows a significant technical defect, a second arterial dissection is undertaken, even if this approach has been criticized.[6]

It is more logical to end the operation by performing a restoration as perfect as possible rather than to wait for a control that is done only in case of postoperative complications.

CONCLUSIONS

Peroperative angiography is a safe and reliable method. It is not time-consuming. It also permits us to correct technical faults and to lower the reoperative rate. Peroperative angiography is the only way to study the natural history of restenosis.

REFERENCES

1. Andersen CH, Collins G, Rich N: Routine operative arteriography during carotid endarterectomy: A reassessment. Surgery 83:67–71, 1978
2. Blaisdell FW, Lim R, Hall A: Technical result of carotid endarterectomy: Arteriographic assessment. American Journal Surgery 114:239–246, 1967
3. Blaisdell FW: Routine operative arteriography following carotid endarterectomy. Surgery 83:114–115, 1978
4. Courbier R: Protection cérébral per operatoire, IN: Arterio athies cérébrales extracraniennes asymptomatiques. R. Courbier (Ed). Editions Médicales Oberval: Marseille 1979, p. 254–263
5. Gaspar MR, Movius HL, Rosental JJ: Routine operative arteriography in carotid artery surgery. Journal of Cardio Vascular Surgery (Special Issue) 477, 1974

6. Hertzer NR, Beven EG, Modie MT: Early patency of the carotid artery after endarterectomy: Digital substraction angiography after two hundred sixty-two operations. Surgery 92:1049–1058, 1982

7. Larson SR, Gaspar MR, Movius HJ, et al: Intra operative arteriography in cerebrovasculars surgery, IN: Cerebrovascular Insufficiency, J. Bergan, J. Yao (Eds). New York: Grune & Stratton, 1983, P. 353–365

8. Rosental JJ, Gaspar MR, Movius HJ: Intra operative arteriography in carotid thromboendarterectomy. Archives of Surgery 106–806, 1973

9. Schutz H, Flemming JFR, Awerbuck B: Arteriographic assessment of carotid endarterectomy. Annals of Surgery 171:509–521, 1970

10. Scott SM, Sethi GK, Bridgmann AH: Peroperative stroke during carotid endarterectomy: The value of intraoperative angiography. The Journal of Cardio vascular Surgery 23:353–358, 1982

11. Turnipseed WD, Berkoff HA, Crummy A: Postoperative occlusion after carotid endarterectomy. Archives of Surgery 115:573–574, 1980

12. Zierler RE, Bandyk DF, Thiele BL, et al: Carotid artery stenosis following endarterectomy. Archives of Surgery 117:1408–1415, 1982

Wilhelm Sandmann
Horst Kniemeyer
and Pierre Peronneau

12

Carotid Bifurcation Doppler Spectrum Analysis at Surgery

The most serious complication of carotid endarterectomy, especially in asymptomatic patients, is a stroke. The explanation for the causes of stroke related to carotid artery surgery are focused on two mechanisms: cerebral ischemia from clamping and cerebral embolism due to manipulation of the vessel at surgery. These different aspects are reflected in the endless discussion of the necessity of an indwelling shunt.[1,2] Since routine shunting has not produced clinical results significantly superior to the nonshunt technique, the assumption of hemodynamic ischemia still remains a hypothesis.[3,4] Because sophisticated brain monitoring techniques and methods affording cerebral protection during thromboendarterectomy are used, it is not surprising that practical explanations like incompleteness of reconstruction and technical failure are generally excluded from the list of reasons that strokes occur in this situation. However, since Blaisdell et al[5] published a 7.5% rate of technical imperfection by intraoperative arteriographic assessment, it has become obvious that palpation and visualisation of the reconstructed vessel cannot provide sufficient information about the restoration of lumen and flow. Minor irregularities, which are not significant in terms of pressure and flow reduction but nevertheless may produce thrombi and emboli due to the development of turbulence, will be missed without an objective method for control.[6] As intraoperative arteriography, which has not made great progress in the past, may be cumbersome in some institutions and can miss smaller details by the one plane technique, we applied the principles of Doppler spectrum analysis for the intraoperative assessment of reconstructed carotid morphology.[7-9] In this study we report our latest experience with "perturbation measurement," which provides indispensable information about the hemodynamic result of reconstruction in terms of local flow. The method guides the surgeon to correct a nonoptimal reconstruction during surgery to avoid neurologic complications.

DIAGNOSTIC TECHNIQUES AND ASSESSMENT
PROCEDURES IN VASCULAR SURGERY

© 1985 Grune & Stratton
ISBN 0-8089-1721-8 All rights reserved

MATERIALS AND METHODS

The measurement of perturbation is based on the idea that any pathologic irregularity of the arterial lumen must produce a deviation of the flow velocity profile. In healthy individuals the flow in the descending aorta and the peripheral arteries is accepted to be nearly laminar, because turbulence resulting from the pulsating heart is damped down by the viscosity of the blood. We have defined the "perturbation index" as the standard deviation of velocity calculated from the frequency distribution of a spectral histogram divided by the mean velocity. In general, perturbation is distortion, disturbance, or turbulence. Beyond an arterial stenosis the degree of diameter reduction is responsible for the level of perturbation, which decreases as the distance from the stenosis increases. For example, the maximum perturbation caused by a stenosis of 30% square area reduction appears at a distance of one diameter behind the stenosis. At a distance of three diameters the perturbation level is already back to normal. Perturbation also varies with pulsatility. Flow acceleration has a stabilizing effect on the velocity profile and reduces perturbation, whereas flow deceleration increases perturbation. The systolic peak flow is a relatively stable moment when perturbation is more dependent on the morphology of the arterial wall and less dependent on the pulsatility. From the abovementioned flow characteristics, it becomes evident that perturbation measurement during a carotid thromboendarterectomy should be performed at the time of systolic peak flow within a distance of no more than one diameter beyond the arteriotomy.

In the glass model it is easy to visualize distortion, disturbance, and turbulence, but how can we measure the degree of perturbation in arteries? "Perturbation" is the result of the various velocities of the blood cells in the flow profile along the arterial diameter. In laminar flow 85% of the blood cells have the same velocity and are located in the center flow. In turbulent flow the velocities are distributed at random in the three dimensions within the lumen of the vessel. The velocity of the blood cells can be measured today by the Doppler ultrasound method while the Doppler spectrum presents the various velocities in the flow. In laminar flow conditions the band width is very narrow and of high density. Increasing perturbation enlarges the frequency spectrum with prominent appearance of high velocities. Turbulent flow is characterized by a broad band width of low density. Two methods are available for the evaluation of the frequencies within the Doppler spectrum: the real time frequency analysis and the Doppler histogram. The latter is based on the time interval readings from the zero crossing detector and has certain limitations (Fig. 12-1). However, it proved to be satisfactory for normal and pathologic flow conditions, which were generated in the hydraulic test bench.[10] The spectral histogram is displayed together with the mean velocity on a dual-beam storage screen. We know from our previous investigations in the hydraulic test bench and in animal experiments that for laminar flow conditions the perturbation index (PI) values are below 20. PI values below 30 represent distortion, above 30 represent disturbance, and above 50 represent turbulence. In carotid endarterectomy PI values above 50 strongly indicate a significant stenosis while values above 30 represent minor or major irregularities.

Immediately after closure of the arterial incision the ultrasound flow probe is placed around the internal carotid artery at a distance of no more than one diam-

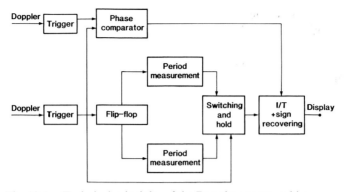

Fig. 12-1. Technical principles of the Doppler spectrum histogram.

eter beyond the arteriotomy. The Doppler spectrum from 10 heart cycles is averaged to overcome physiologic deviations. The averaged values of mean velocity, standard deviation, and PI are plotted by intervals of 10 milliseconds. If PI values are above 40 the bifurcation vessels are immediately clamped again and the arterial incision is reopened. Usually the flow obstacle, which may be an intimal flap, a suture stenosis, or a kinking at the end of the suture line can be identified by the deposition of platelets and fibrin. Appropriate correction is performed until the Doppler spectrum becomes laminar. Techniques such as additional patch grafting, resection of the artery, and shortening by plication have been applied for correction. The overall correction rate in our material due to perturbation measurement was 10%.

RESULTS

From January 1, 1977 to November 23, 1984 we performed 713 carotid endarterectomies on patients who were under general anesthesia for stenosis of the internal carotid artery at the bifurcation: 37.8% were prophylactic operations for critical but asymptomatic stenoses. The stenoses were detected by transcutaneous ultrasound examination in patients undergoing major cardiovascular surgery. In 37.3% one or more transient ischemic attacks were the indication for operation and 24.9% of the patients suffered from residual symptoms of stroke. Until 1981 routine shunting was used for intraoperative brain protection. The stroke rate in 255 patients was 3.1% (Table 12-1). Later shunting was abandoned because it became obvious that

Table 12-1
Neurologic Complications After Surgery for Carotid Artery Stenosis

Type of Protection	No. of Reconstructions	Complications		
		Permanent	Transient	Total
Shunt	255	8 (3.1)	17 (6.7)	25 (9.8)
No shunt	458	5 (1.1)	17 (3.9)	22 (4.0)
Total	713	13 (1.9)	34 (4.7)	47 (6.7)

Note. Data are no. of patients (%) and cover the period January 1, 1977 to November 23, 1984.

the cause of stroke was independent from shunting. The stroke rate in 458 patients without shunting was 1.1%. Routine perturbation measurement was begun in 1979. Of 610 reconstructions measured, 61 were corrected due to the PI compared to 103 previous reconstructions without perturbation measurement. The rate of postoperative technical failure was reduced from 6.8% to 0.6% (Table 12-2). Simultaneously the frequency of permanent neurologic deficits was reduced from 6.8% to 1% (Table 12-3). Because we started perturbation measurement earlier and abandoned shunting later, it was possible to compare a sequential series of 610 patients. In 187 patients where both shunting and perturbation was measured, the stroke rate was 1.1% and the rate of transient deficits was 3.8%. In the subsequent series of 423 patients with hemodynamic control but without shunting, the stroke rate was 0.9% and the rate of transient ischemic attacks was 2.8% (Table 12-4). The difference is not statistically significant but in our material the indwelling shunt was not the

Table 12-2
Technical Failure After Surgery for Carotid Artery Stenosis

		Technical Failure		
Control	No. of Reconstructions	Stenosis	Occlusion	Total
Perturbation	610	2 (0.3)	2 (0.3)	4 (0.6)
None	103	2 (1.9)	5 (4.8)	7 (6.8)
Total	713	4 (0.5)	7 (1.0)	11 (1.5)

Note. Data are no. of patients (%) and cover the period January 1, 1977 to November 23, 1984.

Table 12-3
Neurologic Complications After Surgery for Carotid Artery Stenosis

		Complications		
Control	No. of Reconstructions	Permanent	Transient	Total
Perturbation	610	6 (1.0)	19 (3.1)	25 (4.1)
None	103	7 (6.8)	15 (15.6)	22 (21.4)
Total	713	13 (1.9)	34 (4.6)	47 (6.7)

Note. Data are no. of patients (%) and cover the period January 1, 1977 to November 23, 1984.

Table 12-4
Neurologic Complications After Surgery for Carotid Artery Stenosis

		Complications		
Protection	No. of Reconstructions	Permanent	Transient	Total
Shunt (−), PM (−)	35	3 (8.6)	5 (14.3)	8 (22.9)
Shunt (+), PM (−)	68	4 (5.9)	10 (14.7)	14 (20.6)
Shunt (+), PM (+)	187	2 (1.1)	7 (3.8)	9 (4.8)
Shunt (−), PM (+)	423	4 (0.9)	12 (2.8)	16 (3.8)
Total	713	13 (1.9)	34 (4.7)	47 (6.7)

Note. Data are no. of patients (%) and cover the period January 1, 1977 to November 23, 1984. PM = perturbation measurement.

crucial point for the avoidance of stroke. The technical and neurologic results in our material demonstrate that a sensitive method for intraoperative control and a technically perfect reconstruction under general anesthesia are the most important factors in achieving optimal results.

CONCLUSIONS

Our study demonstrates that even the experienced surgeon needs a reliable method to ensure optimal technical results after carotid thromboendarterectomy. Perturbation measurement proved to be a reliable tool for intraoperative control in carotid endarterectomy. Our results do not support the hypothesis of hemodynamic ischemia or the significance of shunting.

REFERENCES

1. Javid H: Intraluminal shunting during carotid endarterectomy, In Bergan JJ, Yao JJ: Cerebrovascular Insufficiency. Orlando, Fla, Grune & Stratton, 1983, p 309
2. Baker W, Littooy FN, Hayes AC, et al: Carotid endarterectomy without a shunt: The control series. J Vasc Surg 1:50, 1984
3. Ferguson GG: Intraoperative monitoring and internal shunts: Are they necessary in carotid endarterectomy? Stroke 13:287, 1982
4. Sundt TM: The ischemic tolerance of neural tissue and the need for monitoring and selective shunting during carotid endarterectomy. Stroke 14:93, 1983
5. Blaisdell FW, Lim R Jr, Hall AD: Technical results of carotid endarterectomy: Arteriographic assessment. Am J Surg 114:239, 1967
6. Stein PD, Sabbah HN: Measured turbulence and its effect on thrombus formation. Circ Res 35:608, 1974
7. Sandmann W, Peronneau P, Kremer K: Carotischirurgie und Perturbationsmessung. Angio 2:277, 1980
8. Sandmann W: Measurement of blood flow during and after surgery, In: Peronneau P, Diebold A: Cardiovascular Applications of Doppler Echography. INSERM 111:229, 1982
9. Sandmann W, Kniemeyer H, Peronneau P, et al: Improvement of carotid artery reconstruction using intraoperative Doppler spectrum histogram. Stroke 15:190, 1984 (Abstr)
10. Sandmann W, Peronneau P, Ulrich B, et al: Die Messung von Turbulenz mit dem Ultraschall-Doppler Verfahren am Strömungsmodell, am Hund und am Menschen, In: Zeitler E: Hypertonie-Risikofaktor in der Angiologie. Witzstrock 222, 1976
11. Sandmann W, Peronneau P, Gisbertz KH, et al: Untersuchungen zur Turbulenz im normalen und stenotischen Gefäß. Langenb. Arch Klin Chir Suppl 157, 1976

Allan D. Callow

13

The Value of Electroencephalography for Cerebral Protection

The electroencephalogram can assist you in performing carotid endarterectomy by identifying those patients who (1) experience cerebral ischemia during cross clamping of the carotid artery, and (2) may have suffered a stroke during the operation.

The need for temporary shunting during carotid endarterectomy varies from close to zero in the asymptomatic patient with normal collateral circulation to as high as 25% in patients with reduced collateral flow. The latter group includes patients with a history of an old stroke, a computerized tomography (CT) scan positive for cerebral infarct, a residual neurologic deficit at the time of operation, contralateral carotid occlusion or a very high degree of stenosis, and patients with signs and symptoms of coexisting vertebral basilar insufficiency. On occasion the use of a shunt, either upon insertion or removal, produces trauma to the arterial wall and, in addition, with a high lying plaque may make distal dissection of the edge of the plaque more difficult.

With respect to stroke during the course of operation, one need not wait for the patient to awaken from anesthesia but rather one can either immediately reopen the arteriotomy and inspect it for thrombus, usually the white clot or platelet type, or do an immediate intraoperative arteriogram. These two features of continuous electroencephalographic monitoring make it extremely useful, particularly when strenuous effort and meticulous care must be an unremitting constant, to maintain or reduce the present day morbidity and mortality of 1%–2%.

Approximately 15% of the resting cardiac output and 20% of inspired oxygen at rest are appropriated by the brain which does not metabolize free fatty acids to any extent and therefore is essentially dependent on glucose as a source of carbon. The brain consumes the entire output of glucose by the liver in the fasting state and has almost no reserves. Its entire energy consumption is utilized in membrane transport and electrical activity.

A remarkable feature of the cerebral circulation is its ability to regulate itself in an effort to keep brain flood flow constant. Neither increase in cardiac output during exercise nor moderate change in arterial blood pressure is associated with substantial change in brain blood flow. Simultaneous adjustment of resistance of

DIAGNOSTIC TECHNIQUES AND ASSESSMENT PROCEDURES IN VASCULAR SURGERY

© 1985 Grune & Stratton
ISBN 0-8089-1721-8 All rights reserved

small cerebral arteries and arterioles keeps perfusion pressure constant. This complex regulatory mechanism is known as "cerebral autoregulation" and is an energy-dependent process. When autoregulation is functional, cerebral blood flow is relatively free and independent of perfusion pressure. When, however, autoregulation is impaired as in cerebral ischemia,[1] cerebral blood flow is critically dependent on perfusion pressure and to a lesser extent on blood volume and cardiac output. To counteract loss of autoregulation as may happen during carotid endarterectomy, systemic arterial blood pressure should not be permitted to fall below the patient's normal level.

Probably no aspect of carotid surgery is more controversial than the methods for the protection of the brain during carotid cross-clamping and of monitoring cerebral perfusion during the operation. This is true despite the high probability, difficult if not impossible to establish, that perioperative neurologic deficits are more often the consequence of embolization during dissection or after restoration of flow than the result of cerebral hypoxia during endarterectomy.

Routine use of a shunt has several disadvantages, the most important of which is uncertainty as to the completeness of endarterectomy at the distal end of the plaque. Adequate visualization may be difficult with a long, high posterior wall extension of the plaque, and in patients with either a short neck or when the carotid bifurcation is abnormally high as at the level of C-2. Internal carotid back or stump pressure is an indirect measurement of collateral flow; is performed prior to arteriotomy; is a single measurement lacking opportunity for continuous evaluation throughout the operation; and is particularly desirable if there are fluctuations in cardiac rhythm and blood pressure. Lastly, although total cerebral blood flow may be assessed, disturbances in regional cerebral blood flow are not detectable by this method.[2] The duration of ischemic cross-clamping has been reported as directly related to the incidence of neurologic complications[3] (Table 13-1).

Table 13-1
Relation of Occlusion Time to Postoperative Ischemic
Deficits in Patients with P-/ic > 50 mmHg

Occlusion Time (min)	No. of Operations	Postoperative Deficit
< 30	194	0
> 30	30	6*

* Deficit was transient in four patients and prolonged in two patients.

Certainly the most effective endarterectomy is one performed without haste and which is extensive enough to remove all of the atherosclerotic plaque. For surgeons who can perform an adequate endarterectomy with a cross-clamp duration of under 12 minutes and in all patients except those with the most severely compromised collateral circulation, the brain may tolerate hypoperfusion for this limited period. At greater risk are those patients entering the operation with neurologic signs or symptoms, patients with angiographically demonstrable risk factors such as occlusion of the contralateral internal carotid, or tandem lesions, and patients with a history of old stroke or a CT scan positive for cerebral infarct. Recent reports suggesting that an acceptable complication rate can be achieved without monitoring cerebral pressure or flow and without a shunt must be carefully scrutinized (D. Raithel, personal communication),[4] for although many factors other than the use of a shunt affect the outcome of carotid endarterectomy, patient selection is probably the most important. Morbidity and mortality are usually lowest for asymptomatic patients who need the operation least. Whether a shunt is used routinely, selectively, or never may be a matter of personal preference, but to maintain that a shunt is never necessary because cerebral ischemia can never occur suggests a high degree of selectivity in choosing patients for operation, a degree of technical perfection and surgical speed not achieved by most vascular surgeons, or a lack of understanding of the cerebral circulation. We prefer selective shunting as determined by continuous electroencephalographic monitoring.

By way of example, in one series of 289 consecutive carotid endarterectomies in 204 patients in which use of a temporary shunt was based entirely on the electroencephalographic (EEG) changes,[5] evidence of ischemia appeared in 6% of patients despite a carotid stump pressure ≥ 50 mmHg. Patients with a history of completed stroke or with symptoms of vertebral basilar insufficiency in addition to carotid stenosis had a higher incidence of ischemic EEG changes, 24% in each, despite stump pressures of ≥ 50 mmHg. None of these patients had a neurologic deficit during or after operation (Fig. 13-1).[6] A comparison of several methods of management is shown in Table 13-2.

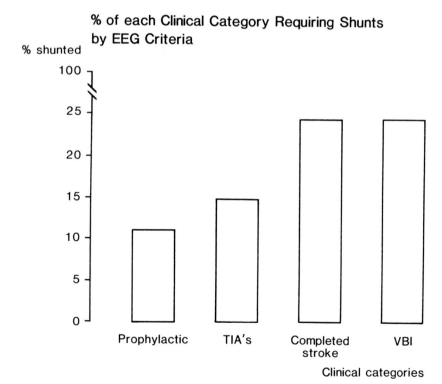

Fig. 13-1. From Callow AD: The Leriche Memorial Lecture. Fact or fancy: A twenty year personal prospective on the detection and management of carotid occlusive disease. J Cardiovasc Surg 21:641, 1980. With permission.

Table 13-2
Perioperative Neurologic Deficit and Method of Monitoring

Method of Monitoring	No. of Patients	CNS Deficits	
		Permanent	Transient
Selective shunting based on EEG	1782	0.9	2
No shunt, general anesthesia, no monitoring	940	1.8	2.2
Contralateral occlusion: stroke	34	9	...
No shunt, no monitoring, general anesthesia, normotensive	1081	1.2	2.0
Stump pressure <25 mmHg, selective shunting, general anesthesia	149	1.4	2.2
No shunt, regional anesthesia		2.2	3.0
Regional anesthesia, selective shunting (awake)	1800	0.3	2.2
No monitoring, routine shunting	1300	0.8	1.4
Routine shunt	1023	0.5	1.9

Note.   Data are expressed as percentage of patients.

For those of you who have little or no interest in cerebral physiology or the theory of electroencephalography, it is recommended that you ignore what immediately follows and proceed to the paragraph beginning, "EEG is totally noninvasive and entirely risk free."

EEG: GENERAL CONSIDERATIONS

The source of the EEG waves are electrical potentials generated by nerve cells in the cerebral cortex lining the surface of the hemispheres (Fig. 13-2).[7] As with other cells, cortical neurons have a resting potential, the difference between the interior of the cell and the extracellular space. Measuring 50–100 mV and negative on the inside of the cell membrane with respect to the outside, it is the result of both passive and active properties of the cell membrane. Passive properties do not require energy. They are the result of unequal permeability to sodium, potassium, chloride, and other ions with sodium and chloride concentrated on the outside and potassium on the inside. This uneven distribution causes a steady difference of electrical potential at rest. Active properties of the neuron are so labeled because energy is required to transport leaking ions against diffusional gradients and thereby restore concentrations appropriate for resting conditions. Most important is the active transport of extracellular sodium and intracellular potassium. Ischemia disrupts cerebral metabolism and reduces or even abolishes the pumping action of the membrane with a resulting reduction of membrane potential. There is increased neuronal excitability which may progress to ultimate collapse of neuronal function.[7]

Rhythmical EEG activity may be due the result of impulses arriving from other neurons and to the projection of periodic impulses from a subcortical pacemaker (Fig. 13-3).[7] Scalp electrodes record principally the summation of changes of potential in the underlying cortex and rarely reflect those produced in distant parts of the brain. Electrical inputs from the scalp electrodes are received at input switches used

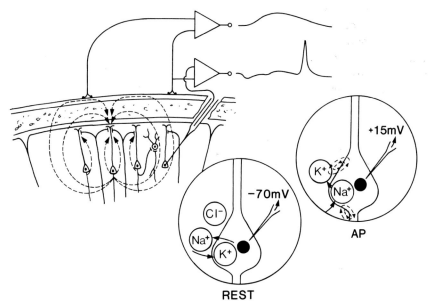

Fig. 13-2. Generation of EEG by cerebral cortex showing uneven distribution of ions across cell membrane (rest). AP = action potention. From Spehlmann R: EEG Primer. Amsterdam, Elsevier North Holland, 1982. With permission.

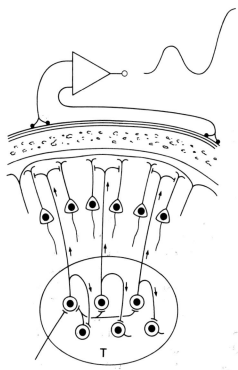

Fig. 13-3. Steps in the production of rhythmical EEG activity in the cortex (C) by impulses from a hypothetical pacemaker in the thalamus (T). See figure legend 13-2.

to select a pair of electrodes or a calibration voltage as the input of each recording channel. The input is connected to differential amplifiers which increase the size of the electrical potential difference between the two electrodes and reject interference simultaneously affecting both. High- and low-frequency filters are used to reduce the size of very slow and very fast potential changes and to emphasize clinically important electrical activity in the medium frequency range. The amplified electrical potentials are used to drive an ink pen or other writing device (Fig. 13-4).[7]

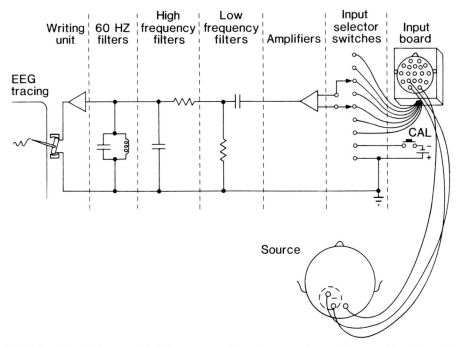

Fig. 13-4. Electrical potential differences on the scalp are registered by recording electrodes. Although most machines have 8 or 16 channels, only one recording channel is illustrated. From Spehlmann R: EEG Primer. Amsterdam, Elsevier North Holland, 1982. With permission.

Electrode Placement

The International 10-20 system of electrode placement (Fig. 13-5)[7] provides uniform coverage of the entire scalp and assures symmetrical, reproducible electrode placements, permitting comparison of EEGs from the same patient. The standard set of electrodes for adults consists of 21 recording electrodes and one ground electrode. Recording electrodes are named with a letter and a subscript. The letter is an abbreviation of the underlying region, prefrontal or frontopolar (Fp), frontal (F), central (C), parietal (P), occipital (O), and auricular (A). Odd numbers refer to electrodes on the left and even numbers on the right side of the head. The subscript z indicates zero or midline placement.

A wide variety of normal EEG patterns (Fig. 13-6)[8] can be seen in different persons at the same age and an even greater variety of normal patterns can occur in different age groups. In addition to the variety of normal patterns, there are a few

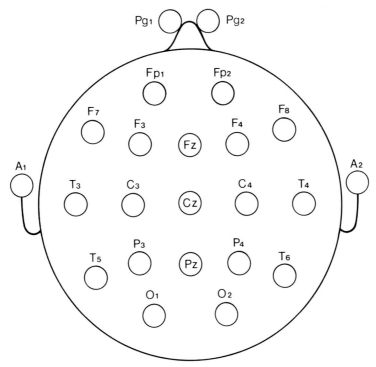

Fig. 13-5. Placement of recording electrodes according to the International 10-20 System. See figure legend 13-2.

EEG components such as spikes and sharp waves, certain slow waves, and amplitude changes that are known to be definitely abnormal in each age group. The normal EEG is often defined more by the absence of abnormal components than by the presence of normal patterns. Frequency refers to the number of times a repetitive wave recurs in one second. A wave completing three cycles in one second is called a wave of 3 Hertz (Hz) or of 3 per sec. The frequency of single or repetitive waves can be determined by measuring the duration of an individual wave, the wave length, and calculating the reciprocal. For instance, a wave lasting 250 msec or 1/4 second is said to have a frequency of 4 Hz regardless of whether or not it repeats (Fig. 13-7).[7]

The frequency of EEG waves is often divided into four somewhat arbitrary bands: (1) delta frequency band: under 4 Hz, (2) theta frequency band: from 4 to 8 Hz, (3) alpha frequency band: from 8 to 13 Hz, and (4) beta frequency band: over 13 Hz (Fig. 13-8).[9]

These four major frequencies were given these Greek letters in the order of their discovery and imply no relationship to importance. The alpha rhythm, a sustained rhythmic activity of 8–13 Hz and usually ranging between 25 to 100 microvolts[10] is the basic and most common symmetric pattern in the adult, and indicates adequate perfusion. Although its true physiologic significance is unknown, it has been suggested that it is related to the visual system and possibly represents an idling rhythm that appears in the absence of specific input to that system. Beta rhythms (Fig. 13-9)[9] are often less easily seen and consist of waves over 13 Hz which appear in a wide distribution. Light to moderate general anesthesia (usually nitrous oxide plus thiopental sodium) produces a 10–20 Hz mixed "alpha-beta" pattern. Diminution of this activity under anesthesia is associated with ischemia and it disappears altogether with severe prolonged ischemia (or hypoxia). Additional signs of ischemia are slow waves of less than 8 Hz, especially significant when the waves are repetitive, frequency, and of wide distribution. These slow waves, the delta band (Fig. 13-10),[7] referred to as slow wave activity,[7,9] have a frequency less than 4 cps. As ischemia or anoxia proceed this may become the dominant rhythm (prior to loss of all activity) coinciding with a decrease of approximately 65%–70% of the cerebral metabolic rate for oxygen. Variations in the depth of anesthesia, changes of $PaCO_2$, and the effect of different anesthetic agents may produce changes other than these characteristic of hypoxia. Frequency thus becomes one of the most important criteria for assessing abnormality in the clinical EEG.

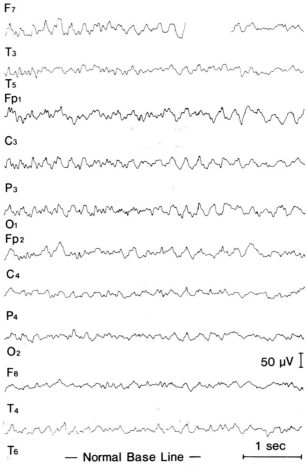

Fig. 13-6. From Callow AD, O'Donnell TF: The detection of cerebral ischemia during carotid endarterectomy by continuous electroencephalographic monitoring, In Greenhalgh RM and Rose FC (eds): Progress in Stroke Research 2. London, Pitman Books, 1983. With permission.

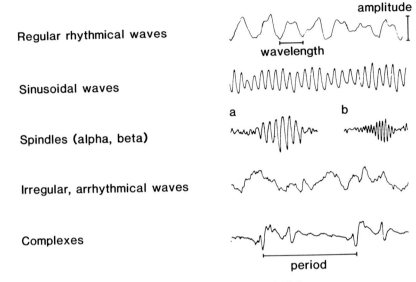

Regular rhythmical waves

amplitude

wavelength

Sinusoidal waves

Spindles (alpha, beta)

a   b

Irregular, arrhythmical waves

Complexes

period

Fig. 13-7.   See figure legend 13-2.

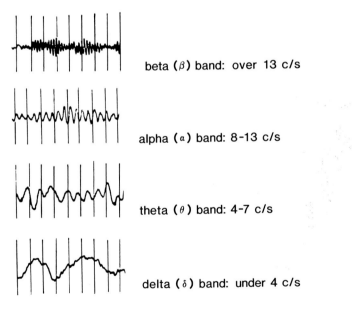

beta (β) band: over 13 c/s

alpha (α) band: 8-13 c/s

theta (θ) band: 4-7 c/s

delta (δ) band: under 4 c/s

(Hess R, EEG Handbook, 1966)

Fig. 13-8.   From Hess R: EEG Handbook. Zurich, Sandaz, 1966. With permission.

137

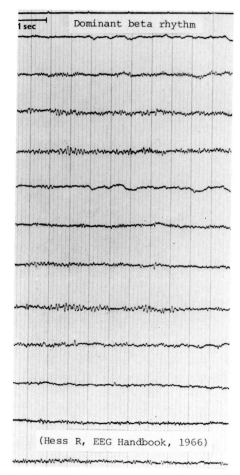

(Hess R, EEG Handbook, 1966)

Fig. 13-9.   From Hess R: EEG Handbook. Zurich, Sandaz, 1966. With permission.

Amplitude is measured in microvolts (μV) and can be expressed in terms of the height of the pen deflection if proper calibrations have been performed. Most often it is described loosely as low ($<20\ \mu$V), medium (20–70 μV), or high ($>70\ \mu$V) (Fig. 13-11).[7] Of great importance, especially when persistent, is the asymmetry that may be recorded simultaneously from corresponding parts of the two hemispheres.

Distribution refers to the occurrence of electrical activity recorded by electrodes positioned over different parts of the head. Terms used to describe it are widespread, diffuse, generalized, lateralized, and focal. The last two are important distinctions especially with regard to abnormal slow waves or loss of a normal component such as beta or fast waves.

An additional characteristic of ischemia, especially when focal or unilateral and progressive, is the development of low amplitude, sometimes referred to as low voltage (Fig. 13-12).[7] Grading of focal slow waves is important as a measure of the degree of abnormality. When marked, and persisting through a large part of the recording, they may consist mainly or entirely of delta waves, an indication of severe cortical ischemia, edema, and acidosis. Occlusion of the carotid artery may result in

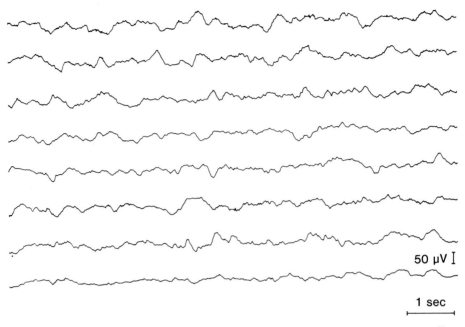

Fig. 13-10. Generalized asynchronous slow waves predominantly delta frequency. From Spehlmann R: EEG Primer. Amsterdam, Elsevier North Holland, 1982. With permission.

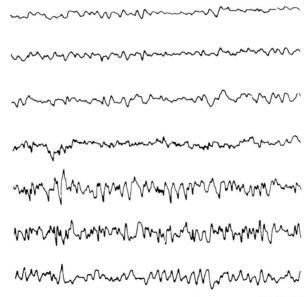

Fig. 13-11. Pattern of local low amplitude. From Spehlmann R: EEG Primer. Amsterdam, Elsevier North Holland, 1982. With permission.

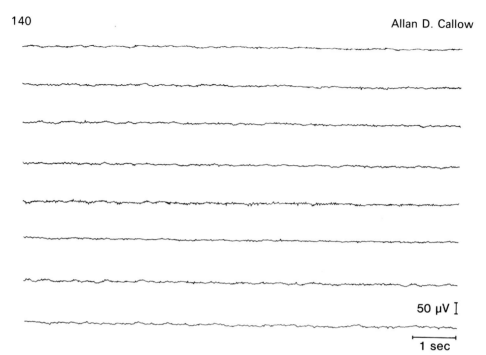

50 μV

1 sec

Fig. 13-12. Pattern of very low amplitude. From Spehlmann R: EEG Primer. Amsterdam, Elsevier North Holland, 1982. With permission.

reduction of cerebral blood flow to a level below that needed to prevent infarction. Imminent infarction may be recognized by the appearance of focal or unilateral slow waves within a few seconds to a few minutes after cross-clamping, often followed by loss of amplitude indicating collateral circulation is inadequate and a temporary shunt is required.

Electroencephalography is totally noninvasive and entirely risk free. Contrary to some opinion, the presence of a neurologist is not required. The EEG console and technician should be easily visible to the surgeon. Significant abnormal changes in the EEG in comparison to normal tracings are readily identifiable.

Correlations of cerebral blood flow measurements with the EEG have been provided by several studies.[11–13] Normal cerebral blood flow is cited as 50–55 mL/100 g/min. Critical flow for the normal brain is approximately 30%–40% of this but it may be much less for the brain previously damaged by ischemia. Occlusion blood flows during carotid endarterectomy measured with radioactive xenon[11] were <5 mL/100 g/min in 2%, 5–9 mL/100 g/min in 5%, 10–14 mL/100 g/min in 11%, and 15–20 mL/100 g/min in 15%. Flows <5 mL/100 g/min produced cerebral infarction within three to four minutes. Tolerance to flows 5–9 mL/100 g/min was not definitely determined and some biologic variation undoubtedly exists. Cerebral blood flow is not homogeneous at these marginal levels. The best available data indicate that a normal animal who has not been given barbiturates can tolerate flows at this critical level for not more than 10 minutes. Ischemic tolerance between 10 and 14 mL/100 g/min is also undetermined, but is probably in the range of 15 and 30 minutes. General anesthesia (depending on depth) may extend this. This variability of the brain to tolerate 10–15 minutes of ischemia may account for the reported disparity in the use of the EEG.

The EEG frequently but not unfailingly reveals signs of vascular insufficiency in patients with a preexisting neurologic deficit or with a history of a previous stroke and in patients with a CT scan positive for cerebral infarct. These patients, therefore, with a history of a preoperative neurologic deficit together with those with contralateral carotid occlusion, severe stenosis, tandem lesions, and a history of a previous stroke are at greater risk. When in doubt a temporary inlying shunt should be utilized. Similarly, patients who are neurologically unstable prior to operation or enter the operation with waxing and waning transient ischemic attacks probably possess a limited collateral circulation and will have a greater incidence of changes in the EEG during cross-clamping. These patients are more likely to require a shunt than patients who are asymptomatic or who have a normal preoperative neurologic status.[14] Thus, the risk of operation and the need for an intraoperative shunt closely correlate with the patient's preoperative neurologic status.

Figure 13-13[15] illustrates the restoration of arterial flow after insertion of a temporary shunt, prompt return of beta activity, and disappearance of slow wave (delta). The change is most marked in the upper four tracings in each panel which are taken from the right hemisphere before, during, and following right carotid cross-clamping. The bottom five tracings are from the left hemisphere. Two electrodes were nonfunctioning in each panel.

If one could be certain that all endarterectomies could be done in no more than 10 minutes cross-clamp time—the so-called "safe period"—then monitoring and temporary shunts probably would be unnecessary.

Critical cerebral blood flow also varies with the anesthetic agent and has been found to be 15–17 mL/100 g/min with halothane, 13–15 mL/100 g/min for ethrane, and 10–13 mL/100 g/min for forane (Fig. 13-14).[7,16]

Barbiturates, especially when given rapidly, produce prominent central or generalized beta activity. At higher blood levels, as for example following intravenous injection during induction, and with an increase in the concentration of an anes-

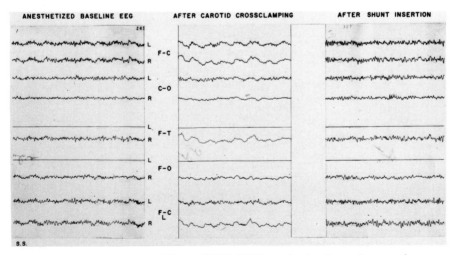

Fig. 13-13. From Callow AD, O'Donnell TF: EEG monitoring in cerebrovascular surgery, In Bergan JJ, Yao JST (eds): Cerebrovascular Insufficiency. Orlando, Fla, Grune & Stratton, 1983. With permission.

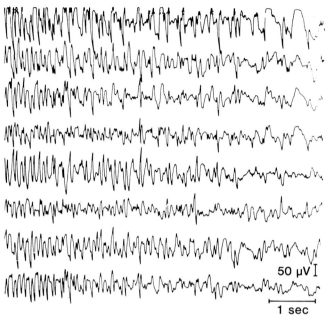

Fig. 13-14. Example of widespread muscular activity seen with induction of anesthesia. From Spehlmann R: EEG Primer. Amsterdam, Elsevier North Holland, 1982. With permission.

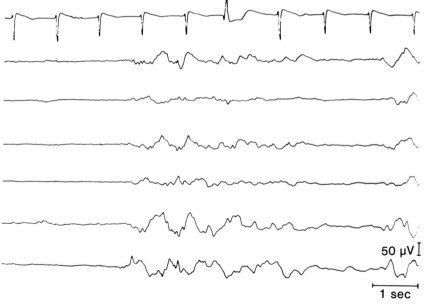

Fig. 13-15. Burst suppression pattern characteristic of barbiturate administration. From Spehlmann R: EEG Primer. Amsterdam, Elsevier North Holland, 1982. With permission.

142

thetic gas, a characteristic pattern described as "burst suppression" evolves. This consists of periods of low amplitude activity or even of complete electrical silence of a few seconds or longer duration which begin to interrupt delta waves at short intervals (Fig. 13-15).[7]

The effects of anesthetic agents on the EEG are variable between classes but usually are predictable and reproducible, ranging from initial cortical excitation and hyperirritability through depression to ultimate isoelectricity. With the exceptions of ketamine class and enflurane, most anesthetic agents are associated with high frequency (beta) desynchronization at low amplitude at subanesthetic doses. This progresses to lower frequencies (alpha) at high amplitudes and through depression with still lower frequencies (theta and delta) and finally to electrical silence—isoelectricity.

The differentiation of ischemic- and anesthetic-induced EEG changes may be made most simply when EEG changes are focal in nature and appear in only one area of the brain. Such focal changes are seldom anesthetic induced but rather related to intracerebral or cerebrovascular pathophysiology. The situation becomes

Table 13-3

Effects of different anesthetic agents on EEG

Drug, Dose	Frequency (Hz)	Amplitude	Comments
Inhalationals			
Halothane			
0.75%	10–20	Low	The frequency of anesthetic-
1.6%	1–5	High	induced EEG activity (SEF) is inversely proportional to the end tidal concentration. Addition of N20 may slightly reduce frequency further.
Isoflurane			
0.75%	15–20	Low	Isoflurane induces isoelectricity
1.6%	0	Low	at a smaller dose than that causing cardiovascular collapse and otherwise resembles halothane.
Enflurane			
1.3%	20–30	Low	Induced seizure activity is further
1.8%	7–12	High	accentuated by hypocapnea. EEG can
3.6%	Spikes		show spike and wave with burst suppression.
Nitrous oxide			
70%	...	...	N20 alone seldom affects the EEG although it may cause slowing in combination with other drugs.
Barbiturates			
Pentothal			
50 mg	25–35	Low	Low doses of barbiturates activate the EEG.
250 mg	1–4	High	High doses are potent depressors of EEG. Burst suppression occurs following an intravenous bolus.

more complicated when global hypoxia must be differentiated from deepening anesthesia for an isoelectric or flat line EEG often produced by severe hypoxia may also be caused by deep hypothermia, large doses of barbiturates greater than those used to induce anesthesia, and isoflurane. Ischemic hypoxia initially causes EEG slowing rather than isoelectricity. The pattern of development of slowing is therefore important. Deep anesthesia requires time to develop; thus, the onset of EEG slowing is gradual. When the transition between adequate and inadequate cerebral oxygen supply is abrupt, as for example following cross-clamping of the carotid, the EEG slowing is also abrupt in onset. Hypocarbia occurring in response to hyperventilation will produce cerebral vasoconstriction. If profound, a hypoxic EEG pattern may result. In addition, enflurane and isoflurane both produce burst suppression in the EEG prior to or together with marked EEG slowing. Burst suppression is not normally a product of acute ischemia.

Another problem is the increasing popularity of narcotic anesthesia. Fentanyl when used as an anesthetic and administered as a bolus may produce abrupt onset of EEG slowing, thus mimicking slowing of hypoxia. The occurrence of such a pharmacologic intervention has to be taken into account when differential EEG alteration is of acute onset. Anesthetic techniques providing a steady depth of anesthesia before and after carotid cross-clamping are preferred if EEG monitoring is of paramount importance (Fig. 13-16).[17,18]

High-dose Fentanyl technique means a large dose is given during induction of anesthesia. EEG stabilizes it with delta waves and no further Fentanyl doses are given. This technique requires postoperative ventilation and is usually not suitable for carotid endarterectomy. Low-dose Fentanyl calls for an initial small bolus for induction and even smaller increments intraoperatively for maintenance. The increments may be substituted by low-dose inhalational anesthesia.

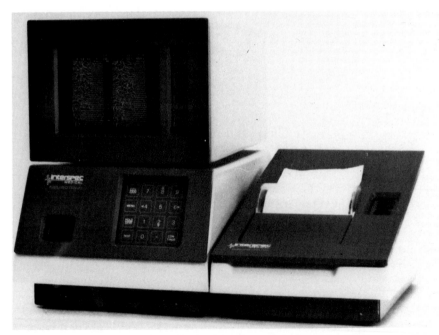

Fig. 13-16. Neurotrac, an EEG Spectral Analyzer, from Interspec. With permission.

There have been numerous inquiries as to the availability of a simplified, compact unit rather than the standard console for possible wider application in the community hospital. Several small computer-based EEG analyzers for routine intraoperative recording and interpretation of the EEG are available for nonspecialists. The limitations created by the size and complexity of conventional equipment, the need for a trained technician, and the difficulty in interpretation of the raw EEG data are reduced or eliminated. A computer processes, compresses, and displays the EEG in a form which is easy to interpret (Fig. 13-17). Analyzing the frequencies of the EEG tracings—spectral analysis—permits an accurate estimation of the depth of anesthesia in the majority of patients and is a reasonably reliable indicator of cerebral ischemia.[20,21] An effective method of displaying the EEG spectral data has been the compressed spectral array (CSA) as described by Bickford et al.[19] The nonspecialist can spot frequency shifts and amplitude changes in the power spectrum by this method. The compressed spectral array begins with a plot of frequency versus power of a segment of EEG; the next segment is pushed beneath the prior segment's data. A "hidden line algorithm" is used to erase the prior trace's sections which would be hidden by the new data and this algorithm gives the display its characteristic three-dimensional effect. A promising development is the calculation and display of what is labeled the spectral-edge frequency and its correlation to depth of anesthesia and cerebral hypoxia (Figs. 13-18, 13-19).[22–29]

In our series of 1713 consecutive carotid operations performed for all indications except the acute progressing or evolving stroke from 1958 to 1984, in which continuous EEG monitoring was used, there were 16 deaths for a mortality of 0.93%. There were 37 transient deficits for an incidence of 2.1% and 18 prolonged or permanent deficits for an incidence of 1%. There were two primary stroke deaths.[8,15] Although some patients with transient ischemic attacks or a history of

Technique used to Generate Compressed Spectra

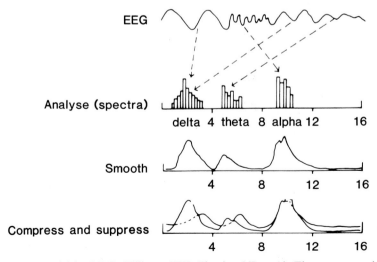

Fig. 13-17. From Bickford RG, Billinger TW, Fleming NI, et al: The compressed spectral array: A pictorial EEG. Proc San Diego Biomed Symp 11:365, 1972.

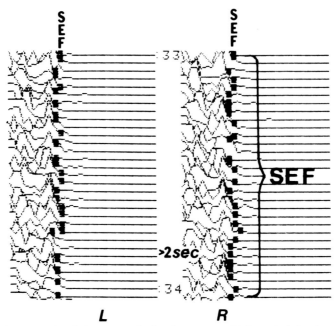

Fig. 13-18. An example of the spectral edge frequency of left and right electrodes. This is defined as a visual marker of the outer or higher edge of the EEG's frequency spectrum and identifies shifts in EEG frequency.

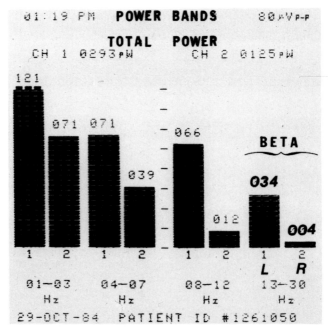

Fig. 13-19. Any of the four frequency bands—1–3, 4–7, 8–12, and 13–30 Hz—selected by the user are displayed as summated powers from each channel, one and two. They are continuously updated. In this example, the marked reduction in beta activity on the right for the right hemisphere, 004, as contrasted to the left, 034, is dramatically illustrated and alerts the surgical team to the occurrence of cerebral hypoxia and the likely need for a temporary shunt.

old stroke demonstrated an abnormal tracing prior to clamping, no prolonged or fixed new deficit occurred without an associated EEG change after clamping. The converse is apparently not true; that is, focal EEG changes in so-called "silent" areas—frontal and temporal lobes, for example—may be seen in the operative EEGs. Such patients may awaken without a readily apparent deficit. Patients with preoperative EEG abnormalities are more vulnerable to reductions in cerebral blood flow than patients with a normal tracing. Such patients as well as those with a cerebral infarction (old or new) as detected by preoperative CT scan, are also more likely to require a shunt during carotid cross-clamping. EEG interpretation in these patients may be more difficult. These patients apparently have a lower ischemic tolerance. Significant transient or permanent ipsilateral EEG changes occurring during or immediately after operation usually indicate thromboembolism from, or thrombosis at, the endarterectomy site. One need not, therefore, wait for the patient to awaken from anesthesia to discover the neurologic deficit. The endarterectomy site can be inspected at the time of occurrence of the EEG abnormality, or a completion arteriogram can be performed.

The EEG permits selective use of a shunt which in the usual distribution of patients (eg, transient ischemic attack, asymptomatic bruits, history of an old stroke, CT scan positive for cerebral infarct, and vertebral basilar insufficiency symptoms superimposed or in association with carotid territory symptoms) are needed in approximately 7% of patients. On a more selective basis (eg, patients with a history of an old stroke, patients with a positive scan for cerebral infarct on the ipsilateral side, and patients with a history or signs and symptoms of coexisting vertebral basilar insufficiency), this number showing ischemic changes by EEG and therefore requiring a shunt increases to approximately 24% in each group. The correlation between need of a shunt is based upon the appearance of changes of ischemia in the EEG. The stump or carotid back pressure is generally high, but unpredictable exceptions have been identified. Inasmuch as the mortality of operation is under 1% and the incidence of permanent neurologic deficit is approximately the same magnitude, the addition of even one stroke in one hundred patients markedly affects this experience, and close monitoring is therefore considered desirable. The same may be said about the fact that even rare instances of trauma associated with insertion or removal of a shunt occur, such misadventures may as well profoundly affect morbidity.

Hence, unnecessary use of a shunt is to be avoided. The EEG thus permits limiting the use of a shunt to a very small number of patients. In addition to the previously stated advantage, EEG also permits better visualization of the distal end of the arteriotomy. There is, therefore, opportunity for a careful, meticulous, and oftentimes lengthy performance of the endarterectomy and arteriotomy closure. The distal end of the plaque is adequately visualized and the removal of those residual tags, which occasionally persist despite what is thought to be an adequate dissection, is sometimes hindered by the presence of the shunt. EEG monitoring provides satisfactory protection for all patients irrespective of changes in the collateral blood flow which may follow upon changes in cardiac function and depth of anesthesia. There is a very close correlation between the electrical activity as visualized in the EEG and the degree or the status of cerebral perfusion. Surveillance is continuous throughout the induction of anesthesia, the operation and various hemodynamic changes occurring with it, changes in the anesthetic agents which are administered, and during the recovery period from anesthesia. One is not forced to rely upon a single measurement of the stump or carotid back pressure available only at the onset of the operation. The disadvantages, we believe, are minor: modest expense and a little added time. Provided the depth of anesthesia does not alter, the EEG is an extremely accurate and reliable indicator of cortical ischemia. This does not, however, diminish the need for a very high degree of cooperation and communication between the surgeon, the anesthesiologist, and the electroencephalographer.

ACKNOWLEDGEMENT

The author is grateful for the assistance provided over many years and in many operations by Kathleen McPeck, Heinrich Wurm, and Bruce Ehrenberg, New England Medical Center.

REFERENCES

1. Toole JF, Patel AN: Cerebrovascular Disorders. New York, McGraw-Hill, 1967
2. Boysen G: Cerebral blood flow measurement as a safeguard during carotid endarterectomy. Stroke 2:1, 1983
3. Wylie EJ, Ehrenfeld WK: Extracranial Occlusive Cerebrovascular Disease. Philadelphia, Saunders, 1970
4. Whitney DG, Kahn EM, Estes JW, et al: Carotid artery surgery without a temporary indwelling shunt. Arch Surg 115:1393, 1980
5. Kelly JJ, Callow AD, O'Donnell TF, et al: Failure of carotid stump pressures. Arch Surg 114:1361, 1979
6. Callow AD: The Leriche Memorial Lecture. Fact or fancy: A twenty year personal perspective on the detection and management of carotid occlusive disease. J Cardiovas Surg 21:641, 1980
7. Spehlmann R: EEG Primer. Amsterdam, Elsevier North Holland, 1982
8. Callow AD, O'Donnell TF: The detection of cerebral ischemia during carotid endarterectomy by continuous electroencephalographic monitoring, In Greenhalgh RM (ed): Progress in Stroke Research 2. London, Pitman Books, 1983, pp 354–375
9. Hess R: EEG Handbook (Sandoz Monographs). EEG Laboratory of University Hospital, Zurich, Sandoz, 1966
10. Westmoreland BF: Normal and benign EEG patterns. Am J EEG Tech 22:3, 1982
11. Sundt TM, Sharbrough FW, Piepgras DG, et al: Correlation of cerebral blood flow and electroencephalographic changes during carotid endarterectomy. Mayo Clin Proc 56:533, 1981
12. Sharbrough FW, Messick JM Jr, Sundt TM Jr: Correlation of continuous electroencephalograms with cerebral blood flow measurements during carotid endarterectomy. Stroke 4:674, 1973
13. Boysen G, Engell HC, Pistolese GR, et al: On the critical lower level of CBF in man with particular reference to carotid surgery. Circulation 49:1023, 1974
14. Thompson JE: Complications of carotid endarterectomy and their prevention. World J Surg 3:155, 1979
15. Callow AD, O'Donnell TF: EEG monitoring in cerebrovascular surgery, In Bergan JJ, Yao JST (eds): Cerebrovascular Insufficiency. Orlando, Fla, Grune & Stratton, 1983, pp 326–341

16. Sundt TM: Electroencephalographic monitoring of carotid endarterectomy. Presented at the ACS Postgraduate Course, Atlanta, October 1983
17. EEG Monitoring—During and After Surgery. Interspec Medical, Interspec, 1–36 (2nd Revision), Conshohocken, Pa, 1983
18. Neurotrac. Compressed Spectral Array. Interspec (brochure), 1983
19. Bickford RG, Billinger TW, Fleming NI, et al: The compressed spectral array: A pictorial EEG. Proc San Diego Biomed Symp 11:365, 1972
20. Saunders D: Editorial: Anaesthesia, awareness and automation. Br J Anaes 38:564, 1973
21. Chiappa KH, Burke SR, Young RR: Results of electroencephalographic monitoring during 367 carotid endarterectomies: Use of a dedicated minicomputer. Stroke 10:381, 1979
22. Rampil IJ, Sasse FJ, Smith NT, et al: Spectral edge frequency: A new correlate of anesthetic depth. ASA Abstracts, Vol 53, No 3, 1980
23. Smith NT, Rampil IJ, Sasse FJ, et al: EEG during rapidly changing halothane or enflurane. Anesthesiology 51:54, 1979
24. Anderson EM, Carney AL, Page L: Carotid and vertebral artery surgery, EEG monitoring and the operating room. Adv-Neurol 30:54, 1981
25. Harris EJ, Brown WH, Pavy RN, et al: Continuous electroencephalographic monitoring during carotid artery endarterectomy. Surgery 62:534, 1977
26. Stockard JJ, Bickford RG, Myers RR, et al: Hypotension-induced changes in cerebral function during cardiac surgery. Stroke 5:730, 1974
27. Trajaborg W, Boysen G: Relation between EEG, regional cerebral blood flow, and internal carotid artery pressure during carotid endarterectomy. Electroencephalogr Clin Neurophysiol 34:61, 1973
28. Epp RL, Negin M, Lee KJ: Performance specification of a microcomputer-based EEG compressed spectral array system. Proc IEEE Fourth Annu Conf EMBS, Philadelphia, 1982, pp 32–39
29. Smith NT, Hoff BH, Rampil IJ, et al: Does thiopental or N20 disrupt the EEG during enflurane? Anesthesiology 51:S5, 1979

Paolo Fiorani, G. R. Pistolese, M. Ventura, E. Sbarigia,
M. Rasura, S. Bastianello, L. M. Fantozzi, and L. Bozzao

14

Predictive Value of CTScan Evaluation in Carotid Surgery

The reability of computerized axial tomography (CT)Scan examination in the diagnosis of patients with neurological deficit is clear.[1,2] In patients with unstable neurological deficit (crescendo TIA, progressing stroke) associated to extracranial carotid lesions, CTScan was useful to ascertain the ischaemic nature of symptoms and the integrity of blood brain barrier, for emergency carotid revascularization.[3,4,5] Our experience with CTScan examination in patients with cerebrovascular insufficiency due to obstructive lesions of carotid axis shows that CTScan may be useful in the evaluation of particular tomographic aspects (size, location and number of ischaemic areas) related to some clinical and angiographic findings.

Furthermore, the aim of this paper is to evaluate if CTScan can be useful in the prognosis of such patients, candidates for carotid endarterectomy (evaluation of risk of cerebral ischaemia due to carotid clamping) and if CTScan may be useful in the evaluation of the late prognosis. For this reason we correlated the results of CTScan (negative or positive) with preoperative clinical and angiographic findings, intraoperative (anatomical and stump pressure measurements), and early and late results of surgical treatment.

Case Material

Six hundred patients affected by cerebrovascular insufficiency due to obstructive lesions of carotid axis were submitted to carotid endarterectomy during the period 1965–1984.

We considered a selected group of 188 patients who underwent CTScan examination and other preoperative non-invasive tests and angiography.

Of 188 patients, 156 were men and 42 were females. The mean age was 58 years ranging between 42 and 75 years. The clinical findings of 188 patients were as follows: 12 patients were asymptomatic (6%), 133 patients suffered from ischaemic attacks (71%), 79 (43%) made a complete recovery (TIA) and 54 (28%) made incomplete recovery (transient stroke). 43 patients showed a severe neurological deficit (23%) (established stroke).

DIAGNOSTIC TECHNIQUES AND ASSESSMENT
PROCEDURES IN VASCULAR SURGERY

© 1985 Grune & Stratton
ISBN 0-8089-1721-8 All rights reserved

Of the 133 patients with TIA or transient stroke, 112 patients (84%) showed focal symptoms as haemiparesis, amaurosis, etc. (hemispheric TIAs), while 21 patients (16%) showed vertebrobasilar symptoms such as vertigo, ataxia, dizziness, etc. (Table 14-1).

Further other non-invasive tests (Doppler examination) were performed pre-operatively; CTScan examination was performed 3–4 weeks after the last episode of cerebral ischaemia. No patient received CTScan in the acute phase. We separated these patients into two groups: The first—one of 84 patients, with a negative CTScan (absence of cerebral infarction) and the second—one of 104 patients with a positive CTScan (presence of cerebral infarction).

In the group of positive CTScan we considered various aspects of the lesions such as size, location and number of the ischaemic areas. The location of the lesions are related to the artery of supply: (1) middle cerebral artery—superficial branches (SM 39 patients); (2) middle cerebral artery—deep branches (DM 13 patients); (3) posterior cerebral artery (P 6 patients); (4) a watershed territory (W 6 patients); or (5) with an aspect of lacunar infarction (L 10 patients).

Concerning the number, the lesions may be single or multiple, mono- or bi-hemispheric (MM 14 patients; MB 16 patients). All patients were submitted to an-giographic examination of the carotid and vertebral arteries by means of direct puncture, or Seldinger technique of the carotid arteries, or digital intravenous angi-ography. The angiographic findings of 82 patients (44%) showed an unilateral lesion, 81 patients showed bilateral lesions (43%), and 20 patients an internal carotid artery stenosis and controlateral occlusion (13%).

All patients were submitted to carotid endarterectomy with general anesthesia by means of neuroleptoanalgesia intravenously and enfluorane inhalation inducing a mild systemic hypertension.

For the evaluation of the risk of cerebral ischaemia due to carotid clamping we used the intraoperative measurement of the stump pressure as an indirect evaluation of collateral cerebral supply. 25–50 mmHg was considered the critical level below which cerebral ischaemia could occur.[6] Intraoperative EEG monitoring was used in the last 50 cases.

In cases of higher risk (low value of stump pressure) an internal shunt was used in 11 cases to assure sufficient cerebral perfusion during carotid clamping.

The anatomical macroscopic aspects of the endarterectomized plaque is evalu-ated on the basis of the surface (smooth or ulcerated) and on the severity of the stenosis (reduction more or less 70% of cross sectional area). The last information was obtained by coupling macroscopic intraoperative and preoperative angio-graphic findings. The early results were calculated on the basis of the analysis of the onset or not of neurological symptoms and operative mortality. The late results were obtained by the analysis of the follow-up by the means of out-patients clinical and non-invasive evaluation.

Results

Correlation Between CTScan and Clinical Findings

Table 14-1 shows our observations after correlating the CTScan results with preoperative clinical findings. Positive CTScans are more frequent in patients with severe neurological deficit (established stroke) (87%), while negative CTScans are

Table 14-1
Correlation Between CTScan and Clinical Findings

			Negative CTScan		Positive CTScan	
			84 patients (42%)		104 patients (58%)	
Asymptomatic	12	(6%)	11	(92%)*	1	(8%)
TIA	79	(43%)	45	(56%)	34	(44%)
Transient stroke	54	(28%)	22	(40%)	32	(60%)
Established stroke	43	(23%)	6	(13%)	37	(87%)*
TIAs and transient strokes	133					
Hemispheric	112	(84%)	52	(43%)	60	(57%)
Vert. basilar	21	(16%)	15	(75%)†	6	(25%)

* $P < 0.001$ † $P < 0.05$

more frequent in asymptomatic patients (92%) or with vertebrobasilar ischaemic attacks (75%).

Considering only the patients with positive CTScan and relating the site and severity of CT infarction to the groups of patients we observe the data shown in Table 14-2.

Table 14-2
Correlation Between CTScan Findings and Severity of Stroke

		TIAs		Transient stroke		Established stroke	
Superficial Small Middle Cerebral Infarction	12	7	(58%)*	—		5	(42%)
Superficial Large Middle Cerebral Infarction	27	8	(30%)	12	(42%)	7	(28%)*
Deep Middle Cerebral Infarction	13	2	(15%)	6	(46%)	5	(39%)
Watershed	6	3	(50%)	1	(16%)	2	(34%)
Lacunar	10	4	(40%)	2	(20%)	4	(40%)
Posterior	6	3	(50%)	1	(16%)	2	(34%)
Multiple monohemispheric	14	3	(22%)	4	(28%)	7	(50%)
Multiple bihemispheric	16	4	(25%)	7	(43%)	5	(32%)

* $P < 0.05$

When the CT infarction area is small, the incidence of severe neurological deficit is low (42%). The increasing of the size of the ischaemic areas (SM2) is related to more severe neurological deficit (transient stroke, established stroke) (70%). In the deep middle cerebral artery territory all patients presented small ischaemic areas, and the rate of TIAs is 15%, while severe neurological deficit are prevalent (85%). Transient and completed stroke are frequent also in multiple mono- or bi-hemispheric areas. In the territory of watershed, lacunar and posterior cerebral artery no differences are noted in the clinical findings.

Correlations Between CTScan and Angiographic Findings

The correlation between CTScan examination and angiographic findings shows in unilateral lesion that CTScan may be positive or negative (Table 14-3). In bilateral stenosis there is a small prevalence of positive CTScan (56%), whereas in the group of stenoses associated with contralateral occlusion there is a prevalence of positive CTScan (72%).

Table 14-3
Correlations Between CTScan and Angiographic Findings

		Negative CTScan	Positive CTScan
Unilat. lesion	82 (44%)	39 (47%)	42 (52%)
Bilat. lesion	81 (43%)	36 (43%)	45 (56%)
Stenosis with contralateral occlusion	25 (13%)	9 (28%)	17 (72%)

Correlation Between CTScan and Intraoperative Macroscopic Aspects of the Lesions (Surface and Severity of the Stenosis)

Correlation between CTScan evaluation and the intraoperative macroscopic findings shows that, concerning the surface of the plaque (smooth or ulcerated) and the severity of the lesion (more or less 70% cross-sectional area reduction), there are not significant differences between the group of positive or negative CTScan (Table 14-4).

Table 14-4
Correlation Between CTScan and Intraoperative
Macroscopic Aspects of the Lesions

		Negative CTScan	Positive CTScan
Smooth	55	14 (26%)	41 (74%)*
Ulcerated	65	30 (47%)	35 (53%)
<70% stenosis	64	24 (38%)	40 (62%)
>70% stenosis	104	47 (46%)	57 (54%)

but it is relevant that in 55 smooth plaques there is a prevalence of positive CTScan (74%).

* $P < 0.05$

Correlation Between CTScan and Intraoperative Stump Pressure Measurements

A correlation between CTScan examination and intraoperative evaluation of cerebral ischaemia due to carotid clamping (stump pressure measurement) shows no significant differences in the incidence of positive and negative CTScan in patients with a sufficient cerebral perfusion and in patients showing a stump pressure value ranging between 25–50 mmHg at the time of carotid surgery (Table 14-5).

Table 14-5
Correlation Between CTScan and Intraoperative Stump
Pressure Measurements

			Negative CTScan	Positive CTScan
> 50 mmHg	118	(55%)	50 (43%)	68 (57%)
25–50 mmHg	49	(40%)	23 (47%)	26 (53%)
< 25 mmHg	10	(5%)	1 (10%)	9 (90%)*
Intraluminal shunt	11		2	9

* P < 0.05

The relevant data is that in patients with very low stump pressure value (25 mm Hg) there is an high incidence of positive CTScan (90%). In 9 patients with positive CTScan and low stump pressure values an intraluminal shunt was used for preventing the cerebral ischaemia; but only two patients had a shunt in the group of negative CTScan.

In the group of patients with positive CTScan the correlation between stump pressure values and the territories of ischaemic areas shows no significant differences.

Correlation Between Early Results of Carotid Endarterectomy and CTScan Examination

The correlation between CTScan examination and the early results of carotid endarterectomy shows no difference of incidence of neurological post operative complications in the groups of negative and positive CTScan (Table 14-6).

Table 14-6
Correlation Between Early Results of Carotid
Endarterectomy and CTScan Examination

	Negative CTScan	Positive CTScan
	84 patients	104 patients
Transient postop. neurol. deficit	5 (5.8%)	3 (2.7%)
Stroke	2 (2.2%)	4 (3.8%)
Total	7 (8%)	7 (6.5%)
Mortality	—	3 (2.7%) (47%)

In the group of negative CTScan postoperative neurological deficit, in the majority of the cases, are less severe with no operative mortality; on the contrary positive CTScan shows more severe postoperative neurological deficit with an operative mortality rate of 2.7% (47% of all postoperative complications).

In the group of positive CTScan the correlation between postoperative complications and the territories of the ischaemic areas show that of four postoperative strokes two occurred in large superficial ischemic areas and two on multiple monohemispheric areas.

Correlation Between Late Results of Carotid Endarterectomy
and CTScan Examination

The late results are obtained in 122 patients submitted to carotid endarterectomy and followed for a period of 4 years (Table 14-7). The correlation between the late results and CTScan shows that the majority of patients are alive and symptom free with no difference between negative and positive CTScan. The deaths are related to myocardial infarction in 4 cases, in 1 case to cancer, and in 1 case to gastrointestinal bleeding. Only 1 patient dead of stroke.

Table 14-7
Correlation Between Late Results of Carotid
Endarterectomy and CTScan Examination

	Negative CTScan	Positive CTScan
	59 patients	63 patients
Deaths	4	3
Alive	55	60
Symptom-free	53 (96%)	57 (95%)
Appropriate TIAs	2	1
Controlateral TIAs	—	2

Discussion

CTScan examination was introduced in 1973 in patients with neurological symptoms to ascertain the nature of clinical findings (ischemic neoplastic or haemorrhagic).[1,2] In patients affected by cerebrovascular insufficiency due to obstructive lesions of the carotid axis documented angiographically, CTScan examination may show an area of cerebral infarction; an episode of cerebral ischemia does not necessarily produce a cerebral infarction documented with CTScan. The usefulness of CTScan was clear especially in patients with acute stroke in whom CTScan was a reliable assessment of the nature of the anatomical damage of the brain, and at the same time of prognostic value. In cases of positive CTScan the integrity of blood brain barrier must be evaluated for the indication to emergency revascularization.[3,4,5] For ascertaining if CTScan may be useful in the prognosis of the risk of cerebral ischemia in patients who must be submitted to carotid endarterectomy, we correlated the CTScan results with preoperative (clinical and angiographic) and intraoperative (anatomical and haemodynamic data) and finally with early and late results of carotid endarterectomy.

Many neuroradiological studies show that in patients with reversible ischemic attacks CTScan examination may be negative or positive. An incidence of 15%–30% of positive CTScan in patients with ischaemic episodes has been reported, but our experience disagrees with these data.[8–14]

The difference between these data may be explained by the fact that our group of patients is a selected one with the presence of angiographically documented lesions of carotid vessels. Furthermore these differences may be explained by different clinical criteria of classification of RIAs.

On the contrary in our experience some patients presenting severe neurological deficit may show a negative CTScan. This agrees with the data of Weisberg and

Miller who explained these cases with the presence of small lacunar infarctions undetected by CTScan.[15,16] Sometimes a CTScan may be negative if performed during the first week after the onset of the neurological deficit; during 14–21 days, CTScan may be negative also for the "fogging" effect.

In unilateral and bilateral lesions there are no differences in the group of negative or positive CTScan. In the group of stenosis and controlateral occlusion there is a high incidence of positive CTScan (72%). In cases of positive CTScan the correlation between the involved territories and the angiographic findings shows that in cases of severe angiographic findings (bilateral or stenosis and contralateral occlusion) only some territories are involved as small superficial middle cerebral artery (75%), watershed (67%), posterior (67%) of monohaemispheric multiple areas (72%).

We performed during carotid endarterectomy the evaluation of the risk of cerebral ischaemia due to carotid clamping by means of intraoperative stump pressure measurement; this technique is easy to perform and very reliable for testing the cerebral perfusion during carotid clamping.[6] Many authors previously tried to select the patients who must be submitted to carotid endarterectomy using an internal shunt by means of preoperative techniques as Doppler or EEG examination associated with digital carotid compression; the result of such studies show that this technique does not seem to be accurate and sensitive;[16,17] on the other hand Hunter suggested that some preoperative clinical findings as a previous stroke could be a useful criteria beside the stump pressure measurement, for internal shunting.[18] The correlation between the CTScan examination and these haemodynamic data shows that the incidence of patients who did and who did not tolerate the carotid clamping is the same in both groups of CTScan (negative and positive). In the negative CTScan 68% of patients show a stump pressure value above 50 mmHg, 30% between 25–50 mmHg and 2% below 25 mmHg; in the patients with positive CTScan 66% show a stump pressure value above 50 mmHg, 26% between 25–50 mmHg, and 8% below 25 mmHg.

On the other hand the majority of patients (90%) with very low stump pressure value, had a positive CTScan. These data suggest that a positive CTScan does not represent by itself a risk factor of postoperative complications due to carotid clamping but only when this finding is associated with a very low stump pressure value ($P < 0.05$). These data agree with a more extensive use of the internal shunt as technique of cerebral protection not only when a very low stump pressure value is present, but also when a finding of positive CTScan is associated.[11,19]

The increased risk of intraoperative cerebral ischaemia in patients with positive CTScan is suggested by the finding that the incidence of postoperative complications in negative and positive CTScan groups of patients is the same but in the group of negative CTScan these complications are more frequently transient and not fatal (2.8%).[11,19]

In the experience of many, the analysis of the postoperative complications shows that the causes may be generally due to: embolism, carotid clamping, and revascularization of ischaemic areas.[20–23]

The analysis of our complications shows that only 50% of postoperative neurological deficit may be related to insufficient cerebral perfusion during carotid clamping while as documented by some, the revascularization of severe ischaemic areas may be invoked.[23] The late results show that there are not significant differences of the two groups of patients (negative and positive CTScan); the majority of cases are free of new symptoms during the follow-up.

In conclusion the correlation between CTScan examination and preoperative (clinical and haemodynamic) data and finally early and late results of carotid endarterectomy shows that: firstly, patients with severe neurological deficit (established stroke), severe angiographic findings (stenosis and contralateral occlusion), very low values of stump pressure (25 mmHg) present a significant prevalence of positivity on CTScan.

The correlation with involved territories shows that this positivity is related with some particular areas of ischaemia. Furthermore, CTScan examination seems to be useful in the evaluation of intraoperative risk of cerebral ischaemia due to carotid clamping; in fact even if generally in positive CTScan there is not a risk of cerebral ischaemia, in patients with insufficient cerebral perfusion during carotid clamping (low values of stump pressure) and positive CTScan an increased risk of postoperative neurological complications is likely, as demonstrated by the higher incidence of severe and fatal complications if compared to the group of negative CTScan.

Finally the correlation between CTScan and late results shows that a positive CTScan does not present risk factor for the late prognosis of patients submitted to carotid endarterectomy and followed-up. In fact the incidence of patients who during the follow-up are still alive and free of symptoms is the same in both the groups of negative and positive CTScan.

REFERENCES

1. Hounfield GN: Computerized transverse axial scanning (tomography) I. Description of the system. Br J Radiol 46:1016, 1973
2. Ambrose J: Computerized transverse axial scanning (tomography) II. Clinical application. Br J Radiol 46:1023, 1973
3. Wylie EJ, Hein MF, Adams JE: Intracranial hemorrhage following surgical revascularization for treatment of acute strokes. J Neurosurg 21:212, 1964
4. Goldstone J, Moore WS: Emergency carotid artery surgery in neurologically unstable patients. Arch Surg 111:1284, 1976
5. Pistolese GR, Ventura M, Speziale F, et al: Emergency carotid surgery. International Surgery 3, 1984
6. Moore WS, Hall AD: Carotid artery back pressure. A test of cerebral tolerance to temporary carotid occlusion. Arch Surgery 99:702, 1969
7. Perrone P, Candelise L, Scotti G, et al: CT evaluation in patients with transient ischaemic attack. Eur Neurol 18:217, 1979
8. Mueller HR: The place of computerized tomography and carotid Doppler sonography in CV episodes. Adv Neurol 25:186, 1979
9. Ladurner G, Sager WD, Iliff LD, et al: A correlation of clinical findings and CT in ischaemic cerebrovascular disease. Eur Neurol 18:281, 1979
10. Bozzao L, Carolei A, Pappatà S, et al: Computerized tomography of the brain and associated risk factors in 240 patients with RIAs. Proceedings of 12th Int Salzburg Conf, 1982
11. Graber JN, Vollman RW, Johnson WC: Stroke after carotid endarterectomy: risk as predicted by preoperative computerized tomography. Am J Surg 147:492, 1984

12. Nicolaides AN, Zukowski A: The significance of silent cerebral infarcts in patients with carotid lesions. Proceeding of the Symposium on Basis for a Classification of Cerebral Arterial Diseases. Marseille 1984

13. Dorndorf W, Horning C: Partial non progressing stroke; clinical criteria and CT-findings. Proceedings of the Symposium on Basis for a Classification of Cerebral Arterial Diseases. Marseille 1984

14. Weisberg LA: Lacunar infarcts; clinical and computed tomographic correlations. Arch Neurol 39:37, 1982

15. Miller VT: Lacunar stroke—A reassessment. Arch Neurol 40:129, 1983

16. Faraglia V, Pistolese GR, Ventura M, et al: Relationship between EEG changes during carotid compression and CBF values carotid surgery. Cerebrovascular Disease Excerpta Medica 276, 1978

17. Ventura M, Laglia P, Spartera C, et al: Valutazione preoperatoria del rischio cerebrale da clampaggio in chirurgia carotidea. Ruolo di una metodica non invasiva. Arch Chir Torac Cardiovasc 4:250, 1982

18. Hunter GC, Sieffert G, Malone JM, et al: The accuracy of carotid back pressure as an index for shunt requirements. Stroke 13:319, 1982

19. Callow AD: Evaluation of operative risk by CTScan and echo B. Proceedings of the Symposium on Basis for a Classification of Cerebral Arterial Diseases. Marseille 1984

20. Thompson JE: Complications of carotid endarterectomy and their prevention. World J Surg 3:155, 1979

21. Towne JB, Bernhard VM: The relationship of postoperative hypertension to complications following carotid endarterectomy. Surgery 88:575, 1980

22. Fiorani P, Pistolese GR, Faraglia V, et al: Valutazione intraoperatoria e risultati a distanza della chirurgia delle carotidi. Proceedings Soc It Chir 107:112, 1982

23. Sundt TM, Sharbrough FW, Piepgras DG: The significance of cerebral blood flow measurements during carotid endarterectomy, in Bergan J, Yao J (eds): Cerebrovascular Insufficiency. Orlando, Florida, Grune & Stratton, 1983, p 287

L. Marosi, H. Ehringer
F. Piza, and O. Wagner

15

Early Postoperative Morphology of the Carotid Artery Following Endarterectomy: Systemic Prospective Studies with a High-Resolution Ultrasound Duplex Real Time Imaging System

The examination of superficial arteries—also of the cerebral arteries—with a high-resolution Ultrasound Duplex real time system (Duplex scanner) permits in a non-invasive way the exact evaluation of the artery wall and spectrum.[1] Plaques can, therefore, be classified as soft or hard and according to position, and morphology (ulcerated or not).[2] With the help of an optic localising Doppler ultrasound ray the influence of the stenosis on the local circulation can be established.[2-14] The intra operative analyses of the flow—measured with the pulsed Doppler Ultrasound—permits the evaluation of the quality of the haemodynamic result and the immediate correction operative deficiency after surgery to the carotid artery.[13,15,16]

Modern high-resolution scanners combined with Doppler make it also possible to observe changes morphologically as well as functionally of the artery wall after the surgical removal of arterial stenosis with thrombendarterectomy (TEA).[17,18]

We used the Duplex scanner to examine:

1. The kind and frequency of the typical changes of the operated carotid artery in the early phase after TEA (up to 2 months after operation).
2. The behaviour of the newly restored artery inner wall and its interaction with the circulating blood.
3. The change of the degree of stenosis as a result of TEA.
4. Continuous post-operative observations concerning the spectral vessel broadening in the area of the operation during the 2 months after the operation.

DIAGNOSTIC TECHNIQUES AND ASSESSMENT
PROCEDURES IN VASCULAR SURGERY

© 1985 Grune & Stratton
ISBN 0-8089-1721-8 All rights reserved

PATIENTS AND METHOD

Fifty operated patients (36 men, 14 women, average age 68, 53–83 years) with stenosis in the area of the internal carotid artery were examined. Carotid endarterectomy was done at the I. Chirurgische Universitäts-Klinik in Vienna (Head: Prof. Dr. A. Fritsch).

Fifty-five (29 right, 26 left) had TEA. Five patients had bilateral operations. Preoperatively, 32 patients were in Grade I of cerebral arterial occlusion (these asymptomatic patients had the TEA before a planned bigger operation usually a vessel reconstruction in the area of the lower extremities). Fourteen patients were Grade II, and 4 in Grade III.

After exact clinical, angiological, and neurological examination the diagnosis was verified on all patients preoperatively by the following non-invasive methods: (1) Carotids–ophthalmic–Doppler–ultrasound examination (continuous wave 10 MHz—probe P95A, bidirectional Doppler Ultrasound Model D9 as well as 2-pen recorders R12A of Medasonics, Mountain View, CA, USA;[2,19] (2) Doppler Ultrasound angiography of the carotid artery on the neck (P2 Ultrasound–arteriograph (pulsed Doppler, 5 MHz) of the firm D. E. Hokanson, Issaquah, WA, USA, combined with the Angioscan frequency analyser of the firm Unigon, Mt. Vernon, NY, USA;[11,20] and (3) Examination of the carotid bifurcation with the Duplex scanner of Biosound, Indianapolis, USA.[21] This examination is the basis of these presented morphological changes of the artery wall of the carotid artery after TEA. The system that was used had a 8 MHz probe, sometimes in addition a 4 MHz probe, and produces on a video monitor a grey scale with 600 lines per second; the image on the video monitor is magnified 6 times; the longitudinal capacity of resolution is 0.3 mm.

Each bifurcation was examined longitudinally on an anterior-posterior (AP), lateral (L), and postlateral (P) plane as well as transversely (T) on the whole section that can be seen from the neck and loaded with a video unit (IVC U-matic, 3/4 inch). The videos were stored for at least 3 months for further studies and analysis. The illustrations of this chapter are polaroid copies of the video. To avoid confusion the left carotid is shown upside down.

The patients were examined with the Duplex scanner a few days before the operation and 2–3 days after operation and again after 1, 2, 4, and 8 weeks. The extent of the stenosis was sectioned in percentage of the reduction of the radius and subdivided into 6 degrees:

Grade 0   (0–5%)
Grade I   (5–24%)
Grade II   (25–49%)
Grade III (50–74%)
Grade IV   (75–99%)
Grade V   (100% = occlusion)

Out of 55 carotid reconstructions, the examination of the early postoperative phase was not possible on two patients because of a haematoma in the area of the operation. In the second postoperative week, all patients except 1 (abscess in the area of the wound) were examined.

Preoperatively, 36 patients had contrast angiography, 14 patients did without this and were operated on solely on the basis of the indicated non-invasive diagnosis. At operation, closure of the arteriotomy was with atraumatic material strength 6–0 or 7–0.[22–26] All patients had a localised rinse of the arteries in the area of the operation with heparin—saline (3000 IE/50 ml) and/or a single i.v. dosage of 5000 IE Heparin was given immediately before the clamping of the artery. None of the patients had a perioperative platelet inhibitory therapy.

The significance of the changes in degrees of stenosis by operation and afterwards was checked with the help of the Wilcoxon paired comparison and the t-test paired comparison.[27] The correlation of the degree of stenosis (see above) before operation and its changes because of operation was checked with the help of the Spearman correlation coefficient.[27]

RESULTS

The typical conditions of the artery wall during examination with the Duplex scanner before and especially after TEA of the carotid artery will be shown on some samples: Figure 15-1 shows a Duplex scan before and Figure 15-2 after carotid surgery (8 weeks). Distally, the newly created inner artery wall is not clearly defined because of the missing intimal layer. The artery wall appears in this area as remarkably thin. In some areas of the new inner wall of the vessel one can see soft, tender deposits in the width of 0.5–1.0 mm (i.e. small arrow as well as distal section of the internal carotid artery). On the real time imaging system the TEA wall of the inter-

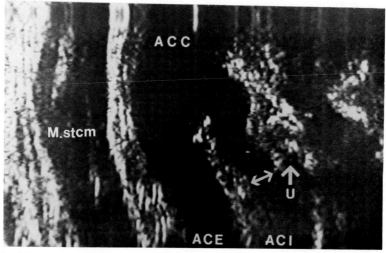

Fig. 15-1. Ultrasound real-time image (8 MHz probe) of a left carotid bifurcation laterally (Pat. K. J., male, 59 years old, left cerebral TIA): In the left hand side of the picture is skin and the sternocleidomastoid muscle (Mstam). The echo poor vessel lumen is shown in black. The carotid bifurcation is shown upside down. The internal carotid leaves as a medial vessel (exit variant). The lumen of the internal carotid artery is narrowed to a high degree of partly hard, partly soft plaques with ulceration. The remaining lumen is 2 mm (arrow). The ACC = common carotid artery. ACI = internal carotid artery. ACE = external carotid artery.

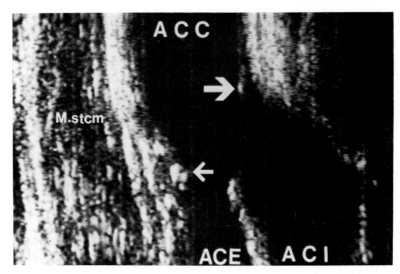

Fig. 15-2. Ultrasound real-time image (8 MHz probe) of the same carotid bifurcation of the patient in Figure 1, 8 weeks after TEA. There is an intimal step (marked with a big white arrow). In the area of TEA the "sonographic intima layer" is missing. Only in a few parts are soft 0.5–1 mm protruding deposits into lumen imaged on the artery inner wall (i.e. small white arrow ACI distal. ACI = internal carotid artery. ACE = external carotid artery.

nal carotid artery showed again strong transverse (cross) pulsation; the "intima lip" in the area of the "intima step" fluttered in the bloodstream quite clearly. Figure 15-3 shows various Duplex scans of a carotid bifurcation 2 weeks after surgery.

The findings of Figure 15-4 were observed from day 4 after operation for 2 months almost without changes; after operation in this patient, the previously transitory symptoms changed to a permanent left cerebral hemisymptomatic. The orig-

Table 15-1
Early Postoperative Changes of the Carotid Artery by Duplex
Scanning

1. On the newly constructed artery wall:
   (a) the "sonographic intima layer" is missing
   (b) structuring and thickness of the artery wall is reduced
   (c) media islands can often be seen
   (d) "soft" thrombotic deposits: 0.5–4.0 mm on the new inner artery wall

2. There is an intimal step proximally always, but not always at the distal end

3. There is a change in calibre through removal of the thickened disease

4. We have noted a "roof-like" protrusion of the artery wall through intramural haematoma and "soft" thrombotic deposits in the area of clamping of the vessel

5. Vessel sutures show as bright dots

6. Strong transverse pulsation are regained

7. The flow is normalized.

inally newly created inner vessel surface (black arrows) on which there are these "soft deposits" is evidently not as smooth as for instance in Figure 15-3.

Sutures can be seen clearly with the Duplex scanner two weeks after surgery (Fig. 15-5).

In Figure 15-6, four days after surgery, the site of the common carotid clamp can be seen.

In Figure 15-7, occlusion was demonstrated and the artery was instantly reexplored. Table 15-1 summarizes the early postoperative changes in the carotid artery.

The newly constructed vessel wall in the area of TEA is characterised through lack of the "sonographic intima layer" (I); this finding stays constant during the observation time of 2 months after operation; the newly constructed inner surface of the vessel wall is sonographically less sharply outlined against the lumen. The vessel wall itself is because of the missing inner layer less structured and thinner. It was not possible to register a change on this matter during the 2 months after operation. In athe area of breakdown of the "sonographic intima layer" there is always a so-called intimal step nearby that was invariably pictured during all of the observation time. The level of this occasionally very abrupt step of the lumen border in longitudinal section depends on the thickness of the disease removed. It can be up to 2 mm per artery wall with correspondingly bigger calibrejumps of the artery in this part (see also Figure 15-3A). A distal intimal step of the internal carotid artery or external carotid artery could only be recorded sonographically in less than 50% of the patients.

The original surface of the newly constructed artery wall gives occasionally the impression of being irregular also as far as the level is concerned in the area of thicker "softer deposits" (see Figure 15-4) media remnants. As shown in part of the data (n = 19) in Table 15-2, at no time was there a significant increase of the thickness of the soft deposits of the endarterectomized wall (p < 0.05). A certain trend towards it occurred with increase in thickness in 19 patients out of 55 patients.

In the longitudinal section, the roof-life finely grained protrusion into the lumen of the common carotid artery away from the area of TEA, is likely to be caused by clamping of the artery. It is caused partly by an intramural haematoma, partly by the mentioned "soft deposits." It was observed in 9 out of 55 carotids (50 patients) it was noticed invariably at the first postoperative control around the third day and subsequently during all of the observation time of 2 months with only a

Table 15-2
Changes of the Thickness of the "Soft Deposits" on the New Inner Artery Wall After Carotid Surgery in the Observation Period

n = 19 $\bar{x} \pm \sigma$ in mm Observation time	2–4 days	After 1 week	After 2 weeks	After 4 weeks	After 8 weeks
Common carotid artery	$\bar{x} = 0.94$ $\sigma = 0.68$	$\bar{x} = 1.22$ $\sigma = 0.73$	$\bar{x} = 1.25$ $\sigma = 0.79$	$\bar{x} = 1.42$ $\sigma = 0.81$	$\bar{x} = 1.42$ $\sigma = 0.79$
Internal carotid artery	$\bar{x} = 0.75$ $\sigma = 0.35$	$\bar{x} = 1.06$ $\sigma = 0.66$	$\bar{x} = 1.08$ $\sigma = 0.62$	$\bar{x} = 1.39$ $\sigma = 1.05$	$\bar{x} = 1.47$ $\sigma = 1.04$
External carotid artery	$\bar{x} = 0.83$ $\sigma = 0.30$	$\bar{x} = 1.06$ $\sigma = 0.57$	$\bar{x} = 1.06$ $\sigma = 0.54$	$\bar{x} = 1.28$ $\sigma = 0.60$	$\bar{x} = 1.25$ $\sigma = 0.58$

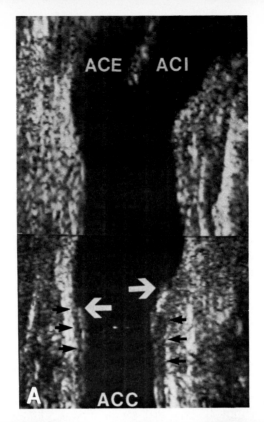

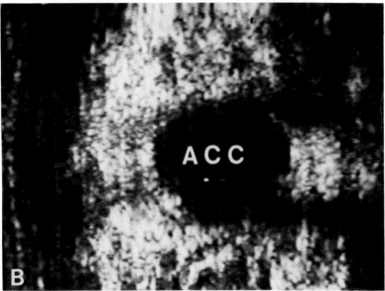

Fig. 15-3(A, B). (A) Ultrasound real-time image (8 MHz probe) of a right carotid bifurcation viewed in AP position 2 weeks after TEA (Pat. G. F., male, 64 years old; right cerebral TIA). Thickening of the "sonographic intima layer." (the border is marked with black arrows, about 1.5 mm thick.) The sonographic intima layer in the area of TEA is missing. The inner lining of the new artery vessel is relatively smooth except where the white arrows show a step. Soft deposits are only recognisable distally of the intima step in the area of the artery back wall (right white arrow). ACC = common carotid artery. ACI = internal carotid artery. ACE = external carotid artery. (B) Transverse section with ultrasound real-time examination of the patient in Figure 15-3A in the area of the right common carotid artery 2 weeks after operation. A "sonographic intima layer" is not recognisable. The surface of the new artery wall is not completely smooth. ACC = common carotid artery.

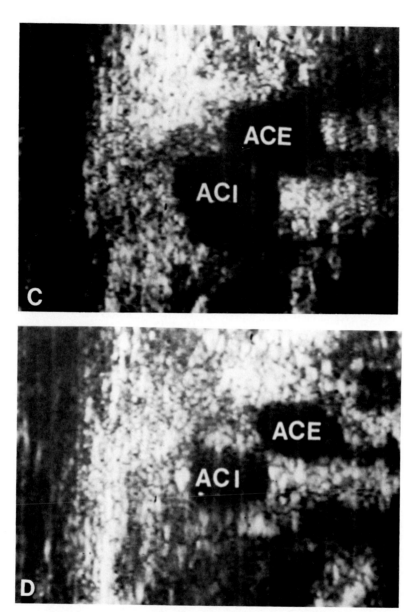

Fig. 15-3 (C, D). (C) Transverse section of the ultrasound real-time examination of the patient in Figure 15-3A in the immediate area of the carotid bifurcation 2 weeks after operation. The "sonographic intima layer" is missing. The new inner border of the artery vessel is not completely smooth. "Soft deposits" are not recognisable. The oval shape of the transverse section is because the plane is not quite vertical. The lumen of the internal and external carotid artery is clear. ACI = internal carotid artery. ACE = external carotid artery. (D) Transverse section of the ultrasound real-time examination of the patient of Figure 15-3A about 1.5 cm off the carotid bifurcation 2 weeks postoperatively. The sonographic intima layer is missing. The new inner border of the artery wall is not completely smooth. "Soft deposits" are not recognisable. Oval shape of the transverse section because done through a not quite vertical plane. The lumen of the internal (ACI) as well as external (ACE) is free flowing.

167

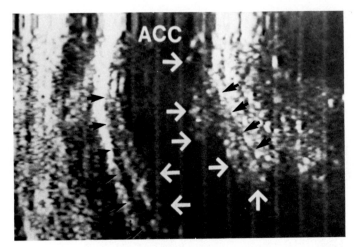

Fig. 15-4. Ultrasound real-time image (8 MHz probe) of a left common carotid artery (ACC) as far as into the area of bifurcation, (upside down) laterally, 2 weeks after TEA (Pat. K. L., female, 79 years old, postoperative left cerebral hemi symptomatic). On the operated artery inner wall (marked with black arrows) there are irregularly defined finely grained structured thrombotic soft deposits (white arrows) that clearly narrow down the lumen. They are to be found in the whole area of the artery inner wall adjoining the proximal intima step that has been affected by TEA.

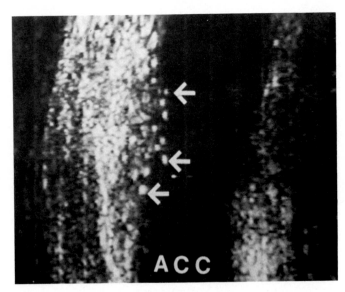

Fig. 15-5. Ultrasound real-time image (8 MHz probe) of a right common carotid artery laterally, 2 weeks after TEA (Pat. K. J., male, 62 years old). Apart from other findings of TEA here the lengthwise sutures (white arrows) are especially pronounced. ACC = common carotid artery.

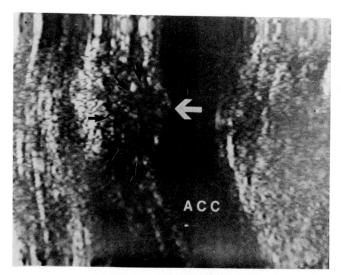

Fig. 15-6. Ultrasound real-time image (8 MHz probe) of a right common carotid artery (ACC) view AP 4 days after TEA (Pat. Sch. V., male, 64 years old). In the area of the white arrow there is a longitudinal section a "roof-like" protrusion of the anterior artery wall into the lumen; somewhat less also on the opposite side. This is the area where the clamp was placed on the artery and presumably, bleeding in the artery wall occured and there are soft deposits at the clamping site. The remaining radius of the common carotid artery in the area of the roof-like stenosis is 4.5 mm.

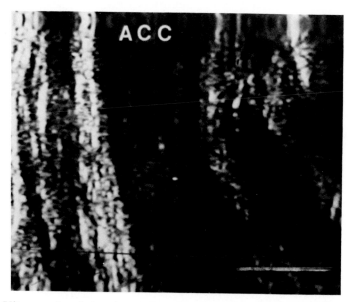

Fig. 15-7. Ultrasound real-time image (8 MHz probe) of a right common carotid artery (ACC) AP view 2 days after TEA (Pat. St. H., male, 62 years old). The "sonographic intima layer" is not visible. The lumen is filled in the upper part with finely grained substances. The Doppler flow signal and the transverse pulsation of the wall were missing in this area. This occlusion was corrected at a second operation on the same day and the patient recovered completely.

very slight tendency to recede. Since this "roof-like" deposit can protrude into the artery, it can cause in isolated cases a certain stenosis of the lumen (see Figure 15-6).

After surgery the artery wall shows also a strong cross pulsation. At the first check-up 2–4 days after the operation this was not yet very marked because of the extent of the wound haematoma, but later it became apparent and the Doppler ultrasound signals of the carotid artery showed a clear tendency to normalisation.[28]

It was noticeable that the degree of stenosis had slightly increased between the first postoperative check-up (2–4 days) and the check up 2 months by an average $+0.27 \pm 0.68$ (p < 0.0005) (Table 15-3). This was caused by a considerable increase of thickness of the soft deposits in the new inner artery wall in only some of the patients (see also Figure 15-4), which can be seen in the great scattering (B–C, Table 15-3).

Table 15-3
Degree of Stenosis of the Internal Carotid Artery Before and
After TEA

	n	Degree of Stenosis $\bar{x} \pm \sigma$	Change of Degree of Stenosis $\bar{x} \pm \sigma$	p*
A Before operation	55	3.00 ± 0.87		
			A–B	
B After operation (2–4 days)	55	1.27 ± 0.45	-1.73 ± 1.12	<0.0001
			A–C	
C After operation (8 weeks)	55	1.54 ± 0.69	-1.46 ± 1.09	<0.0001
			B–C	
			$+0.27 \pm 0.68$	<0.005

* Wilcoxon pairing comparison, t-test pair comparison.

Out of 55 carotid endarterectomies on 50 patients, a neurological deficit was noted, 7 times. Twice it reversed and 5 times a hemiplegia occurred, which disappeared practically completely in two patients after further surgery on the same day. On two more patients, the hemiplegia was improved quickly and on a fifth patient there was a slow and incomplete reduction.

None of the patients in this group died during the observation period.

DISCUSSION

The described typical morphological image of the artery wall in the area of TEA of the internal carotid artery is well explained by the operating technique. After removal of the stenosis with the thickened intima and part of the media the artery wall is thinner.[29]

The following findings from a clinical point of view are possible with the Duplex scanner:

1. Smoothness of the scooped out layer
2. Residue media islands
3. Intima lips

4. Intima steps
5. Vessel geometry
6. Intramural haematoma and dissection of the artery wall
7. Artery sutures at the arteriotomy area
8. Postoperative cross pulsation
9. Local flow behaviour

"Intima steps" namely in the area of the common carotid artery are a help for the pinpointing of the layer in which the scooping out of the intima-media cylinder by the surgeon has been done (see Figure 15-3). The bigger the intima step is the more it is likely to cause the emergence of flow turbulence with its negative consequences for the encouragement of localised thrombosis.[3] It is perhaps not by chance that postoperatively thrombotic, sonographic "soft" deposits are found in this area especially regularly (see Figure 15-3). Since with the help of the Duplex scanner practically the whole of the artery circumference in longitudinal and transverse section can be examined it is also possible to show whether the scooped out cylinder tore off circularly in the same transverse section and equally clearly, as wanted, or whether there are referring to this area differences in the artery circumference, as the example in Figure 15-2 shows (intima lip only on the medial circumference).

The clinically important artery geometry, distortions, kinking, i.e. local dilatation after operation or the postoperative removal of such changes can be evaluated precisely with the Duplex scanner as well as its influence on the flow reaction of the carotid artery.[13,15,16] Also intramural haematoma of the artery wall and dissection in the area of operation can easily be recognised by an experienced examiner with the help of a Duplex scanner (see Figure 15-6).

They are caused as a consequence of traumatisation[24,25] in the area of the clamping of the artery and in the area of the sutures and from manipulation of the intima media cylinder when removed. Intramural haematoma can be found especially where the artery had been clamped intraoperatively. This can also apparently injure the intima, partly with tearings, so that there can also be found the sonographic "soft deposits" brought about by thrombotic secretions. The haematoma with the mentioned sonographic criteria is often also present in the periarterial area. The mentioned consequences of clamping evidently play a part in the emergence of immediate relapse (haematoma, endothelium damage, thrombosis) and of so called early relapse up to two years after operations. These investigations are clearly of importance to the surgeon who must use the most atraumatic occlusion instruments that he can find.

REFERENCES

1. Marosi L, Ehringer H: Die extracranielle A. carotis im hochauflösenden Ultraschall-Echtzeitdarstellungssystem: morphologische Befunde bei Gesunden jungen Erwachsenen. Ultraschall 5 (1984) 174
2. Marosi L, Ehringer H, Samec P: Carotis-Diagnostik mittels hochauflösendem Ultraschall-Real-Time-Scan: Vergleich mit Angiographie. In: Bildgebende Ultraschallverfahren in der Angiologie: Ehringer H., Marosi L. (Hrsg.) Thieme Stuttgart 1984 (im Druck)
3. Blackshear W, Phillips D, Thiel B: Detection of carotid occlusive disease by ultrasonic imaging and pulsed Doppler spectrum analyses. Surgery 86 (1979) 698

4. Breslau PJ, Fell G, Phillips DJ, Thiele BL, Strandness DE: Evaluation of carotid bifurcation disease. Arch. Surg. 117 (1982) 58

5. Cooperberg P, Robertson W, Fry P, Sweeney V: High resolution real-time ultrasound of the carotid bifurcation. Clin. Ultrasound 7 (1979) 13–17

6. Crew JR, Dean MJ: Intimal visualization: the imaging barometer. Presented at the San Diego Symposium on noninvasive diagnostic techniques in vascular disease, October 1982

7. Dunnick N, Schuette W, Shawker T: Ultrasonic demonstration of thrombus in the common carotid artery. Am. J. Radiol. 133 (1979) 544–545

8. Edward JH, Kricheff II, Riles R, Imparato A: Angiographically undetected ulceration of the carotid bifurcation as a cause of embolic stroke. Radiology 132 (1979) 2

9. Hirschl M, Ehringer H, Marosi L: Flußmessung der A. carotis communis mit einem vielkanaligen gepulsten Doppler-Ultraschallgerät: Normalwerte, Patienten mit Stenosen der extracraniellen Arteria carotis interna, Einfluß operativer Therapie. In: Therapie der peripheren arteriellen Verschlußkrankheit. Müller-Wiefel H., Barras J. P., Ehringer H., Krüger M. (Hrsg.) Witzstrock, Baden-Baden, Köln, New York, 1979, 436–440

10. Hokanson DE, Mozersky DJ, Sumner DS, McLeod FD, Strandness DE Jr: Ultrasonic arteriography: a noninvasive method for arterial visualization. Radiology 102 (1972) 435

11. Konecny U, Mühlgassner A, Marosi L, Ehringer H: Doppler-Ultraschall-Angiographie (Statischer Angioscan) der A. carotis am Hals mit instantaner Audiofrequenzanalyse: Ergebnisse bei Gesunden. In: Bildgebende Ultraschallverfahren in der Angiologie. Ehringer H., Marosi L. (Hrsg.) Thieme Stuttgart 1984 (im Druck)

12. Mozersky DJ, Hokanson DE, Baker DW, Sumner DS, Strandness DE Jr: Ultrasonic angiography. Arch. Surg. 103 (1971) 663

13. Roederer GO, Langlois Y, Chan ATW, Breslau P, Phillips DJ, Beach KW, Chikos PM, Strandness DE Jr: Postendarterectomy carotid ultrasonic duplex scanning concordance with contrast angiography. Ultrasound in Med. & Biol. 9 (1983) 73

14. Ringelstein EB, Kolmann HL, Zeumer H: Carotis B-Scan: Konkurrenz oder Ergänzung der Ultraschall-Dopplersonographie. Dtsch. med. Wschr. 107 (1982) 928–933

15. Zierler ER, Bandyk DF, Thiele BL, Strandness ED: Carotid artery stenosis following endarterectomy. Arch. Surg. 117 (1982) 1408

16. Zierler RE, Bandyk DF, Berni GA, Thiele BL: Intraoperative pulsed doppler assessment of carotid endarterectomy. Ultrasound in Med. & Biol. 9 (1983) 65

17. Marosi L, Ehringer H, Piza F, Wagner O, Kretschmer G: Frühe Postoperative Veränderungen nach Carotis-Desobliteration: Untersuchung mit einem hochauflösenden Ultraschall-Real-Time-Duplex-Scanner. Angio Archiv. 5 (1984) 73

18. Sandmann W, Kremer K, Hennerici M, Freund HJ: Hämodynamische Qualitätssicherung in der rekonstruktiven Arterienchirurgie. Angio Archiv 5 (1983) 79

19. Marosi L, Ehringer H, Ingerle H, Hirschl M, Minar E, Ahmadi R, Piza F, Wagner O, Klausberger W: Ophthalmica-Doppler-Ultraschallbefunde vor und nach operativer Rekonstruktion von Stenosen der Extracraniellen A. carotis interna. Vasa Supplement 8 (1981) 62

20. Ehringer H, Mühlgassner A, Marosi L, Samec P, Konecny U, Minar E: Doppler-Ultraschall-Angiographie (Statischer Angiosan) der A. carotis am Hals mit instantaner Audiofrequenzanalyse: Vergleich mit der Angiographie bei Patienten mit Stenosen, Verschlüssen und Schlingenbildung. In: Bildgebende Ultraschallverfahren in der Angiologie. Ehringer H., Marosi L. (Hrsg.) Thieme Stuttgart, 1984 (im Druck)

21. Biosound—Produktinformation

22. Carrea R, Molins M, Murphy G: Surgical treatment of spontaneous thrombosis of the internal carotid artery in the neck. Carotid-carotideal anastomosis. Report of a case. Acta Neuro. Latinamer. 1 (1955) 71

23. Don Santos JC: Sur la desobstruction des thromboses arterielles anciennes. Mém. Aca. Chir. 73 (1947) 409

24. Piza F: Zur Problematik der Endarteriektomie. Klin. Medizin 11 (1964) 497–503
25. Piza F: Erfahrungen mit der Endarteriektomie. Langenbecks Arch. f. klin. Chir. 313 (1965) 823
26. Thompson JE, Talkington CM: Carotid endarterectomy. Ann. Surg. 184 (1976) 1
27. Documenta Geigy. Wissenschaftliche Tabellen. 7. Auflage, 1968
28. Minar E, Ehringer H, Marosi L, Piza F, Wagner O, Kretschmer G, Polterauer P: Doppler-Ultraschall-Angiographie der A. carotis mit instantaner Audiofrequenzanalyse: Postoperative Ergebnisse. In: Bildgebende Ultraschallverfahren in der Angiologie: Ehringer H., Marosi L. (Hrsg.) Thieme Stuttgart 1984 (im Druck)
29. Imparato AM, Bracco A, Kim GE, Zeff R: Intimal and neointimal fibrous proliferation causing failure of arterial reconstructions. Surgery 72 (1972) 1007

PART III

Aortic Aneurysms and Renal Ischaemia

Lars Norgren

16

Population Screening for Abdominal Aortic Aneurysms

The ruptured aortic aneurysm is a disaster with a mortality rate of 50% or more in most materials. This was true in the material presented by De Bakey et al[1] and is still valid, e.g., in a Norwegian multicenter study published in 1983,[2] presenting 173 patients with a ruptured aneurysm. Their mortality rate was 59%.

From Houston, Lawrie et al[3] reported improved results, and a mortality of only 14.8% in ruptured aneurysms. The difference between their material and at least most European investigations seems to be the ratio between ruptured and nonruptured aneurysms. They only had an incidence of 4.4% ruptured aneurysms. In the Norwegian material the corresponding figure was 40%, and in a recently presented Italian paper the frequency was 31%.[4]

In our own service there has been a slow decline in the proportion of ruptured aneurysms and a steady increase in elective cases (ratio 1 : 3). Still, the mortality rate in ruptured aneurysms is about 40% after having been more than 60% during the period of 1975–1979.[5]

There is not only this high mortality rate to take into consideration, but also the fact that a majority of these patients die in a rather violent and sometimes not very short postoperative course with fulminant organ failure.[6] On the contrary, in elective surgery the mortality rate is in different materials between 1 and 4%. It therefore seems to be extremely important to identify the abdominal aortic aneurysm before the rupture. Consequently two questions are raised: (1) Are there risk-factors that could be screened for in the population? and (2) Are there simple examinations, useful as screening tools?

POSSIBLE RISK FACTORS

If certain risk factors could be determined, this should be a practicable way to find the aneurysm in an early stage. The incidence of aortic aneurysms increases with age, a well-known factor, which does not give much aid in identifying risk patients.

DIAGNOSTIC TECHNIQUES AND ASSESSMENT
PROCEDURES IN VASCULAR SURGERY

© 1985 Grune & Stratton
ISBN 0-8089-1721-8 All rights reserved

There is a common coexistence of systemic hypertension, aneurysms, and other cardiovascular diseases.[7,8] Hypertension and age have been evaluated by our group as possible risk factors in a population based study (see below).

Is arteriosclerosis per se a risk factor? Factors determining arterial occlusive disease or aneurysmatic dilatation are still essentially unknown. Using ultrasonography in arteriosclerotic patients, Cabellon et al[9] found 9.6% abdominal aortic aneurysms. This incidence seems to be higher than expected in the total population.

Heredity has been suggested[95] a possible factor in the development of aortic aneurysms. Among other family case histories Clifton[10] described three brothers with ruptured aneurysms. In a systematic analysis of all aneurysms treated in Umeå, Sweden, Norrgård et al[11] found that abdominal aortic aneurysms occurred in the families of 18% of the patients. Tilson and Seashore[12,13] discussed possible genetic factors in the pathogenesis of aortic aneurysms. They suggested one possible X-linked and one possible autosomal dominant form of the disease.

There may be a possibility to screen for aortic aneurysm due to inheritance but it seems premature to be discussed yet, and reasonably only a limited proportion of aneurysms will be found that way. Factors such as lipoproteins, bloodgroups, and haptoglobins have been evaluated,[14–18] partly with contradictory results. Cannon et al[19] reported an increase in serum proteolytic activity in smokers with abdominal aortic aneurysms, which was not found in patients with arteriosclerotic occlusive disease. Decreased hepatic copper levels in patients dying with aortic aneurysms were described by Tilson et al.[20] Other biochemical abnormalities and atherosclerotic aneurysms were discussed by De Palma.[21] The association between malignancy and aortic aneurysm was reported by Tilson et al.[22] suggesting explanations such as immunological mechanisms. All the factors described may be more or less important. They are, however hitherto difficult or impossible to use as predictors for aortic aneurysm.

To complete, the well-known relationship between aortic aneurysm and Marfan's syndrome as well as Ehler-Danlos' syndrome must be mentioned. There is also a higher incidence of aortic aneurysm in patients with polycystic kidneys.[23] Even in homocystinuria aortic aneurysm has been described.[24] Finally, a considerable group of patients with aortic aneurysm even have signs of retroperitoneal fibrosis.[25] Most of them should however be classified as inflammatory aneurysms or periaortic fibrosis.[26]

POSSIBLE EXAMINATIONS

Since most aortic aneurysms are asymptomatic, these patients are not aware of their condition! Physical examination, including careful palpation of the abdomen may give a suspicion of an aortic aneurysm. The examination is, however, not always easy since a considerable number of patients are obese. On the other hand, a palpable aorta may be a more or less regular finding in thin persons. Cabellon et al[9] reported 2.6% aneurysms found by physical examinations in patients with arteriosclerosis, while ultasonography revealed 9.6%.

We have previously described ultrasonographic findings in patients referred due to suspected aortic aneurysms.[27] Among 92 patients with a pulsating abdominal mass, referred from different outpatient services, 52% showed to have an abdominal aortic aneurysm, 5% had another lesion ventral to the aorta, and 43% had no pathological explanation.

Besides ultrasonography, the most commonest examination procedures are aortography and computer tomography (CT). It has been shown that ultrasonography is almost as relevant as CT in the evaluation of aortic aneurysm.[28] For screening purpose ultrasonography seems to be the easiest and cheapest radiological method.

POPULATION STUDIES

In a Swedish autopsy study from 1964 Carlsson and Sternby[29] found that 1.3% of the cases had abdominal aortic aneurysms. The common figure reported from autopsies is 1–6%.[30,31] In a review of 12 autopsy studies including 145,000 cases, Gore and Hirst[32] reported an incidence of abdominal aortic aneurysm of 1.2%. In men in their sixth decade the incidence was 6%, increasing by age to 14% in the ninth decade. Male/female ratio was 5/1 and aneurysms usually were not found until the age of 40.

Few studies have been reported on the incidence of abdominal aortic aneurysm in the living population. Recently, however, Melton et al[33] reported on a changing incidence in the Rochester population between 1951 and 1980. The overall incidence in 1971–1980 was 36.5 per 100,000 people per year. This was a seven-fold increase since the 1950s.

In our service we operate on about 30 abdominal aortic aneurysms each year, which appears to give a somewhat lower incidence than in the Rochester study. We have had an impression that most of our patients had a systemic hypertension, which was the reason for the study described below.

The "Dalby-Study"

The purpose of the study was to estimate the prevalence of abdominal aortic aneurysms in patients aged 50–70 years suffering from systemic hypertension.[34]

All hypertensives born in the period 1912–1931 visiting the Dalby Health Centre in 1980 were invited to a medical examination including ultrasonography of the abdominal aorta. Of the 264 patients, 253 attended the clinical examination and 245 the ultrasonographic one. The patients were identified by means of the statistical computer scheme for patient-care in the Dalby primary care district. They comprised 9% of all inhabitants in this age group. The scheme can be described as an individually based computer system for the processing of statistical information about inhabitants and their contacts with health and medical care services.[35] The patients comprised 70–85% of all known hypertensives aged 50–69 years and did not differ when compared with those treated outside the Health Centre.[36,37]

First of all a clinical examination was performed, including blood pressure measurement and abdominal palpation. Secondly ultrasonography was performed, whereby the abdominal aorta was scanned longitudinally and transversely. The transverse scans were made at intervals of 2 cm covering the area from the diaphragm to the aortic bifurcation. The diameter of the aorta was measured at the level of the renal arteries and the left renal vein. The abdominal aorta was considered normal when its diameter at the aortic bifurcation was identical with or smaller than that at the renal arteries. Relevant information was obtained from all 245 patients.

In Figure 16-1, the size of the abdominal aorta for males and females is shown. Among the 245 patients only one case (0.4%) of abdominal aortic aneurysm was found! This abdominal aortic aneurysm was not diagnosed at the clinical examination. Two clinically suspected cases of aortic aneurysms were negative at the ultrasonography.

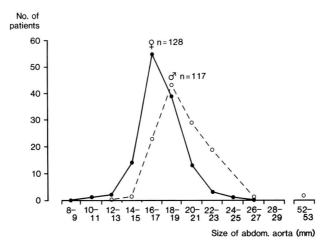

Fig. 16-1.   Ultrasonographic measurement of lumbar aorta, disclosing one aortic aneurysm among 245 patients.

In order to establish the prevalence of abdominal aortic aneurysm in hypertensives, a large group of patients must be examined. The number depends on the prevalence and the degree of certainty that is required. Regarding the problem of carrying out ultrasonography on several thousands of patients we selected in this study hypertensives in a geographically defined population. By statistical means it can be shown that our extremely low incidence of aortic aneurysm in the material implies a very low probability (below 5%) that the true prevalence in this risk group is as high as 2%.

There may be several explanations for the low prevalence in this study. One is that it comprises only patients cared for under a primary health care scheme, another is that other studies show too high figures as they are based on selected autopsy materials. It has been shown previously that the hypertensive group described here is representative of all known hypertensives in the population.[36,37] The risk for cerebro-cardiovascular disease in the patient group was high as described in these studies. In the age group 40–59 years, 21% of the male and 8% of the female hypertensives had suffered from stroke, coronary heart disease, or intermittent claudication. Corresponding figures for those aged 60–69 years were 36 and 14% respectively. Therefore, the low incidence of abdominal aortic aneurysms in this "risk" group seems to be relevant.

CONCLUSIONS

The classical study of Szilagyi clearly shows that there is a benefit from surgical treatment of abdominal aortic aneurysms, especially above the size of 6 cm. With the knowledge of an extremely high mortality rate in ruptured aneurysms and a very low mortality rate in elective cases, even in the elderly population, it should be of utmost importance to find as many aortic aneurysms as possible before they rupture. This has also economical aspects, such as expensive emergency surgery and expensive intensive care.

Is there any possibility to screen population groups in order to find these aneurysms electively? The survey given and the study presented does not show any simple and safe possibility to find the risk population. As ultrasonography is a simple and noninvasive method it may naturally be used on all elderly persons but that seems almost impossible to work through. The population study described did not reveal a reasonable chance to find the risk patient among hypertensives in the age group 50–69 years.

For the surgeon it is still to be expected that most patients will be referred due to a suspicion of an aortic aneurysm on palpation of the abdomen, or they will appear due to symptoms, from slight abdominal discomfort to fulminant symptoms of a rupture. Thus, the only "screening" procedure that is beneficial seems to be a careful abdominal palpation followed by ultrasonography if there is the slightest suspicion of an aortic aneurysm.

A final question is whether it is of interest to the surgeon to find the small (< 6 cms) asymptomatic aneurysm. By using screening methods, and by recommending careful abdominal examinations in older patients, the number of small aneurysms discovered may increase. It is evident for all vascular surgeons that ruptures appear even in small aneurysms. Despite the knowledge from Szilagyi[38] that the risk of rupture is lesser in such cases it therefore seems valuable to find even these patients and investigate them with surgical treatment as an aim, if contraindications are not present.

ACKNOWLEDGMENT

For the presentation of the Dalby study, the author gratefully acknowledges the cooperation with Lars Lindholm M.D., Ph.D., Lillemor Forsberg M.D., Ph.D., and Göran Ejlertsson Ph.D.

REFERENCES

1. De Bakey ME, Crawford ES, Cooley DA, et al: Aneurysm of abdominal aorta. Ann Surg 160:622, 1964
2. Søreide O, Lillestøl J, Christensen O, et al: Abdominal aortic aneurysms: Survival analysis of four hundred thirty-four patients. Surgery 91:188, 1982
3. Lawrie G, Morris G, Crawford ES, et al: Improved results of operation for ruptured abdominal aortic aneurysms. Surgery 85:483, 1979.
4. Botta GC, Contini S, Adorni A: Abdominal aortic aneurysms: Some controversial points. J Cardiovasc Surg 24:481, 1983

5. Norgren L, Andersson H, Einarsson E, Ribbe E: Aortic aneurysms in Lund 1975–1979. Acta Chir Scand suppl. 506:12, 1981

6. Christenson J, Eklöf B, Gustafson I: Abdominal aortic aneurysms: Should they all be resected? Br J Surg 64:767, 1977

7. Spittell JA: Hypertension and arterial aneurysm. J Am Coll Cardiol 1:533, 1983

8. Roberts W: The hypertensive diseases. Evidence that systemic hypertension is a greater risk factor to the development of other cardiovascular diseases than previously suspected. Am J Med 59:523, 1975

9. Cabellon S, Moncrief CL, Pierre DR, et al: Incidence of abdominal aortic aneurysms in patients with atheromatous arterial disease. Am J Surg 146:575, 1983

10. Clifton MA: Familial abdominal aortic aneurysms. Br J Surg 64:765, 1977

11. Norrgård Ö, Rais O, Ängquist KA: Familial occurrence of abdominal aortic aneurysms. Surgery 95:650, 1984a.

12. Tilson MD, Seashore MR: Fifty families with abdominal aortic aneurysms in two or more first-order relatives. Am J Surg 147:551, 1984a

13. Tilson MD, Seashore MR: Human genetics of the abdominal aortic aneurysm. Surg Gynecol Obstet 158:129, 1984b

14. Norrgård Ö, Ängquist KA, Johnson O: Familial aortic aneurysms—serum concentrations of triglyceride, cholesterol, HDL-cholesterol and (VLDL + LDL)-cholesterol. In print 1984b

15. Norrgård Ö, Cedergren B, Ängquist KA, et al: Blood groups and HLA antigens in patients with abdominal aortic aneurysms. Human Hered 34:9, 1984c

16. Norrgård Ö, Fröhlander N, Beckman G, et al: Association between haptoglobin groups and aortic abdominal aneurysms. Human Hered 34:166, 1984d

17. Morris T, Bouhoutsos J: ABO blood groups in occlusive and ectatic arterial disease. Br J Surg 60:892, 1973

18. Morris T, Bouhoutsos J: The Rhesus factor in occlusive and ectatic arterial disease. J Cardiovasc Surg 15:647, 1974.

19. Cannon J, Casteel L, Read RC: Abdominal aortic aneurysm, Lerich's syndrome, inguinal herniation, and smoking. Arch Surg 119:387, 1984

20. Tilson MD, Davis G: Deficiencies of copper and compound with ion-exchange characteristics of pyridinoline in skin from patients with abdominal aortic aneurysms. Surgery 94:134, 1983

21. De Palma RG: Biochemical abnormalities and atherosclerotic aneurysms, In Bergan JJ, Yao JST (eds): Aneurysms Diagnosis and Treatment, New York, Grune & Stratton, Inc, pp 45, 1982

22. Tilson MD, Fieg EL, Harvey M: Malignant neoplasia in patients with abdominal aortic aneurysms. Arch Surg 119:792, 1984c

23. Chapman JR, Hilson AJW: Polycystic kidneys and abdominal aortic aneurysms. Lancet 1:646, 1980

24. Almgren B, Eriksson I, Hemmingsson A, et al: Abdominal aortic aneurysm in homocystinuria. Acta Chir Scand 144:545, 1978

25. Sethia B, Darke SG: Abdominal aortic aneurysm with retroperitoneal fibrosis and ureteric entrapment. Br J Surg 70:434, 1983

26. Baskerville PA, Blakeney CG, Young AE, et al: The diagnosis and treatment of periaortic fibrosis ('inflammatory' aneurysms) Br J Surg 70:381, 1983

27. Treugut H, Karp W, Norgren L: Ultraschalldiagnostik beim nicht aneurysmatischen pulsierenden Abdominaltumor. Chirurg 51:506, 1980

28. Eriksson I, Hemingsson A, Lindgren P: Diagnosis of abdominal aortic aneurysms by aortography, computer tomography and ultrasound. Acta Radiol Diag 21:209, 1980

29. Carlsson J, Sternby N: Aortic aneurysm. Acta Chir Scand 127:466, 1964

30. Darling R, Messina C, Brawster R: Autopsy study of unoperated abdominal aortic aneurysms. Circulation 56: suppl II 161, 1977

31. Kagan AR, Sternby NH, Uemur K, et al: Atherosclerosis of the aorta and coronary arteries in five towns. Bull WHO 53, 1976

32. Gore J, Hirst AE: Arteriosclerotic aneurysms of the abdominal aorta. A review. Prog Cardiovasc Dis 16:113, 1973

33. Melton LJ, Bickerstaff LK, Hollier LH, et al: Changing incidence of abdominal aortic aneurysms: A population-based study. Am J Epidemiol 120:379, 1984

34. Lindholm L, Ejlertsson G, Forsberg L, Norgren L: Low prevalence of abdominal aortic aneurysm in hypertensive patients a population-based study. Submitted Br Med J; 1984a

35. Ejlertsson G: Production and consumption of health care services in a defined population. Lund: Studentlitteratur; 1981. Thesis.

36. Lindholm L, Schersten B, Thulin T: Hypertension in elderly people in a Swedish primary care district. Scand J Prim Health Care 3–4:120, 1983

37. Lindholm L, Ejlertsson G, Schersten B: High risks of cerebrocardiovascular morbidity in well treated male hypertensives. Acta Med Scand 216:251, 1984b

38. Szilagyi DE, Smith RF, DeRusso FJ, et al: Contribution of abdominal aortic aneurysmectomy to prolongation of life. Ann Surg 164:678, 1966

Averil O. Mansfield

17

Imaging Aneurysms

Clinical examination is usually all that is needed to establish a diagnosis of abdominal aortic aneurysm. The well-established routine of inspection and palpation will first alert the clinician who notes a visible pulsation and mass and subsequently feels it. Apart from population screening, asymptomatic aneurysm is a chance finding. Even when the opportunity for abdominal palpation is presented, the diagnosis may be missed, perhaps because the clinician's hand did not pause long enough to feel the pulsation or because obesity made examination difficult. Sometimes the diagnosis is made apparent by radiologic investigation, such as a roentgenogram of the lumbar spine in a patient with backache, or a barium study in a patient with abdominal pain or constipation. When the clinician is made aware of the aneurysm, it is often easy to feel. When clinical abdominal examination leaves some uncertainty, a plane roentgenogram or ultrasound examination can often resolve the doubt. The plane abdominal radiography may show a rim of calcification, the lateral view being the most conclusive. Radiography may also demonstrate additional aneurysms in the pelvis, but it is not as helpful in evaluating the upper extent of the aneurysm.

ULTRASOUND

Ultrasound will determine dimensions of the aneurysms with accuracy; one of the most valuable uses of ultrasound is in monitoring enlargement of a small aneurysm. Again, the main limitations are at the upper end where there may be confusion concerning the level at which the renal and intestinal vessels arise. A chest radiograph is also valuable in alerting the clinician to dilatation or frank aneurysm formation in the thoracic aorta.

Clinical examination, perhaps supported by plane roentgenogram and/or ultrasound examination, reveals that there is an aneurysm. Is anything more required? If, on examination, you can get between the aneurysm and the costal margin, and if the chest roentgenogram is normal, then probably you can manage without anything else.

DIAGNOSTIC TECHNIQUES AND ASSESSMENT
PROCEDURES IN VASCULAR SURGERY

© 1985 Grune & Stratton
ISBN 0-8089-1721-8 All rights reserved

It has always been my practice to determine the site and function of the kidneys and the course of the ureters. The intravenous urogram (IVU) will provide this information. It will determine that both kidneys are working and how well. It will determine the normality of the renal architecture and position and will warn of the important anomalies, such as the pelvic kidney and the horseshoe kidney, both of which make aneurysm surgery more difficult and may indicate the need for preoperative angiography to determine the position and number of the renal arteries.

Marked difference in function of two kidneys may point to the possibility of renal artery stenosis, and again may lead to further investigations prior to operation. An isotope scan will usually determine the differential function of the two kidneys; perhaps an angiogram should be performed if the scan is abnormal.

Particular attention is directed towards the ureters in patients with aneurysms because of the occasional occurrence of retroperitoneal fibrosis in association with aneurysms. In this disease the ureters will be displaced medially with some hold-up in the ureters. Normally situated ureters may be partially obstructed as they pass over iliac aneurysms, further valuable preoperative information.

If all of these investigations reveal an aneurysm and no other abnormality, and if there is no clinical suggestion of renal artery or intestinal artery involvement, the next step may well be the operation.

COMPUTERIZED AXIAL TOMOGRAPHY

This investigation has only become available to me in the last two years and yet already I look upon it as a valuable and desirable preliminary examination. In my own practice it is now routine, but the straightforward case can certainly be managed without it. If a computerized tomography (CT) scan is to be a routine examination, then the IVU is omitted because the contrast-enhanced CT scan provides the same information. The particular advantages are accurate preoperative knowledge about the aneurysm itself. A typical CT scan of an abdominal aortic aneurysm is shown in Figure 17-1. In addition, totally unexpected and unrelated pathology may be revealed, a not unusual occurrence in the age group with which we are dealing. The CT scan demonstrates accurately the extent and dimensions of the aneurysm. There are one or two exceptions which are discussed later.

Most surgeons are worried by the prospect of unexpectedly discovering during an operation that the aneurysm extends above the renal arteries. This finding not infrequently results in the declaration that the aneurysm is inoperable, whereas with preoperative warning and a planned approach (probably a different incision) such involvement will still allow operative correction.

If the upper aorta is not aneurysmal (Fig. 17-2) and the coeliac, superior mesenteric, and renal vessels can be seen arising from this undilated aorta, then one can be certain that there is no problem.

Aortic bifurcation is usually seen well and the involvement of the iliacs by aneurysmal disease can be determined, thus allowing prospective prediction of whether a tube or a bifurcation graft will be needed. The aorta can easily be divided into its three components: lumen, thrombus, and wall. The first two are not of much clinical significance but the wall thickness is of great importance. The so-called

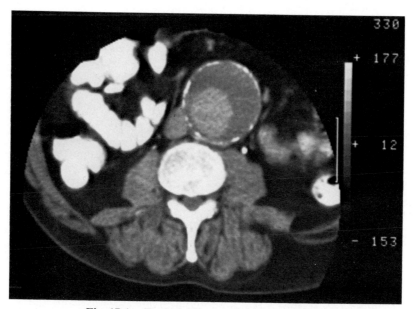

Fig. 17-1. Typical CT scan of aortic aneurysm.

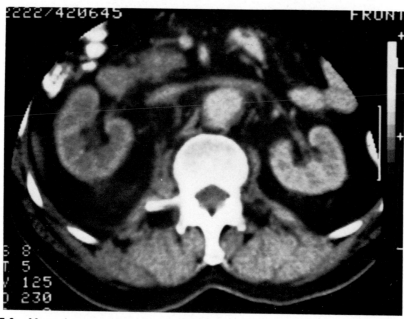

Fig. 17-2. Normal aorta and renal veins. With permission of St. Mary's Hospital Medical School, London.

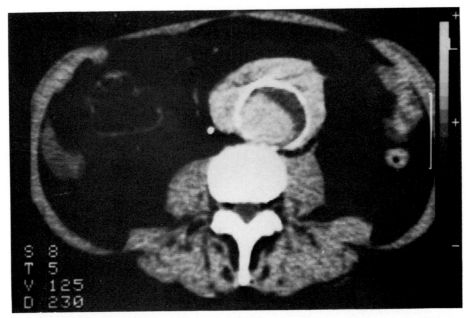

Fig. 17-3. Thick wall of "inflammatory" aneurysm with deficient posterior wall. With permission of St. Mary's Hospital Medical School, London.

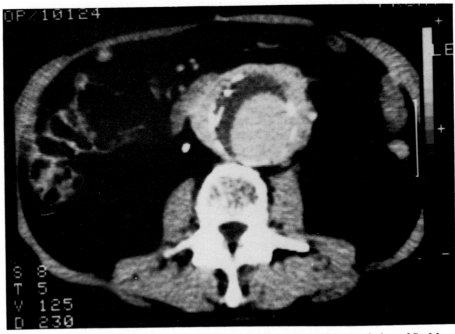

Fig. 17-4. Ureters visualised. Left one in the wall of the aorta. With permission of St. Mary's Hospital Medical School, London.

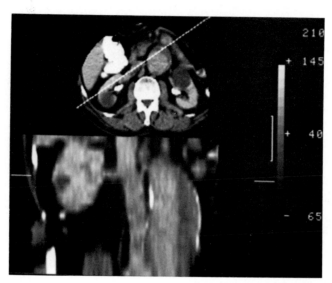

Fig. 17-5. Reconstructed CT scan showing aortic aneurysm and IVC and kidney.

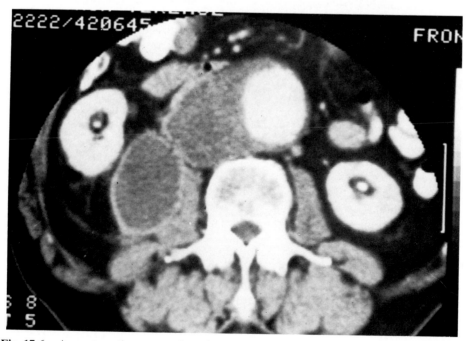

Fig. 17-6. Asymptomatic rupture of aortic aneurysm. With permission of St. Mary's Hospital Medical School, London.

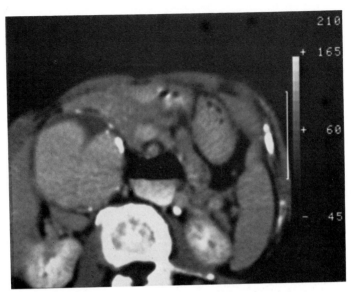

Fig. 17-7.   This appearance may indicate dissection.

inflammatory aneurysm may have a very thick wall, and an interesting feature of the thick wall is its distribution. Those who believe that the thick wall prevents rupture should look at the posterior wall (Fig. 17-3), which is usually thin even in those with extensive retroperitoneal fibrosis or "inflammation." An additional observation of great clinical importance is the course of the ureter, which in these cases may be found embedded in the thick wall or surrounding dense tissues (Fig. 17-4).

A tortuous aorta can sometimes provide difficulties of interpretation but the improving reconstructed views may solve this problem of whether it is an aneurysm or tortuosity. At the present time the CT scan appearance which suggests that the renal arteries rise from the aneurysm, can sometimes be the results of tortuosity of the aorta in an anterior-posterior direction (Fig. 17-5). Angiography is required to resolve the direction.

Unexpected findings, such as a previous rupture (Fig. 17-6), a double lumen from dissection (Fig. 17-7), or a false aneurysm may be valuable preoperative warnings. Retroperitoneal gas shadows may provide the clue to the presence of an aorto-intestinal fistula.

NUCLEAR MAGNETIC RESONANCE (NMR)

NMR provides a new dimension in scanning, requiring neither contrast nor exposure to irradiation. It can provide accurate visualisation of the aorta as the example shows (Fig. 17-8). This figure shows a young man with Bechet's disease in whom the use of contrast was undesirable. My personal experience with this exciting new technique is very limited.

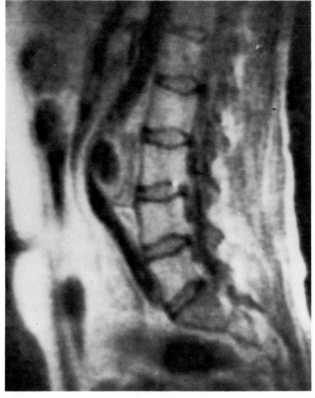

Fig. 17-8. Nuclear magnetic resonance to show false aneurysm of aorta. With permission of St. Mary's Hospital Medical School, London.

ANGIOGRAPHY

As with most investigations in vascular surgery, the angiogram remains a vital tool. It is only required in those cases where there are complicating features or questions that remain unanswered by the other modes of examination. This is principally the question of involvement of the intestine and renal vessels from the aneurysm itself. When the aneurysm appears on CT scan to extend higher than the renal arteries, then a catheter angiogram should be performed, enabling the visualisation of the origins of the vessels, and their relationship to the aneurysm defined.

Angiography outlines only the lumen, hence the outline of the aneurysm itself may not be easy to define, and often the angiogram and the CT scan have to be examined together. Oblique or lateral views are usually required to define all the vessels because of the distortion and tortuosity associated with aneurysmal disease. Careful attention should be paid to the origins of the renal vessels and, particularly, to determining the number of renal vessels when these arise from the aneurysm. When the aneurysm extends into the chest, it is of great value to know exactly where the aneurysm begins in relationship to the left subclavian artery. This cannot

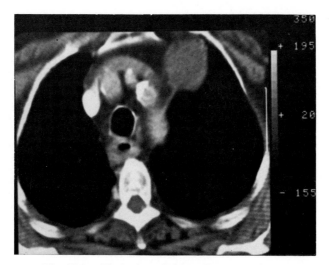

Fig. 17-9. Thoracic aneurysm. Great vessels seen.

clearly be determined from these two CT scans (Figs. 17-9 and 17-10). Essentially the aim of angiography is to divide aneurysms into three groups: those that can be dealt with in the abdomen entirely, those that require a thoracoabdominal approach, and those that require cardiopulmonary bypass because the arch is involved. These three approaches are so radically different from one another that careful preoperative investigation is essential so as to know with certainty that the left carotid need not be clamped and secondly where there is a need to revascularise the kidneys and the intestines.

I believe there is one more image most surgeons dealing with the more complex aneurysms would like, and that is to know the dominant source of supply to the

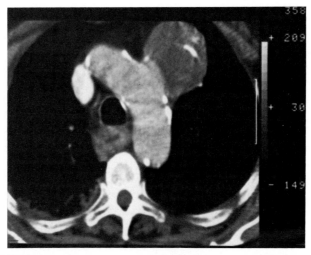

Fig. 17-10. Thoracic aneurysm. Difficult to relate to origins of great vessels.

spinal cord so that it can be protected or revascularised as need be. At the moment interpretation of angiograms with regard to the spinal cord blood supply is, at best, guess work and I can give no assurance in this area.

In summary, many aneurysms require only minimal investigation for safe management. When CT scanning is available it removes most of the guess work from interpretation of clinical and ultrasound examinations and the IVU. Angiography remains a valuable investigation in the small percentage of aneurysms thought to extend above the renal arteries or into the thorax. Accurate preoperative assessment and surgical planning are needed for these more complex aneurysms if we are to achieve good results.

John A. Mannick, Herbert B. Hechtman,
Anthony D. Whittemore, and Nathan P. Couch

18

Hemodynamic Studies in Patients Undergoing Abdominal Aneurysm Repair

About a decade ago it became apparent that the operative mortality from repair of abdominal aortic aneurysms had declined from levels of 10% or more in the 1960s to about 5% in the 1970s.[1-3] This residual operative mortality was almost exclusively cardiac in origin. In 1972 we began hemodynamic investigation of patients on our service who underwent abdominal aortic aneurysm surgery to test the hypothesis that a further reduction in operative mortality might be obtained if optimum circulating blood volume and normal blood pressure could be maintained throughout the perioperative period.[4]

We inserted radial artery cannulas and thermister-tipped Swan-Ganz pulmonary artery catheters in 10 consecutive patients undergoing elective abdominal aortic aneurysm repair. We made observations of cardiac index, mean arterial pressure, pulmonary artery wedge pressure, and heart rate at the time of the induction of anesthesia, 30 minutes after clamping of the abdominal aorta, at the time of declamping, and at the time of completion of wound closure. These observations demonstrated that there was a significant drop in cardiac index at the time of aortic declamping, which was associated with a fall in mean arterial pressure and a considerable rise in pulmonary artery wedge pressure (Fig. 18-1, left). This suggested that the patients as a group had a temporary period of left ventricular failure associated with aortic declamping. Hypotension at the time of release of the aortic cross-clamp had been noted for many years by vascular surgeons and had been termed "declamping shock."

The fact that the pulmonary artery wedge pressure in these patients undergoing aneurysm repair was quite low at the beginning of the operative procedure suggested that they were coming to the operating room without an adequate circulating plasma volume despite apparently normal urinary output and normal blood pressure. We therefore investigated (preoperatively) a series of 23 patients scheduled for abdominal aortic aneurysm repair. These patients also had radial arterial cannulas and Swan-Ganz catheters inserted on the evening prior to surgery. Cardiac index and pulmonary artery wedge pressure were measured at intervals following incremental intravenous boluses of 12.5 g of albumin or 250 mL of Ringer's lactate solu-

DIAGNOSTIC TECHNIQUES AND ASSESSMENT
PROCEDURES IN VASCULAR SURGERY

© 1985 Grune & Stratton
ISBN 0-8089-1721-8 All rights reserved

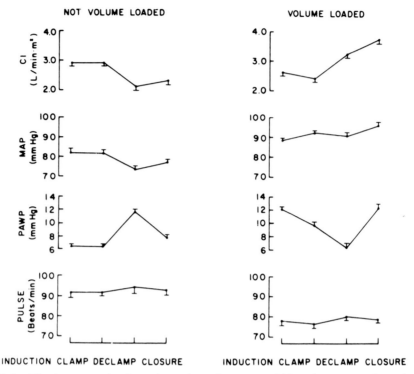

Fig. 18-1. The intraoperative hemodynamic performance of 10 patients not volume loaded is compared with that of 23 volume-loaded patients. Cardiac index (CI), mean arterial pressure (MAP), pulmonary artery wedge pressure (PAWP), and pulse were measured during induction of anesthesia, 30 minutes following aortic cross-clamping, 5 minutes after declamping, and during closure of the abdominal incision. Vertical bars indicate the SEM. In contrast to patients not volume loaded preoperatively, the volume-loaded group demonstrated improved cardiac performance as evidenced by the increased CI, stable MAP, and diminished PAWP following declamping. This improvement was observed in the absence of pharmacologic manipulation. With permission of the Annals of Surgery.

tion which raised the pulmonary artery wedge pressure in step-wise fashion. This allowed the construction of individual left ventricular performance curves as demonstrated in Figure 18-2. It was found that most patients had performance curves of the sort demonstrated by patient A in Figure 18-2 with a progressive rise in cardiac index with increase in pulmonary artery wedge pressure. Some patients, however, had preoperative ventricular performance curves of the sort manifested by patient B with an initial rise in cardiac index with increase in pulmonary artery wedge pressure, and then a fall in cardiac output as the wedge pressure was further increased. A few patients had preoperative ventricular performance curves of the sort demonstrated by patient C in Figure 18-2 with a fall in cardiac index with increase in pulmonary artery wedge pressure. It seemed logical that a pulmonary artery wedge pressure should be selected for each patient which was associated with a satisfactory cardiac index, and that the patients should be maintained at that pulmonary artery wedge pressure by appropriate volume administration during the perioperative period.

The group of 23 patients was managed in this fashion during abdominal aneurysm repair and hemodynamic measurements were again made at the time of induction of anesthesia, 30 minutes after aortic cross-clamping, five minutes after the release of the cross-clamp, and at the time of wound closure. As shown in the right half of Figure 18-1, this group of patients responded quite differently to the release of the aortic cross-clamp with maintenance of mean arterial pressure, a prompt rise in cardiac index, and a fall in pulmonary artery wedge pressure. All patients were monitored carefully postoperatively and pulmonary artery wedge pressure was carefully maintained during the first 48 hours after surgery. Careful attention was also paid to ensuring adequate oxygenation by repeated measurements of arterial blood gases.

It was apparent that optimally volume-loaded patients had far less difficulty in maintaining normal hemodynamics during aortic surgery than individuals who had been managed without preoperative assessment of volume status and cardiac performance. We postulated that careful monitoring of pulmonary artery wedge pressure might lead to a reduction in postoperative mortality from myocardial infarction and other cardiac causes. In a subsequent series of 227 patients undergoing elective and urgent abdominal aortic aneurysm repair, this method of hemodynamic monitoring was utilized routinely. The 30-day operative mortality for the entire group was 1.3%, which suggests but does not prove that this method of perioperative management had resulted in the desired effect on operative mortality.

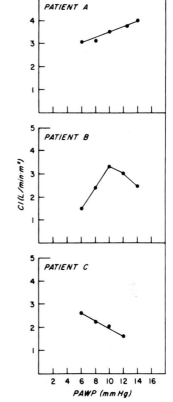

Fig. 18-2. Three types of preoperative myocardial performance curves are illustrated. During volume infusion, patient A increased cardiac output with each increment in PAWP. In contrast, patient B had a peak in cardiac output such that with further increases in PAWP, output decreases; patient C demonstrated a steady decline in cardiac performance. Volume therapy is designed to raise the PAWP to the point at which cardiac output peaks, or if this does not occur, to a maximum of 12–14 mmHg with a cardiac index of >2.5. With permission of the Annals of Surgery.

While falls in the cardiac index during aortic surgery could be minimized in patients who were adequately volume loaded, it was apparent that there was nevertheless a significant fall in cardiac index at the time of aortic cross-clamping in most of these individuals. Because of experimental work that suggested that levels of prostaglandins were elevated in the plasma in patients undergoing aortic clamping and declamping,[5] we set out to investigate the effects of aortic surgery on circulating levels of prostacyclin and thromboxane A_2, which are respectively potent vasodilating and vasoconstricting agents. It was further known that thromboxanes directly or indirectly have cardiodepressant activity'[6]

Twenty-two patients undergoing abdominal aneurysm repair were studied in a randomized fashion:[7] 11 received 650 mg of aspirin orally 10 hours prior to operation and 11 received a placebo. Hemodynamic monitoring was carried out as usual with pulmonary artery wedge pressure and cardiac output monitored preoperatively and intraoperatively. As is shown in Figure 18-3, the administration of aspirin preoperatively blunted the drop in cardiac output associated with aortic cross-clamping and did not prevent the prompt rise in cardiac index with declamping. Neither aspirin nor placebo had any significant effect on pulmonary artery wedge pressure in these patients. Measurements of 6 keto-PGF1 and thromboxane B_2 in the plasma of these patients by a double antibody radioimmunoassay technique[8] demonstrated that there was a prompt rise in 6 keto-PGF1, the stable metabolite of prostacyclin, immediately following the induction of anesthesia and then a gradual decline in patients who received placebo. Aspirin administration lowered baseline levels of 6 keto-PGF1 and inhibited the rise associated with surgery (Fig. 18-4). As shown in Figure 18-5, aortic cross-clamping led to a rise in thromboxane B_2, the stable metabolite of thromboxane A_2 in the placebo group. Aspirin administration reduced preoperative thromboxane concentration and maintained low levels during surgery.

We also studied the effect of patient plasma obtained preoperatively and 30 minutes after aortic clamping on the contractility of rat papillary muscle in vitro.

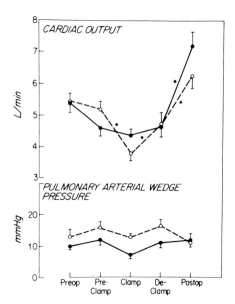

Fig. 18-3. Aortic cross-clamping was associated with a significant decline in CO, an event prevented with aspirin. The PAWP was not altered by surgery or aspirin. *$P < .05$. †Comparison between placebo and aspirin groups where $P < .05$. ($\bigcirc$ --- $\bigcirc$) = placebo, ($\bullet$ --- $\bullet$) = aspirin, and I = SEM. With permission of the Annals of Surgery.

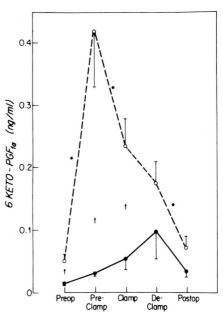

Fig. 18-4. Thirty minutes after the start of surgery, 6-keto-PGF$_1$ concentrations rose significantly and then declined. Aspirin lowered baseline levels of 6-keto-PGF$_1$ and inhibited any rise with surgery. *$P < .05$ comparing adjacent study periods. †Comparison between placebo and aspirin groups were $P < .05$. (○ --- ○) = placebo, (● --- ●) = aspirin, and I = SEM. With permission of the Annals of Surgery.

Plasma was used to bathe the rat papillary muscle to detect the presence of a humoral negative inotropic agent. Developed tension (Tpd) at constant pre-load was measured with an isometric force transducer (Harvard Apparatus, Millis, Mass). The preoperative plasma sample was always reapplied at the end of each experiment to confirm the ability to reverse any decrease in Tpd. As shown in Figure 18-6, during aortic cross-clamping plasma contained a negative inotropic agent in the patients receiving the placebo as shown by the fall in Tpd of rat papillary muscle bathed with this plasma. Aspirin administration again inhibited this decline in contractility, suggesting that thromboxane release in the placebo group was responsible for this negative inotropic effect and that this effect might very well be important in the clinically observed reduction in cardiac output during aortic cross-clamping in the placebo group.

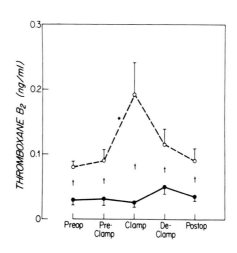

Fig. 18-5. Aortic cross-clamping led to a rise in T × B$_2$. Aspirin-reduced preoperative Tx concentration and maintained low levels during surgery. *$P < .05$ comparing adjacent study periods. †Comparison between placebo and aspirin groups were $P < .05$ (○ --- ○) = placebo, (● --- ●) = aspirin, and I = SEM. With permission of the Annals of Surgery.

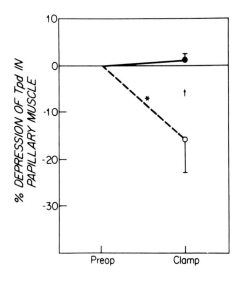

Fig. 18-6. During aortic cross-clamping, plasma contained a negative inotropic agent(s) as shown by the fall in Tpd of a rat papillary muscle bathed with this plasma. Aspirin inhibited the decline in contractility. *$P < .05$ comparing adjacent study periods. †Comparison between placebo and aspirin groups where $P < .05$ (O---O) = placebo, (●---●) = aspirin. With permission of the Annals of Surgery.

A similar study was again carried out on 26 consecutive patients under-going abdominal aortic aneurysm repair. These patients were randomized into a group of 11 patients who, in double-blind fashion, received the cyclooxygenase inhibitor ibuprofen (12 mg/kg by mouth). Fifteen patients received a placebo by mouth prior to surgery. As before, blood was drawn for prostaglandin assays before anesthesia, 30 minutes after incision, 30 minutes after aortic cross-clamping, 5 minutes after removal of the clamp, and 24 hours after surgery. As in the prior study, ibuprofen totally prevented the rise in circulating 6 keto-PGF1, which occurred in the placebo group following surgical incision (Fig. 18-7). Ibuprofen also inhibited the rise in thromboxane levels seen following aortic clamping (Fig. 18-8). It was found in studying arterial values of these prostaglandin metabolites and those found in mixed venous blood that both prostaglandins were principally released in the lung. This is demonstrated in Figure 18-9.

As in the previous study, it is apparent that the plasma from the control group had a negative inotropic effect on rat papillary muscle, whereas plasma from the ibuprofen-treated group had no discernible negative inotropic effect (Fig. 18-10).

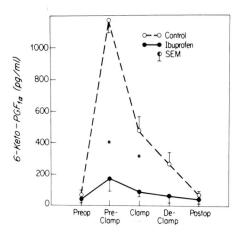

Fig. 18-7. A marked rise in circulating levels of 6-keto-PGF$_1$ occurred 30 minutes after surgical incision, indicating an increased production of PGI$_2$. With permission of the Annals of Surgery.

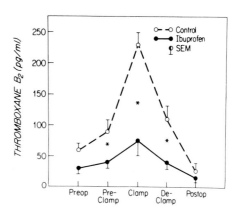

Fig. 18-8. Increase in TxB₂ levels coincided with aortic cross-clamping and lower-limb ischemia in the placebo group. Ibuprofen maintained this prostanoid at baseline levels.
With permission of the Annals of Surgery.

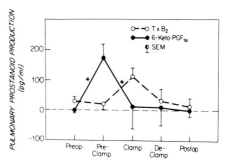

Fig. 18-9. In patients treated with placebo, aterial values of 6-keto-PGF₁ and TxB₂ were higher than those in mixed venous blood 30 minutes after incision (preclamp), and 30 minutes after aortic clamping (clamp), respectively. This indicates pulmonary synthesis.
With permission of the Annals of Surgery.

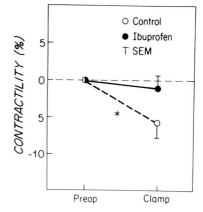

Fig. 18-10. Cyclooxygenase inhibition prevented the formation of a negative inotrope as measured by the in vitro rat papillary heart muscle bioassay. With permission of the Annals of Surgery.

As a chance occurrence in this study, five patients in the ibuprofen group were not adequately volume-loaded during the aortic surgery and their pulmonary artery wedge pressures were maintained at suboptimal levels. As shown in Figure 18-11, these suboptimally volume-loaded patients were not protected from the decline in cardiac output during aortic cross-clamping by ibuprofen administration. Thus, it appears that to prevent a drop in cardiac output following aortic cross-clamping, both adequate volume-loading and a blockade of thromboxane of synthesis are needed.

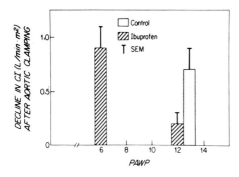

Fig. 18-11. Only patients in the ibuprofen group with preoperative pulmonary artery wedge pressures ≥ 10 exhibited cardiac stability during clamping. With permission of the Annals of Surgery.

These studies of prostaglandin metabolism offer an explanation for the fall in cardiac output seen with aortic cross-clamping. However, there was no difference in clinical outcome between the groups of patients who received cyclooxygenase inhibitors and those who received placebos. Thus, the clinical importance of these observations remains in doubt. However, it seems likely that in individuals with borderline cardiac function, prophylactic administration of modest doses of cyclooxygenase-inhibiting agents might be helpful in maintaining normal hemodynamics during abdominal aortic surgery.

REFERENCES

1. Baker AG Jr, Roberts B, Berkowitz HD, et al: Risk of excision of abdominal aortic aneurysm. Surgery 68:1129, 1970
2. Hicks GL, Eastland MW, DeWeese JA, et al: Survival improvement following aortic aneurysm resection. Ann Surg 181:863, 1975
3. Thompson JE, Hollier LM, Patman RD, et al: Surgical management of abdominal aortic aneurysms. Ann Surg 181:654, 1975
4. Whittemore AD, Clowes AW, Hechtman HB, et al: Aortic Aneurysm Repair. Reduced operative mortality associated with maintenance of optimal cardiac performance. Ann Surg 192:414, 1980
5. Graham LM, Stanley JC, Gewertz BL, et al: Prostaglandin E_{2a} attenuation of aortic declamping hyperemia and hypotension. J Surg Res 20:413, 1976
6. Karmazyn M, Dhalla NS: Thromboxane B_2: A cardiodepressant of isolated rat hearts and inhibitor of sarcolemma Na^+-K^+ stimulated ATPase activity. Prostaglandin Med 3:81, 1979
7. Utsunomiya T, Krausz MM, Dunham B, et al: Maintenance of cardiodynamics with aspirin during abdominal aortic aneurysmectomy (AAA). Ann Surg 194:602, 1981
8. Levine L, Alam I, Langone J: The use of immobilized ligands and ^{125}I protein A for immunoassay of thromboxane B_2, prostaglandin D_2, 13,14-dihydro-prostaglandin E_2, 5-6-dihydro-prostaglandin I_2; 6-keto-prostaglandin F_{1a}, 15-hydroxy-9_a, 11_a (expoxymethanol) prosta-5,13-dienoic acid and 15-hydroxy-11_a, 19_a (epoxymethano) prosta-5,13-denoic acid. Prostagland Med 2:177, 1979
9. Huval WV, Lelcuk S, Allen PD, et al: Determinants of cardiovascular stability during abdominal aortic aneurysmectomy (AAA). Ann Surg 199:216, 1984

William K. Ehrenfeld
and Linda M. Reilly

19

The Assessment of Renal Ischemia Prognosis Following Operative Treatment of Renovascular Hypertension

Since the first report of surgical cure of hypertension by nephrectomy in 1937[1], the simple and reliable identification of hypertensive patients who would benefit from operative treatment has remained an elusive goal. This is because the diagnosis of renovascular hypertension (RVH) is essentially a retrospective one, and can only be definitively made when there is permanent relief of hypertension after renal revascularization or nephrectomy. The inaccuracies of selecting operative candidates, the difficulty in performing many of the diagnostic tests, the poor early results of surgical treatment, and the increasingly successful medical control of blood pressure have all resulted in restricted use of surgical correction. Recently, however, three developments have again focused attention on the role of correction of renal artery stenosis in the management of renovascular hypertension. The first is the use of venous digital subtraction angiography to detect renal artery lesions and the second is the emergence of transluminal angioplasty to correct the stenosis. Thirdly, and perhaps most significant, is the increasing realization that renovascular hypertension is a manifestation of an ischemic end-organ (the kidney) and that successful blood pressure control does not reduce, but may in fact worsen, renal ischemia. Thus, in spite of optimal medical control of blood pressure, in the presence of renal artery stenosis one may see silent progression of the stenosis,[2-5] loss of renal mass,[6-8] and loss of renal function.[9-12] The recognition of hypertension as a symptom and renal ischemia as the disease, combined with safer methods of diagnosis and treatment, makes the diagnosis of renovascular hypertension urgent.

The diagnostic problem is two-fold. First, renovascular disease and renovascular hypertension are not synonymous. Therefore, it is necessary to establish the functional significance of any renal artery disease that is present. The finding of renal artery stenosis in normotensive patients, especially among older patients, is not uncommon and may be as high as 35–50%.[13-15] Conversely, patients with essential hypertension may have coincidental renal artery stenosis.[13,16,17] Secondly, it is necessary to identify which patients with renovascular hypertension will be cured or improved by surgery. Although the operative result is influenced by patient

DIAGNOSTIC TECHNIQUES AND ASSESSMENT
PROCEDURES IN VASCULAR SURGERY
© 1985 Grune & Stratton
ISBN 0-8089-1721-8 All rights reserved

age, type of renal artery disease, and presence of symptomatic non-renal atherosclerosis,[18-25] the single most important determinant of a favourable response to surgery is the functional status of the kidney at the time of operation. This assessment has proved to be most difficult. Since the outcome of operative treatment of renovascular hypertension has been assessed almost completely in terms of cure or control of blood pressure, little data is available to determine the effect of revascularization on the preservation of normalization of renal function in comparison to the preoperative level of function.

A variety of tests have been used to diagnose renovascular hypertension and predict operative response, including rapid sequence intravenous urography, isotope renography, split renal function studies, peripheral and renal vein renin activity, angiotensin antagonist tests (saralasin infusion), and renal angiography. However, no single test or combination of tests is consistently sensitive and specific for the diagnosis of RVH.[9,26] It is the purpose of this chapter to outline our approach to the management of these patients, the basis for differences between this approach and that of others, and the functional results of operative treatment obtained by following this diagnostic and therapeutic regimen.

METHODS OF ASSESSING RENAL ISCHEMIA

Patients admitted to our unit with hypertension with or without renal insufficiency have frequently completed an evaluation for a renovascular etiology prior to admission and have been selected for aortorenal angiography prior to a decision regarding surgery. Pertinent admission laboratory data include bilateral supine and upright blood pressure measurements, serum creatinine and urea nitrogen, and creatinine clearance measurements. These serve principally as a baseline for comparison with postoperative results.

Clinical features that are significant in determining the presence of renovascular hypertension include a white patient, younger than 30 years or older than 50 years at the onset of hypertension; hypertension of short duration, resistant to medical treatment, or with a recent marked deterioration of medical control. The patient usually is not obese, has a history of other vascular disease, but no family history of hypertension. The only discriminating physical findings are the presence of an abdominal or flank bruit and arteriospastic retinal vascular changes.

Intravenous and Isotope Urography

Rapid-sequence intravenous pyelography or hypertensive urography (HTU) is not routinely obtained on our patients. Although this test can provide important data on kidney size, its ability to diagnose RVH or predict the result of surgical correction remains limited. Coincidentally, when the IVP is used as a screening test, a significant difference in kidney size (greater than 2 cm) may be the first indication of possible renovascular hypertension. The false negative rate of rapid-sequence IVP in diagnosing unilateral RVH is 20–30%[19,26-31] and for bilateral disease approaches 45%.[32] The incidence of true positive tests is discouragingly low[33-35] and the occurrence of false negative HTU studies among patients subsequently cured or improved by surgery is also striking, varying between 30% and 50%.[35]

Therefore as a diagnostic or prognostic modality, HTU is an inadequate basis for any therapeutic decision. For those patients who will undergo renal angiography, an accurate assessment of kidney size can be obtained during this study without requiring an additional IVP contrast load.

Renal isotope scanning tests have essentially the same results, although a lower false negative rate is often seen (Table 19-1). To date this test has not been proved to have any important clinical role in the assessment of RVH.[36] However, renal scanning does offer a relatively non-invasive, non-nephrotoxic method for the early postoperative assessment of reconstruction patency. We often use renal scanning in this manner, but rarely as a component of the preoperative assessment.

Table 19-1
Hypertension Screening with Isotope Renography

		False Positive	False Negative
(1)	Hunt et al	5	—
(2)	Johnson and Odum	5	6
(3)	Kaufmann and Maxwell	10	—
(4)	Kennedy	7	1
(5)	McNeil et al	15	10
(6)	Morris et al	12	—
(7)	Taplin	5	25
(8)	Wax and McDonald	6	24

Split Renal Function Studies

Determination of individual kidney function (split renal function studies, SRF) classically identifies impaired renal function by comparing one kidney with the other. The test is invasive, requiring brisk intravenous hydration as well as cystoscopy with ureteral intubation. Certain anti-hypertensive medications must be stopped before the procedure and not all patients can tolerate the volume load or the hyperosmolarity resulting from urea infusion. The existence of several methodologies for performing SRF studies has resulted in different interpretation criteria[37–39] and varying clinical results. Dean et al have shown that results using the classic criteria have an unacceptably high false negative rate (Table 19-2). This can be markedly improved by the use of lateralizing changes rather than absolute changes in urine volume, creatinine and PAH concentration, but only at the expense of test sensitivity (Table 19-2). In addition, the presence of bilateral disease, which is

Table 19-2
Results of Split Renal Function Studies
Using Various Interpretation Criteria

Criteria	False Positive	False Negative
Classic	2%	50%
Half classic	2%	28%
Lateralizing	10%	8%

common with either atherosclerosis or fibromuscular disease, causes a reduced sensitivity of SRF studies. Dean et al, using their liberalized criteria for a positive test (Table 19-3), found only a 67% lateralization in the setting of bilateral disease.[19] Nonetheless Dean feels that split renal function studies have been accurate predictors of a favourable response to operation among patients with RVH and are especially useful when renal function is severely compromised.[39,40] They feel that the arteriographic demonstration of a suitable distal vessel without branch stenosis and the finding of hyperconcentration of urea and PAH on split renal function studies means that the kidney is salvageable and that renal function will improve after revascularization.

Table 19-3
Criteria for Interpretation of Split Renal Function
Studies[39]

Criteria	Positive Test
Classic	40% ↓ in urine volume
	50% ↑ in creatinine concentration
	100% ↑ in PAH concentration
Half classic	25% ↓ in urine volume
	25% ↑ in creatinine concentration
	50% ↑ in PAH concentration
Lateralizing	consistent lateralization × 3 measurements with ↓
	urine volume and ↑ creatinine and PAH concentrations

We are in agreement with most authors who feel that the invasive nature of SRF studies and the resultant complication rate (major—3 to 5%, minor—30%)[39,41] and the high false negative rate for bilateral disease, makes split renal function studies a poor diagnostic modality for renovascular hypertension. However, the ability to identify patients who are candidates for renal revascularization to preserve or retrieve renal function, rather than nephrectomy, makes this an important tool in choosing the most beneficial operative approach once the diagnosis of RVH has been made.

Renin Measurements

The delineation of the role of the renin-angiotensin system in the control of blood pressure has resulted in the use of renin measurements to identify patients with renovascular hypertension and to predict operative curability. Although the hypersecretion of renin in response to decreased renal perfusion should be diagnostic of curable RVH it has become increasingly clear that the relationship between renin activity elevation and hypertension is not a simple one. Currently, renin determinations are performed in one of three ways: (1) peripheral plasma renin activity (PRA), (2) renal vein renin ratios (RVRR), and (3) renal vein renin/systemic renin indices (RSRI). Accurate renin measurements pose several significant problems. First, patient preparation is critical. All antihypertensive medications must be stopped for a period of 2 weeks, which is not feasible in many patients. The sodium profile is important and mild salt depletion is necessary prior to renin sampling;

changes in posture and acute reductions in blood pressure also influence renin measurements. In addition, there are several variations in technique of specimen sampling and methodology that result in varying data and interpretation criteria. Many investigators ascribe the different results reported in the literature to these difficulties with renin measurement. While this is meant to reassure the physician of the validity of the test, it makes the comparison of results difficult and the problem of accurate renin measurement remains unsolved.

Peripheral PRA is felt by some to be elevated in most patients with RVH.[42,43] However a literature review reported only a 44% incidence of elevated PRA among RVH patients[44] and Grim et al noted only a 27% incidence in his patient group.[26] In addition, 15% of patients with essential hypertension have high peripheral PRA.[45] Also, in the setting of bilateral renal artery disease an elevated peripheral plasma renin activity will not identify the responsible lesion. These observations, plus the difficulty in performing accurate renin measurements, makes peripheral PRA measurement a poor diagnostic test for renovascular hypertension. The authors do not use this modality for diagnosis or prognosis of operative result.

To improve the sensitivity of PRA some investigators now combine it with the saralasin infusion test. If PRA is a static test, saralasin infusion is then a functional test of the extent to which the renin-angiotensin system contributes to the patient's hypertension. Using this competitive inhibition of angiotensin II to induce a blood pressure drop, several groups of investigators have reported false negative and false positive rates of 5 to 8%.[46-51] However, others report false negative rates of 40 to 50%.[26,52] The lower sensitivities (higher false negative rates) were observed in studies that used blood pressure improvement following surgical revascularization as the "gold standard" for diagnosing renovascular hypertension. In contrast, the higher sensitivities occurred in studies using renal vein renin ratios or peripheral PRA to diagnose RVH. Finally, both groups have reported a 15 to 25% depressor response in patients with essential hypertension.[26,48,49] Thus, the collective data from these studies and from a subsequent cooperative study[53] demonstrate a sensitivity of 65% to 75%, with a false positive rate of 15%. These results are not much different from the sensitivity of hypertensive IVP[26,27,54] and indicate significant limitations in the use of saralasin infusion to diagnose RVH or to predict operative curability.

A second approach to the use of renin measurements is the determination of renal vein renin ratios (RVRR), comparing the ischemic with the normal kidney. Typically a ratio exceeding 1.5 : 1 is considered positive. Although the cure rate of patients with a positive test approaches 95%, the false negative rate is impressive. Russell reported 35% of patients with negative RVRR were cured or improved by operation.[55] Dean and Foster reported a 21% false negative rate;[56] Marks and Maxwell showed that 57% of 155 patients with non-lateralizing RVRR were cured or improved by revascularization[57] and Foster noted failure to lateralize in 35% of patients with RVH.[29] In addition, Stanley noted no difference between the RVRR of cured patients and improved patients in a group of 85 patients who were revascularized[58] and that overall 16% of patients who benefitted from operation had a RVRR of less than 1.5.[59] He concluded that the RVRR needs to be in excess of 1.89 to diagnose excessive renin secretion and is a poor indicator of the revascularization response. Stanley's group has found the renal vein renin to systemic renin index (RSRI) to be a more reliable prognosticator of operative response.[58] The ischemic kidney RSRI was significantly greater than the contra-lateral kidney RSRI in both cured and improved patient groups but it was the degree of contralateral suppression of renin production (RSRI of the "normal" kidney) that discriminated between patients who were subsequently cured and those who were only improved by revascularization.

The authors emphasize that elevation of renin activity does not imply that the renin-angiotensin system is the sole mediator of the patient's hypertension. Con-versely, the high false negative rate of renin determinations either implies that the methodology of renin measurement is too insensitive or that there is a non-renin dependent form of renovascular hypertension that may exist in 15–20% of patients.[50,52,60]

At the present time then, the role of renin measurement in the evaluation of renal ischemia can be summarized as follows: In the setting of unilateral disease when there is an elevated peripheral plasma renin activity, contralateral suppression of renin production, and lateralization of increased renin production to the ischemic kidney (RVRR > 1.5 : 1 or RSRI > 0.48) there is a reasonable likelihood that reno-vascular hypertension is present and a beneficial response from revascularization is probable. However, if the test is negative there is still a significant possibility that RVH is present and that the patient will benefit from surgical correction of the appropriate renal artery lesion. Combining test modalities increases the sensitivity but does not eliminate false negative results. Bilateral disease significantly reduces the diagnostic accuracy and prognostic reliability of all of these modalities. For these reasons, the authors do not base the decision for or against operation on these test results. Given the appropriate clinical setting, such as recent onset of moderate to severe hypertension, sudden deterioration of previously controlled hypertension, deterioration of renal function in a hypertensive patient, a mid-abdominal systolic/diastolic bruit, and an appropriate renal artery lesion, renal revascularization would be recommended.

Angiography

Aortorenal angiography continues to be the definitive study in the evaluation of renovascular hypertension. It provides accurate and reliable diagnosis of the pre-sence of any renal artery disease, as well as the extent of the disease and its morpho-logic characteristics. Aortography is necessary to detect juxtarenal aortic atherosclerosis, while selective renal artery injections are required to assess the renal artery branches and the intraparenchymal vessels. The disadvantages of convention-al arteriography are two-fold. First, it is an invasive test requiring hospitalization, and exposes patients to the risks of arterial cannulation and contrast-related com-plications. Secondly, it diagnoses renovascular disease, not renovascular hyper-tension, and when renal revascularization is based solely on the finding of a renal artery stenosis, less than 50% of patients will have a reduction in blood pressure.[39] Thus, although the sensitivity of angiography in detecting RVH is nearly 100%, its specificity (false positive rate) is only 50%.

Nonetheless we use the patient's clinical setting and the arteriographic findings to determine the patient's operative candidacy. The presence of the clinical features discussed earlier greatly increases the specificity of angiography, and allows for sel-ection of appropriate patients for study. This approach also prevents missing a significant renal artery lesion in a patient without the clinical features of classic RVH, or with a false negative IVP, renal scan or renin measurement. Data obtained from other tests for renal ischemia, performed prior to angiography, is considered supportive but not definitive. If the clinical setting is appropriate, the patient's operative risk acceptable, and if the patient is willing to undergo surgery when renal artery disease is found, then angiography will be recommended.

Recent progress in digital imaging techniques has prompted the use of venous digital subtraction angiography (DSA) as both a screening test and the definitive test for renovascular hypertension.[61-63] This approach is attractive since venous DSA can be performed as an outpatient, is almost non-invasive, requires no special patient preparation, and is economical. However, DSA is not as good as conventional angiography in the assessment of the size of a lesion, in depicting small collateral vessels and in visualizing the renal parenchymal circulation. In spite of these disadvantages, DSA is increasingly used as the definitive imaging modality in the assessment of a hypertensive patient. The benefit of this is that fewer significant lesions will be overlooked because of concerns about the risk of angiography. The challenge will still be the proper selection of these patients for revascularization.

RESULTS OF OPERATIVE TREATMENT

The clinical results of surgical treatment of renovascular hypertension in patients selected by using the assessment protocol discussed above have been encouraging (Table 19-4). Among patients treated for fibromuscular disease 98% were cured or improved with no operative mortality. Late assessment of treatment results in 39 patients of this study group, evaluated more than 5 years postoperatively showed continued cure or improvement of hypertension in all patients. Renal artery reconstruction for renal atherosclerosis was associated with a slightly higher mortality (2.0%), but we have observed, as have others, a steady decline in operative mortality, attributable to improved surgical techniques and anesthetic management. Cure or control of hypertension was achieved in 80% of these patients (80 of 105), the higher incidence of failures probably resulting from operation on some patients with non-renovascular hypertension or combined essential and renovascular hypertension. Finally, patients with diffuse, generalized atherosclerosis who required combined aortorenal reconstruction have the highest operative mortality (9.0%), but the beneficial effect on blood pressure control was similar, with 84% of patients cured

Table 19-4
UCSF Results of Surgical Treatment of Renovascular Hypertension
Blood Pressure Control

Renal Artery Pathology	Number of Patients	Treatment Result (%)			Operative Mortality (%)
		Cured	Improved	Failed	
Fibromuscular disease	77	66	32	2	0
Renal atherosclerosis	105	44	36	19	2.0
Renal and aortic atherosclerosis	90	84		16	9.0

or improved and a 16% failure rate. Of 74 patients evaluated to determine late hypertension status, 85% remained cured or improved and 15% were unchanged from their preoperative status. These results are comparable to the treatment results obtained at other centers with a significant experience in the surgical treatment of renovascular hypertension (Tables 19-5 and 19-6).

The patient group with generalized atherosclerosis who underwent combined aortorenal reconstruction were also evaluated to determine the effect of reconstruction on renal function, both acutely and at late follow-up evaluation (Table 19-7). At discharge 73% of patients had normal or improved renal function. At late follow-up 98% of patients had the same or better renal function than prior to surgery. Thus, during a mean 3 year follow-up period, only 1 of 74 patients experienced significant renal function deterioration. This is in contrast to the course of patients treated medically as reported both in Hunt's study comparing medical and surgical treatment of RVH,[7] and in the preliminary data from the Vanderbilt cooperative study.[10]

Table 19-5
Results of Surgical Treatment of Renovascular Hypertension
Fibromuscular Dysplasia[25]

Study	Number of Patients	Treatment Result (%)			Operative Mortality (%)
		Cured	Improved	Failed	
Stanley et al	144	55.0	39.0	6.0	0
Lawrie et al	113	43.0	24.0	33.0	0
Hunt & Strong	63	66.0	24.0	10.0	?
Foster et al	44	72.0	24.0	4.0	2.3

Table 19-6
Results of Surgical Treatment of Renovascular Hypertension
Atherosclerosis[25]

Study	Number of Patients	Treatment Result (%)			Operative Mortality (%)
		Cured	Improved	Failed	
Lawrie et al	360	34	31	35	2.5
Stanley et al	135	29	52	19	4.4
Novick et al	78	40	51	9	2.0
Foster et al	63	50	45	5	9.0
Lankford et al	52	31	61	8	5.8

Table 19-7
UCSF Results of Surgical Treatment of Renovascular
Hypertension Preservation of Renal Function

	Normal/Improved	Unchanged	Worse
Discharge	60	19	3
	(73%)	(23%)	(4%)
Late Follow-up	49	24	1
	(66%)	(32%)	(2%)

SUMMARY

The assessment of renal ischemia remains a difficult clinical problem. Although the pathophysiology of renovascular hypertension is now more clearly defined, knowledge of these mechanisms has not been easily translated into accurate clinical modalities for the diagnosis of RVH and identification of operative candidates. We continue to use primarily the patient's clinical history and the results of aortorenal angiography to determine if the renal artery lesion is reconstructable and if the patient is likely to benefit from the operative repair. Although positive results of tests used to assess renal ischemia identify patients with a high likelihood of a good blood pressure response following revascularization, a negative test should not be used to exclude the patient from consideration of surgical treatment. Variations in patient preparation, test methodology, data collection and result interpretation make the assessment of renal ischemia too insensitive to be the sole basis of a decision for therapy. Advances in anesthetic management have reduced the patient group whose operative risk would previously have precluded surgery. Operative technical advances have greatly increased patency rates, thus expanding the spectrum of lesions that are anatomically appropriate for reconstruction. Thus, if the clinical setting is appropriate, the renal artery lesion technically reconstructable and the operative risk acceptable, revascularization should be undertaken.

The additional consideration of renal function preservation suggests that even some "asymptomatic" renal artery stenoses, especially those observed to progress over time, will require correction, to prevent loss of renal mass and function. In fact, the presence of any hemodynamically significant renal artery lesion, whether clinically silent or associated with either renovascular or essential hypertension, warrants serious consideration of reconstruction to prevent renal function deterioration, even if no effect on hypertension is anticipated. The ability to detect non-invasively a reduction in blood flow across such a lesion may greatly aid the selection of patients for operation. Magnetic resonance imaging and Doppler ultrasound studies both are promising modalities for the non-invasive diagnosis of abnormal renal blood flow. For the present, continued study of the long-term effects of medical and surgical treatment of renovascular hypertension is mandatory in order to define the optimal role of each modality in the management of this varied and challenging disease.

ACKNOWLEDGEMENT

This work has been supported in part by the Pacific Vascular Research Foundation, San Francisco, California.

REFERENCES

1. Butler AM: Chronic pyelonephritis and arterial hypertension. J Clin Invest 16:889, 1937
2. Wollenweber J, Sheps SG, Davis GD: Clinical course of atherosclerotic renovascular disease. Am J Cardiol 21:60, 1968
3. Schreiber MJ, Novick AC, Pohl MA: The natural history of atherosclerotic and fibrous renal artery disease. Kidney Int 19:175, 1981

4. Stewart BH, Dustan HP, Kisen WS, et al: Correlation of angiography and natural history in evaluation of patients with renovascular hypertension. J Urol 104:231, 1970

5. Meany TF, Dustan HP, McCormack LJ: Natural history of renal arterial disease. Radiology 91:881, 1968

6. Brewster DC, Buth J, Darling RC, et al: Combined aortic and renal artery reconstruction. Amer J Surg 131:457, 1976

7. Hunt JC, Sheps SG, Harrison EG Jr, et al: Renal and renovascular hypertension. A reasoned approach to diagnosis and management. Arch Int Med 133:988, 1974

8. Dean RH, Kieffer RW, Smith BM, et al: Renovascular hypertension. Anatomic and renal function changes during drug therapy. Arch Surg 116:1408, 1981

9. Ying CY, Tifft CP, Gavras H, et al: Renal revascularization in the azotemic hypertensive patient resistant to therapy. N Engl J Med 311:1070, 1984

10. Dean RH, Hollifield JW, Oates JA: Medical versus surgical treatment of renovascular hypertension. In Stanley JC, Ernst CB, Fry WJ (eds): Renovascular Hypertension. Philadelphia, W. B. Saunders Co, 1984, p 354

11. Hricik DE, Browning PJ, Kapelman R, et al: Captopril-induced functional renal insufficiency in patients with bilateral renal-artery stenoses or renal-artery stenosis in a solitary kidney. N Engl J Med 308:373, 1983

12. Curtiss JJ, Luke RG, Whelchel JD, et al: Inhibition of angiotensin-converting enzyme in renal transplant recipients with hypertension. N Engl J Med 308:377, 1983

13. Dustan HP, Humphries AW, deWolfe VG, et al: Normal arterial pressure in patients with renal arterial stenosis. JAMA 187:138, 1964

14. Holley KE, Hunt JC, Brown AL, et al: Renal artery stenosis. Am J Med 37:14, 1964

15. Hunt JC, Strong CG: Renovascular hypertension. Mechanisms, natural history and treatment. Am J Cardiol 32:562, 1973

16. Gifford RW Jr: Epidemiology and clinical manifestations of renovascular hypertension. In Stanley JC, Ernst CB, Fry WJ (eds): Renovascular Hypertension. Philadelphia, W. B. Saunders Co, 1984, p 77

17. Eyler WR, Clark MD, Garman JE, et al: Angiography of the renal areas including a comparative study of renal artery stenosis in patients with and without hypertension. Radiology 78:879, 1962

18. Franklin SS, Young JD Jr, Maxwell MH, et al: Operative morbidity and mortality in renovascular disease. JAMA 231:1148, 1975

19. Dean RH, Oates JA, Wilson JP, et al: Bilateral renal artery stenosis and renovascular hypertension. Surgery 81:53, 1977

20. Novick AC, Straffon RA, Stewart BH, et al: Diminished operative morbidity and mortality in renal revascularization. JAMA 246:749, 1981

21. Ernst CB, Stanley JC, Marshall FF, et al: Renal revascularization for arteriosclerotic renovascular hypertension: Prognostic implications of focal renal arterial vs. overt generalized arteriosclerosis. Surgery 73:859, 1973

22. Shahian DM, Najafi H, Javid H, et al: Simultaneous aortic and renal artery reconstruction. Arch Surg 115:1491, 1980

23. Brewster DC, Buth J, Darling RC, et al: Combined aortic and renal artery reconstruction. Amer J Surg 131:457, 1976

24. Stoney RJ, Skioldebrand CG, Qvarfordt PG, et al: Juxtarenal aortic atherosclerosis: Surgical experience and function result. Ann Surg 200:345, 1984

25. Stanley JC, Ernst CB, Fry WJ: Surgical treatment of renovascular hypertension: Results in specific patient subgroups. In Stanely JC, Ernst CB, Fry WJ (eds): Renovascular Hypertension. Philadelphia, W. B. Saunders Co, 1984, p 363

26. Grim CE, Luft FC, Weinberger MH, et al: Sensitivity and specificity of screening tests for renal vascular hypertension. Ann Int Med 91:617, 1979

27. Bookstein JJ, Abrams HL, Buenger RE, et al: Radiologic aspects of renovascular hyper-

tension: Part 2. The role of urography in unilateral renovascular disease. JAMA 220: 1225, 1972

28. Maxwell MH, Bleifer RH, Franklin SS, et al: Cooperative study of renovascular hypertension: demographic analysis of the study. JAMA 220:1195, 1972

29. Foster JH, Dean RH, Pinkerton JA, et al: Ten years experience with the surgical management of renovascular hypertension. Ann Surg 177:755, 1973

30. Kaufmann JJ, Marks LS, Maxwell MH: Renovascular hypertension—1979. Surg Ann 11:313, 1979

31. Novick AC, Stewart BH: The surgical treatment of renovascular hypertension. Curr Probl Surg 16:8, 1979

32. Bookstein JJ, Maxwell MH, Abrams HL, et al: Cooperative study of radiologic aspects of renovascular hypertension. Bilateral renovascular disease. JAMA 237:1706, 1977

33. Bailey SM, Evans DW, Fleming HA: Intravenous urography in the investigation of hypertension. Lancet 2:57, 1975

34. Lewis PJ, Bulpitt CJ, Sherwood T, et al: Routine intravenous urography in the investigation of hypertension. J Chron Dis 29:785, 1976

35. Thornbury JR, Stanley JC, Fryback DG: Hypertensive urogram: a nondiscriminatory test for renovascular hypertension. Am J Roentgenol 138:43, 1982

36. Blaufox MD: Isotopic renography in renovascular hypertension—commentary. In Stanley JC, Ernst CB, Fry WJ (eds): Renovascular Hypertension. Philadelphia, W. B. Saunders Co, 1984, p 133

37. Howard JE, Connor TB: Hypertension produced by unilateral renal disease. Arch Int Med 109:8, 1962

38. Stamey TA, Nudelman IJ, Good PH, et al: Functional characteristics of renovascular hypertension. Medicine 40:347, 1961

39. Dean RH, Rhamy RK: Split renal function studies in renovascular hypertension. In Stanley JC, Ernst CB, Fry WJ (eds): Renovascular Hypertension. Philadelphia, W. B. Saunders Co, 1984, p 135

40. Dean RH, Lawson JD, Hollifield JW, et al: Revascularization of the poorly functioning kidney. Surgery 85:44, 1979

41. Dahl DS, O'Connor VJ Jr, Walker CD, et al: The morbidity of differential renal function studies: Analysis of 271 studies. JAMA 202:857, 1967

42. Vaughan ED Jr, Buhler FR, Laragh JH, et al: Renovascular hypertension: Renin measurements to indicate hypersecretion and contralateral suppression, estimate renal plasma flow, and score for surgical curability. Am J Med 55:402, 1973

43. Vaughan ED Jr, Carey RM, Ayers CR, et al: A physiologic definition of blood pressure response to renal revascularization in patients with renovascular hypertension. Kidney Int 15:S83, 1979

44. Marks LS, Maxwell MH: Renal vein renin value and limitations in the prediction of operative results. Urol Clin North Am 2:311, 1975

45. Vaughan ED Jr: Peripheral and renal vein renin activity in renovascular hypertension. In Stanley JC, Ernst CB, Fry WJ (eds): Renovascular Hypertension. Philadelphia, W. B. Saunders Co, 1984, p 146

46. Streeten DHP, Anderson GH, Freiberg JM, et al: Use of an angiotensin II antagonist (saralasin) in the recognition of "angiotensinogenic" hypertension. N Engl J Med 292:657, 1975

47. Baer L, Parra-Carrillo JZ, Radichevich I, et al: Detection of renovascular hypertension with angiotensin II blockade. Ann Int Med 86:257, 1977

48. Wilson HM, Wilson JP, Slaton PE, et al: Saralasin infusion in the recognition of renovascular hypertension. Ann Int Med 87:36, 1977

49. Marks LS, Maxwell MH, Kaufman JJ: Renin, sodium and vasodepressor response to saralasin in renovascular and essential hypertension. Ann Int Med 87:176, 1977

50. Streeten DHP, Anderson GH: Angiotensin antagonists and angiotensin-converting enzyme inhibitors in renovascular hypertension. In Stanley JC, Ernst CB, Fry WJ (eds): Renovascular Hypertension. Philadelphia, W. B. Saunders Co, 1984, p 161

51. Keenan RE, Horne ML, Conklin VM: Angiotensin II blockade. N Engl J Med 297:52, 1977

52. Tucker RM, Strong CG, Brennan LA Jr: Renovascular hypertension. Relationship of surgical curability to renin-angiotensin activity. Mayo Clin Proc 53:373, 1978

53. Horne ML, Conklin VM, Keenan RE: Angiotensin II profiling with saralasin: summary of Eaton Collaborative Study. Kidney Int 15:S115, 1978

54. Krakoff LR, Roberior RB, Gorkin JU, et al: Saralasin infusion in screening patients for renovascular hypertension. Am J Cardiol 45:609, 1980

55. Russell RP: Renal hypertension. Surg Clin North Am 54:349, 1974

56. Dean RH, Foster JH: Criteria for the diagnosis of renovascular hypertension. Surgery 74:926, 1973

57. Marks LS, Maxwell MH, Varady PD, et al: Renovascular hypertension: does the renal vein renin ratio predict operative results? J Urol 115:365, 1976

58. Stanley JC, Gewertz BL, Fry WJ: Renal: systemic renin indices and renal vein renin ratios as prognostic indicators in remedial renovascular hypertension. J Surg Res 20:149, 1976

59. Stanley JC, Whitehouse WM Jr, Graham LM, et al: Operative therapy of renovascular hypertension. Br J Surg 69(Suppl):S63, 1982

60. Marks LS, Maxwell MH, Kaufman JJ: Non-renin-mediated renovascular hypertension: a new syndrome? Lancet 1:615, 1977

61. Hillman BJ, Ovitt TW, Capp MP, et al: The potential impact of digital video subtraction angiography on screening for renovascular hypertension. Radiology 142:577, 1982

62. Hillman BJ, Ovitt TW, Nudelman S, et al: Digital video subtraction angiography of renovascular abnormalities. Radiology 139:377, 1981

63. Osborne RW Jr, Goldstone J, Hillman BJ, et al: Digital-video subtraction angiography: Screening technique for renovascular hypertension. Surgery 90:832, 1981

PART IV

Vascular and Microvascular Reconstruction

Ken A. Myers

20

Preoperative Assessment of Lower Limb Ischaemia

Since the first vascular laboratories were established 20 years ago, many techniques have been introduced to study the morphologic and haemodynamic changes in peripheral arterial disease. This review describes various techniques, discusses their validity and limitations, and indicates how they can help select the best management for lower limb ischaemia.

Problems involved in making clinical decisions are illustrated by the outcome of 1500 operations performed in our unit for chronic lower limb ischaemia. Surviving patients were followed up for at least one year to determine cumulative graft patency and limb salvage rates. In addition, the Doppler ankle pressure index was measured before and again 4–6 weeks after reconstruction in many patients to assess the early response to surgery. Until recently, whether to operate and what procedure to perform were decided on the clinical features and arteriogram alone, with no special investigations other than Doppler ankle pressure index. The clinical response and ankle pressure index changes were used to evaluate how good or bad were these decisions and whether other investigations might improve clinical decision-making.

Specific investigations help to make specific decisions—whether to advise conservative treatment, transluminal dilation, arterial reconstruction, sympathectomy or amputation, and how best to perform these procedures. The most useful investigations should be those that are most accurate; in practice, those that are least expensive and most easily performed are most widely used. It helps if the surgeon understands the investigation, but some recent techniques sorely try this ability. Different groups dispute which test is best and what is an "abnormal" result. It is not surprising, then, that many surgeons rely solely on their clinical judgement, but unfortunately this can be unreliable.

Our clinical evidence suggests that there are some groups of patients, particularly claudicants with isolated aorto-iliac disease or superficial femoral occlusion alone, who are managed very well using clinical assessment alone, and other groups, particularly those with disease at multiple levels, for whom special investigations should be most helpful.

DIAGNOSTIC TECHNIQUES AND ASSESSMENT
PROCEDURES IN VASCULAR SURGERY

© 1985 Grune & Stratton
ISBN 0-8089-1721-8 All rights reserved

EVALUATION OF SPECIAL INVESTIGATIONS

Statistical correlation between a new investigation and a standard of reference does not necessarily establish whether the new test helps clinical decision-making. Ideally, a test should have two values that are clearly "normal" and "abnormal." If most results fall between these values, then the test will rarely help and should be discarded.

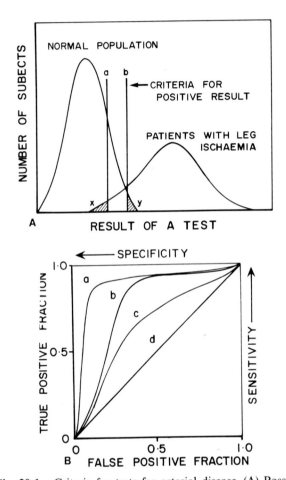

Fig. 20-1. Criteria for tests for arterial disease. (A) Possible distribution of tests. a)—an appropriate criterion for a patient with critical ischaemia; there is a small number of false negatives (x). b)—an appropriate criterion for claudicants; there is a small number of false positives (y). (B) Receiver operating characteristic curves constructed from a range of criteria. a)—an excellent test. b)—a test with good sensitivity above a certain criterion but with poor specificity, as with many tests for aorto-iliac disease in the presence of a superficial femoral occlusion. c)—a test that is inferior to a) because of poor sensitivity and specificity. d)—a theoretical level at which the test has no relation to the disease.

In practice, the utility of a new investigation is best tested by establishing a single criterion, on either side of which the result is probably normal or abnormal. This can determine the sensitivity and specificity of the new technique by comparing it with an old "reliable" technique which then acts as a standard of reference. The criterion can be set at any level, but the most appropriate level depends on "penalty" paid for a false result.[1] For example, a test might be intended to detect "significant" aorto-iliac disease. If the patient has critical ischaemia, it might be as well to set the criterion nearer to normal values to increase the sensitivity of the test; the positive predictive value may be low but the penalty for rejecting an effective operation because of a false negative result might be amputation. For a claudicant, on the other hand, perhaps the criterion should be set further from normal values to increase specificity; the positive predictive value is then high and false negatives are not too much of a worry, for otherwise the penalty might be a major operation that proves to be ineffective and unecessary (Fig. 20-1A).

The optimal criterion level can be selected by plotting several threshold values for sensitivity and specificity to construct a receiver operating characteristic (ROC) curve[2] (Fig. 20-1B). This also must be related to the clinical circumstances. For example, the optimal criterion from ROC curves for Doppler pulse wave studies in aorto-iliac disease depends on whether the superficial femoral artery is patent or occuluded.[3,4]

Unfortunately, the standard of reference may itself be difficult to validate. A study may finish up comparing one intangible with another. For example, Doppler techniques to assess aorto-iliac disease might be compared with arteriographic grading[3,5,6] or intra-arterial pressure studies[4,7-9] before operation, or with change in ankle pressure after operation,[5,10] but these may not truly reflect disease nor relate to the symptomatic improvement (which is impossible to measure accurately).

CLINICAL EVALUATION

A surgeon must start by relying on the history and examination to determine the presence, site, and severity of disease, and the site of occlusion should be confirmed by arteriography if intervention is contemplated. In many patients, these are adequate for decision-making but in others, particularly patients with disease at multiple sites, clinical assessment is unreliable.

Early disease can go unnoticed. Over 450 diabetics were investigated by noninvasive pressure studies.[11] More than one-half were considered to have no evidence of lower limb ischaemia from the history and physical examination. Of these, one-third who were asymptomatic and one-fifth considered to have a normal physical examination in fact had appreciable arterial disease. A similar study of 100 asymptomatic "second legs" in patients with unilateral claudication[12] showed that more than one-half had lower limb ischaemia, yet less than one-third of these had abnormal physical signs. Presumably few, if any, of these patients had disease severe enough to warrant intervention.

If a patient has thigh or buttock claudication, then it is likely that there is significant aorto-iliac disease, although thigh claudication can be caused by profunda stenosis alone and buttock claudication by internal iliac disease. However, most patients with aorto-iliac disease do not have proximal claudication; of a group of patients who gained clinical benefit from aorto-femoral bypass, 65% had calf claudication alone.[13]

A committee convened to define critical ischaemia[14] felt that surgeons' clinical assessment of rest pain and the relation between gangrene and ischaemia were often too lax, necessitating an objective criterion. If the pulse is absent then it is reasonable to assume that the occlusion above this level is significant. It is when the pulse is apparently reduced that its significance is most difficult to assess. While it is important to feel the pulse pressure and to listen for a bruit, both at rest and with exercise, these can be unreliable. A normal pulse at rest does not exclude proximal disease; of a group of patients who gained clinical benefit from aorto-femoral bypass, 45% were considered to have normal femoral pulses.[13] We found considerable interobserver variability between six surgeons asked to classify the femoral and popliteal pulses as being normal, reduced, or absent.[15] A femoral bruit does not mean that there is significant aorto-iliac disease, as assessed by arteriography[16]; artery compression tests suggested that about two-thirds of femoral bruits are due to profunda femoris or proximal superficial femoral artery stenosis.

Conventional uniplanar arteriography is not accurate. Atheromatous plaques often are eccentric. In the iliac arteries, disease usually starts on the back wall and can be missed when viewed en face. Eleven observers were asked to classify disease into four grades from uniplanar arteriography,[17] and their agreement for the aorta, iliac, and profunda femoris arteries was not much better than that provided by chance. We found that the correlation between femoral and popliteal pulse assessment and the arteriographic grading was poor. Even when biplanar arteriography was compared with intraarterial pressure measurement to detect aorto-iliac disease,[18] the sensitivity was less than 70% and specificity less than 80%. Furthermore, in a critically ischaemic leg, arteries are poorly defined below the occlusion, so that even the best arteriogram is unreliable.

ALTERNATIVE INVESTIGATIONS TO SHOW MORPHOLOGY

Since conventional preoperative arteriography is not accurate and is also unpleasant, occasionally dangerous, time-consuming, and expensive, alternative techniques are being explored. As yet, none has been extensively used to assess lower limb ischaemia.

Digital Subtraction Angiography (DSA)

DSA to evaluate arteries to the legs can supplement or even supplant conventional arteriography.[19] It is safer, less painful, and cheaper, but each injection shows only a limited segment. Intravenous studies (IV DSA) defined the aorto-femoral segment as well as conventional arteriography in 90% of cases[20] and can detect recurrent stenosis after reconstruction or transluminal dilation (Fig. 20-2A). Intra-arterial studies (IA DSA) often demonstrate distal arteries better than does conventional arteriography,[19] particularly in the critically ischaemic leg (Fig. 20-2B). A fine catheter is used and less contrast medium is required.

Intra-operative Arteriography

A static arteriogram can be obtained by injecting the common femoral artery[21] or cannulating the popliteal or tibial arteries[22] at the start of an operation. This defines arteries distal to a femoro-popliteal occlusion better than conventional arteriography. It reveals arteries that can be used for a bypass graft, and shows whether the pedal arch is patent, which in turn influences long-term femoro-tibial graft patency.[23]

Ultrasound Techniques

Doppler ultrasound examination can reveal patent common femoral or profunda femoris arteries below an occluded aorta, patent tibial arteries in the leg, the peroneal artery over its anterior lateral malleolar branch, and the pedal arch over the first metatarsal space.[24] The arteries can be displayed by B-mode ultrasound, and this can be linked to pulsed range-gated Doppler ultrasound with spectral analysis to sample points within the arteries. This combination comprises the "Duplex scan," which can be used to assess the common femoral, profunda femoris, and popliteal arteries.

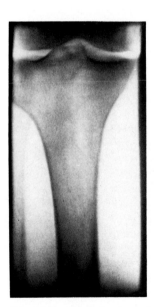
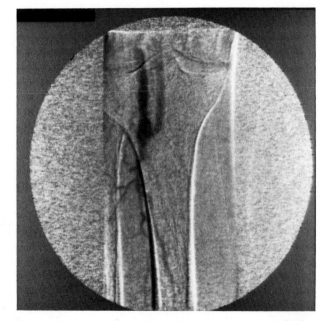

Fig. 20-2. Digital subtraction angiogram. (A) An intravenous study showing a stenosis that has developed at the lower end of a femoro-popliteal vein graft with poor run-off. (B) An intra-arterial study to show good definition of tibial arteries below a femoro-popliteal occlusion causing critical ischaemia.

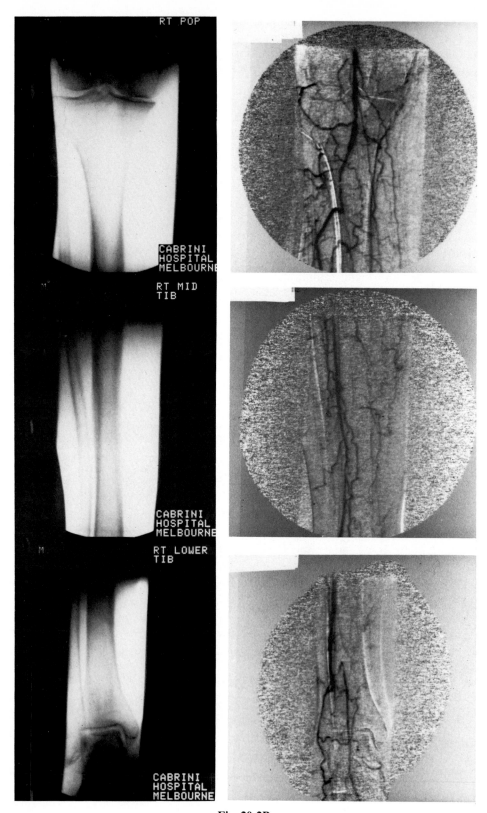

Fig. 20-2B

INVESTIGATIONS TO SHOW HAEMODYNAMIC CHANGES

Although morphologic studies show whether an artery is stenosed or occluded, they do not show how much this restricts blood flow.

Intra-arterial Pressure Studies

Theoretically, the systolic pressure difference between two points in an artery is proportional to flow reduction caused by a stenosis in the segment.[25] However, it is very difficult to prove that this is true in clinical practice. The pressure difference may only be revealed by manouevres that simulate exercise, such as the injection of Papaverine[8] or induction of reactive hyperaemia.[26] Femoral artery pressure studies can disclose aorto-iliac disease. Needles inserted into each common femoral artery record pressures that can be compared to the brachial artery pressure, either before[8,25] or during operation. Multiple pressures can be measured through a catheter during arteriography, while withdrawing the catheter from the aorta to the common femoral level.[27] This better defines the relative effect of multiple stenoses. A 10 mm Hg difference at rest or 25 mm Hg difference during hyperaemia[9] or a femoral/arm index less than 0.7 or fall of this index by more than 15–20% with hyperaemia[8,27] have been taken to indicate significant aorto-iliac disease.

Intra-arterial pressure measurements have been compared with femoral pulse examination and arteriographic grading.[26] It was considered that either the pulse was diminished or the arteriogram showed moderate to severe disease in one-third of patients whose pressure studies were normal, and that the femoral pulse was normal and the arteriogram showed no more than mild disease in one-quarter of patients whose pressure studies were abnormal. It is hard to know which is the more reliable assessment.

Noninvasive Pressure Studies

The systolic pressure can be measured using a cuff placed on the thigh, calf, ankle, or toe, listening over tibial arteries with a Doppler probe[28] or using plethysmography.[29] The absolute pressure or leg/arm pressure index (PrI) is measured. The pressure can be obtained at rest and then at intervals following exercise, walking on the flat or on a treadmill, or using a foot pedal. Reactive hyperaemia tests are a poor substitute.[30]

Theoretically, pressure is reduced proportional to resistance from any stenoses or collaterals around occlusions above the cuff, but in practice there are several potential errors.[31] The systemic pressure can fluctuate and may differ in each arm. There is a cuff artefact due to the limb thickness. The calf arteries may be too rigid to be compressed, a problem in about 25% of diabetics.[32] Reactive hyperaemia occurs if the cuff is deflated slowly and this causes the measured pressure to be less than the true pressure. While the cuff is inflated above arterial pressure, flow is reduced and there is less pressure gradient across a resistance so that the first pressures recorded as the cuff is deflated tend to be higher than the true pressure.[25] These artefacts are greatest for thigh and least for toe pressure studies,[29] but the latter are influenced more by laboratory conditions.

Thigh Pressure Measurements

An arm to thigh pressure difference or reduced thigh pressure index (TPrI) should reflect aorto-iliac resistance and predict whether proximal arterial reconstruction or dilation will improve blood flow. Comparing the arm-thigh and thigh-ankle pressure differences should define the relative effect of proximal and distal disease.

Calf Pressure Measurements

This technique may help to predict whether a below-knee amputation is likely to heal—the absolute level is more helpful than a pressure index.[33] However, others found that calf pressure had no predictive value for amputation.[34]

Ankle Pressure Measurements

This test, developed by Yao,[28] is the study most widely used in most vascular laboratories. This test has a coefficient of variation less than 10%.[31] A change of more than 0.15 is considered significant.[35] APrI reliably distinguishes normal from diseased arteries, as judged by arteriography,[36] but does not relate well to symptoms nor site of disease (Fig. 20-3). An abnormal result does not indicate which patients require intervention nor what procedure to advise, but a normal result in the contralateral leg determines whether intervention is required for just one leg or both.[12] A preoperative measurement gives a baseline to assess the early and late response to intervention.[37]. APrI can be used as a standard of reference to validate new techniques.[5,10]

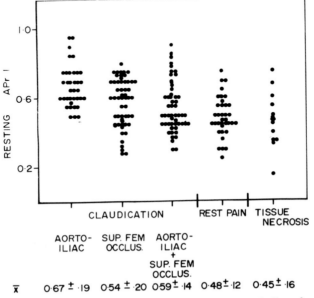

Fig. 20-3. Distribution of resting ankle pressure indices for claudicants, according to site and extent of disease, and for patients with critical ischaemia.

Toe Pressure Measurements

These appear to relate to symptoms better than does APrI. A toe systolic pressure less than 30 mm Hg is a reliable index for critical ischaemia.[23,29,38]

Doppler Pulse Wave form Analyses

The shape of the pulse wave signal can show whether the artery is diseased. The normal triphasic signal is lost and the systolic component becomes flatter and wider. Mathematical techniques can analyse the pulse wave components so as to measure these changes. Three techniques have been studied—pulsatility index, Laplace transform to provide a damping factor, and principal component analysis. These methods have been used particularly to detect aorto-iliac disease. The measurements are obtained at rest so that they must be sensitive enough to detect a stenosis that becomes significant only during exercise. Spectral analysis can show increased turbulence caused by scattering of sound into the centre of the tracings, and spectral broadening can be quantified, the velocity spectra ratios along the segment giving a "stenosis index."

Pulsatility Index (PI)

Femoral PI falls with increasing aorto-iliac stenosis. Some studies report that PI accurately detects significant aorto-iliac disease.[4,7] However, others show a poor diagnostic efficiency, particularly with combined aorto-iliac and superficial femoral disease.[5,6,9] One study reports that the optimal criterion is 7.6 if the superficial femoral artery is patent and 5.0 if it is occluded.[3] We studied PI in 80 patients.[39] The coefficient of variation was less than 10%. PI was independent of age, blood pressure, and risk factors for atherosclerosis, but usually was increased only if the artery diameter was reduced by more than 70%.

Laplace Damping Factor (LDF)

LDF rises with increasing arterial stenosis—the value ranges from 0 to 1.0. We studied 65 patients.[40] LDF had a coefficient of variation less than 10%. It was very sensitive for detecting preclinical disease related to risk factors for atherosclerosis. The mean value for normal subjects was 0.35 and the criterion for early clinical disease was approximately 0.60. Bench experiments suggested that LDF is independent of both distal stenosis and variations in artery wall compliance. The technique is convenient for clinical studies.[41]

Principal Component Analysis (PCA)

PCA seems to detect less severe iliac disease and to give better discrimination between grades of disease than PI or LDF, as gauged by comparison with intra-arterial pressure measurements, particularly in patients with a superficial femoral occlusion.[9]

Other Techniques

Skin temperature does not correlate well with flow. Transcutaneous oxygen tension correlates well with ischaemia. It can be used to follow the patient's course and to predict whether an amputation is likely to heal.[42,43] Isotope clearance following subdermal injection, using Xenon (Xe^{133}), Technicium (Tc^{99}), or Iodine (I^{125}) specifically measures skin capillary blood flow.[44] Histamine can be added to induce hyperaemia and an overlying cuff can then be inflated to measure skin perfusion pressure.[45] Isotope clearance has been used to demonstrate increased capillary blood flow after sympathectomy[46] and to predict whether amputation is likely to heal.[44,45]

ASSESSMENT FOR MANAGEMENT OF THE ASYMPTOMATIC LEG

For patients with unilateral claudication or critical ischaemia due to aorto-iliac disease, most surgeons perform aorto-bifemoral reconstruction. We measured APrI before and after such operations. It was considered that improvement had occurred if APrI rose by an arbitrary level of more than 0.15. This criterion for success is probably lenient. Nevertheless, only 30% of the "second legs" showed improvement (Fig. 20-4) suggesting that aorto-iliac disease did not cause or even contribute to ischaemia on the asymptomatic side in many patients. It now seems logical to use APrI and TPrI to exclude appreciable disease in the second leg. However, for increased sensitivity exercise resting is essential.[12] In such patients we now perform unilateral extraperitoneal ilio-femoral reconstruction whenever possible, for this should reduce surgical morbidity and mortality. Prophylactic reconstruction for these second legs might seem to be justified if they were destined soon to develop severe symptoms, but of 37 patients treated by unilateral reconstruction alone, only 4 later needed iliac reconstruction on the other side. However, if transperitoneal aortic reconstruction is required, it might as well be bilateral. A similar policy is appropriate for the second leg after femoro-popliteal bypass. The response to one

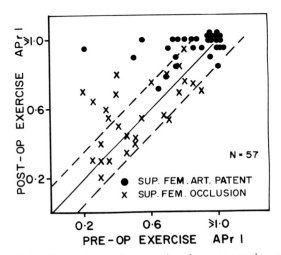

Fig. 20-4. Comparison of pre- and early postoperative exercise ankle pressure indices in the "second leg" of claudicants treated by aorto-femoral reconstruction. ●—patent superficial femoral artery. x—occluded superficial femoral artery. Only 30% showed increase of APrI by more than an arbitrary level of 0.15.

minute of exercise at 4 km/hr on a 10% slope was measured in 100 patients before femoro-popliteal bypass[12]; one-half had normal pressure response in the other leg at the time of bypass, although serial studies revealed that on-half of these became abnormal within three years.

ASSESSMENT OF PATIENTS WITH SEVERE INTERMITTENT CLAUDICATION

The decision that claudication is severe enough to warrant intervention depends on the patient's mental attitude, the general physical condition, and the extent of disease in the leg. Each patient's subjective assessment of claudication should be checked by measuring the distance, walking on a treadmill or on a level stretch in time to a metronome. Although the claudication distance is not highly reproducible[36], no other objective assessment helps to make the decision whether or not to advise intervention. APrI correlates poorly with walking distance.[31] If arterial dilation or reconstruction are to be performed, arteriography is required, but the best technique varies with the clinical circumstances. Our results suggest that haemodynamic studies may be helpful for patients with combined aorto-iliac and superficial femoral disease, but that clinical judgement alone is sufficient for patients with isolated aorto-iliac or superficial femoral disease.

Transluminal Dilatation (TLD)

TLD is a cost-effective alternative to reconstruction for limited disease and probably is the best treatment if arteriography shows a localised iliac stenosis or stenosis in a bypass graft, is good treatment for a single femoral stenosis, and is feasible for multiple stenoses or an occlusion less than 5 cm long in the superficial femoral artery. Late patency rates after TLD are only one-half of those for reconstruction, but since TLD enables surgery to be deferred or even avoided, it may be the preferred initial treatment in up to 40% of patients,[47] a level that depends on how far one is tempted to treat claudicants not sufficiently disabled to require reconstruction.

Increase in post-dilation APrI correlates well with intra-arterial pressure studies and the clinical response.[48] Technical success is not necessarily equivalent to clinical success; claudication persists and APrI remains abnormal in up to 40% of technically successful TLD's.[49,50]

Clinical suspicion that a lesion is suitable for TLD can be confirmed by DSA. In future, the Duplex scan may be found to detect suitable patients. Some surgeons rely on the radiologist's discretion to proceed to TLD at the time of conventional arteriography, but this makes for a longer and more risky procedure.

Arterial Reconstruction

If it is decided that reconstruction is required, it is necessary to localise the predominant lesion, demonstrate patent arteries above and below, and identify significant disease at other levels. This information is usually gained from conventional arteriography. However, the morphologic and haemodynamic studies described can give more precise information.

Aorto-Iliac Disease Alone

We performed 68 aorto-femoral reconstructions in claudicants with aorto-iliac disease and a patent superficial femoral artery. The patency rate at 2 years was over 90% (Fig. 20-5). Technical success almost invariably led to complete, lasting relief of symptoms.[51] It was rare for disease to progress elsewhere so as to require further surgery. Exercise APrI measured before and after aorto-femoral reconstruction for claudicants with aorto-iliac disease alone (Fig. 20-6A) showed the clinical assessment usually was accurate, for exercise APrI increased by more than 0.15 in every case. Thus, if disease is localised to the aorto-iliac segment, a claudicant can be assured of a good result.

Certainly, haemodynamic studies are very accurate in this group, but since clinical assessment is apparently reliable, it seems that these further investigations are not required for decision-making. Intra-arterial pressure studies can accurately predict the response to reconstruction.[8,26,27] Pressure measurements at operation can define the relative significance of iliac and profunda stenoses.[52] Disease in the aorto-iliac segment is accurately detected by TPrI[53] or Doppler pulse wave studies.[3,6,7,9] The specificity is higher than for patients with associated superficial femoral occlusion[4] so that there are few false positives.

The aorto-iliac lesion almost invariably ends above the common femoral or profunda femoris arteries and either will accept a bypass graft. It is tempting to define these by IV DSA alone. In the future it may be found that the Duplex scan is a good method to show whether the distal anastomosis should be onto the common femoral or profunda femoris arteries.

Femoro-Popliteal Disease Alone

We performed 124 femoro-popliteal bypass grafts for intermittent claudication. The patency rate at 2 years only 76% (Fig. 20-5). Further surgery was required for progressive proximal disease or stenosis in the graft or anastomoses in 41 patients

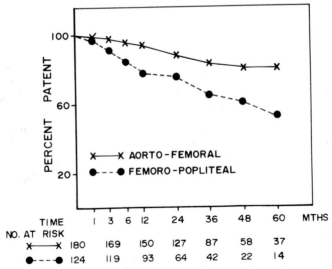

Fig. 20-5. Cumulative patency rates for aorto-femoral reconstruction and femoro-popliteal bypass for intermittent claudication.

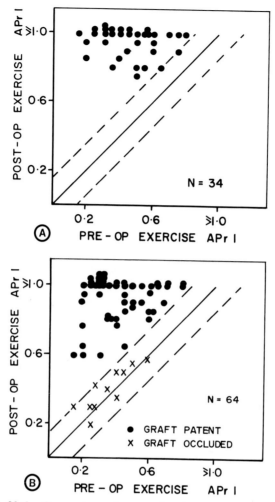

Fig. 20-6. Comparison of pre- and early postoperative exercise ankle pressure indices in claudicants; A—with aorto-iliac
disease alone, treated by aorto-femoral reconstruction, and
B—with superficial femoral occlusion alone, treated by
femoro-popliteal bypass. Almost all patients showed improved
APrI by more than an arbitrary level of 0.15 if the reconstruction was technically successful.

and 4 patients eventually required amputation. It is for these reasons that many
units are reluctant to perform femoro-popliteal bypass for claudication alone.
However, technical success almost invariably gave complete symptomatic relief and
increase in the exercise APrI by more than 0.15 (Figure 20-6B). If proximal disease
can be excluded, it would seem that haemodynamic studies have little further to
offer and that the simplest morphologic studies sufficient to define the anatomy are
all that is required.

The best site for the distal anastomosis can be shown by IA DSA or intraoperative arteriography. The run-off is also shown, although we found that this did
not influence long-term patency rates for femoro-popliteal bypass in claudicants.

It is possible that minor to moderate aorto-iliac disease that is not yet sufficient to reduce flow can progress and later compromise a femoro-popliteal bypass. Correcting these early lesions might improve long-term patency but combining aorto-iliac and femoro-popliteal reconstructions simply to protect distal bypass seems over-enthusiastic. IV DSA combined with TPrI or Doppler pulse wave studies help to exclude proximal disease.[53]

Aorto-Iliac Disease with Superficial Femoral Artery Occlusion

This is one of the most difficult problems in vascular surgery. Aorto-femoral reconstruction will improve claudication only if proximal resistance during exercise is appreciable compared to the collateral resistance around the distal occlusion. Many patients will be disappointed unless they fully accept the daunting proposition that proximal reconstruction may not suffice and that a secondary femoro-popliteal bypass may be necessary, perhaps on both sides. A policy to perform more extensive reconstruction at the one operation might be expected to increase morbidity and mortality, but a more conservative approach might lead to a higher incidence of failure and the risks from multiple operations.

We performed 180 aorto-femoral reconstructions for claudication in patients with combined proximal and distal disease. A femoro-popliteal bypass was added at the same time in only 5 patients, and a secondary femoro-popliteal bypass was used in only 4 more. At one year, almost 90% were patent (Fig. 20-5) yet only 75% of patients gained appreciable symptomatic improvement at this time.[51] Exercise APrI measurements before and after aorto-femoral reconstruction in claudicants who were shown on arteriography to have combined proximal and distal disease (Fig. 20-7A) showed that APrI increased by more than 0.15 in only 35% of legs. These results highlight the need to use newer techniques to identify appreciable proximal disease.

Although we try to define the two sites by DSA, frequently we need to resort to conventional arteriography. The arteriogram merely hints at the haemodynamic significance of proximal disease. Intraoperative pressure measurements suggest that the iliac or profunda femoris artery diameter needs to be decreased by up to 70% to reduce flow[52] although this may be less for multiple stenoses.

The femoral/brachial intra-arterial pressure index accurately predicted the response to surgery in 95% of legs, as judged by APrI, in one study,[8] and abnormal femoral artery pressure studies almost invariably predicted symptomatic relief from proximal reconstruction alone in another,[26] although clinical improvement apparently also occurred in about 45% of patients who had normal pressure studies before surgery.

Many interested groups have used various noninvasive techniques to show the importance of aorto-iliac disease. The studies appear to have been meticulous, yet the results are often widely divergent. The following summarizes several reports. Normal thigh pressure index reliably excluded proximal disease,[53] but abnormal TPrI or thigh/ankle pressure difference did not relate well to symptomatic improvement or postoperative increase in APrI after aorto-femoral bypass.[10] Reports comparing pulsatility index with intra-arterial pressure studies, selecting optimal criteria by ROC curves, revealed a sensitivity and specificity of more than 90% at an optimal PI of 5.4 in one study[4] but less than 70% at an optimal PI of 2.5 in another.[5] One group combined PI with intra-arterial pressure measurements to

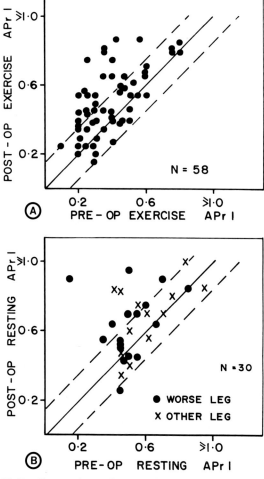

Fig. 20-7. Comparison of pre- and early postoperative ankle pressure indices in patients treated by aorto-femoral reconstruction for aorto-iliac disease combined with superficial femoral occlusion. (A) Exercise APrI in the worse leg of claudicants. (B) Resting APrI in the worse leg (●) and other leg (x) in patients with critical ischaemia. Only 35% and 40% respectively showed increase of APrI by more than an arbitrary level of 0.15.

improve specificity.[7] If the PI was more than 4, no pressure gradient was found at arteriography in any patient and it was safe to perform distal reconstruction alone. If the PI was less than 4 (about 70% of legs), there were abnormal pressure differences in about one-half, and these were treated by proximal reconstruction. Prospectively they advocate intra-arterial pressure studies only if PI is less than 4. Good correlation between the Laplace damping factor and arteriography for aorto-iliac disease has been reported[6] with a sensitivity and specificity more than 85% at an optimal criterion of 0.6, but others report that LDF gives no more information than PI as judged by arteriography[3] or intra-arterial pressure studies.[9] Principal component analysis has been said to give better results than either PI or LDF, as judged by intra-arterial pressure studies.[9]

Many surgeons would feel that more agreement is required before these techniques can be recommended for routine clinical use. However, our clinical results in this group give no cause for complacency and suggest that some form of objective assessment is required to improve clinical decision-making.

ASSESSMENT FOR TREATMENT OF CRITICAL ISCHAEMIA WITH DISEASE AT MULTIPLE LEVELS

In our experience, most patients with rest pain, ischaemic ulceration, or gangrene have a superficial femoral or popliteal artery occlusion, associated either with significant aorto-iliac disease or appreciable tibial artery disease, in about equal proportions. APrI less than 0.6 has been proposed to define critical ischaemia[14] and we found this to be a reasonable definition although many claudicants had APrI less than 0.6 (Fig. 20-3).

Arterial Reconstruction

Because disease is more extensive in patients with critical ischaemia than in claudicants, there is a dilemma. Investigation may disclose widespread disease in arteries to the legs, but the patient's general condition may not safely allow an extensive operation. The surgeon must decide whether to risk combined proximal and distal surgery, whether to hope that dealing with the proximal lesion alone will suffice, whether to ignore proximal disease and perform a distal reconstruction, or whether simply to advise primary amputation. Our primary amputation rate rose from 15% in the first half of this study to 21% in the second half. Ideally, investigations should not only help select the most appropriate procedure but should also indicate when attempted reconstruction is likely to be a lost cause. To date there have been few reports that address this problem. Patients with critical ischaemia are considerably more difficult to investigate than claudicants, but the penalties for wrong decisions are worse.

Aorto-Iliac Disease with Superficial Femoral Occlusion

For patients with critical ischaemia, we performed 232 proximal reconstructions. The procedure was usually technically successful, yet the operation failed to relieve rest pain or heal necrotic tissue, with the subsequent need for major amputation in spite of a patent graft, in about 10–15% (Fig. 20-8A). Proximal reconstruction alone may not increase flow at all; resting APrI measurements before and after aorto-femoral reconstruction for critical ischaemia showed an increase of more than 0.15 in only 40% of legs (Fig. 20-7B). Even if flow is increased, it may not be sufficient to heal tissues; postoperative increase of APrI does not correlate well with limb salvage.[10] Further, distal perfusion through thigh collaterals increases over several weeks[10] and this may be too slow for the patient with severe pain.

The limb salvage rate might have been improved by adding a femoro-popliteal bypass, but in fact combined reconstructions were rarely performed. We now believe that if morphologic or haemodynamic studies strongly suggest that the "second leg"

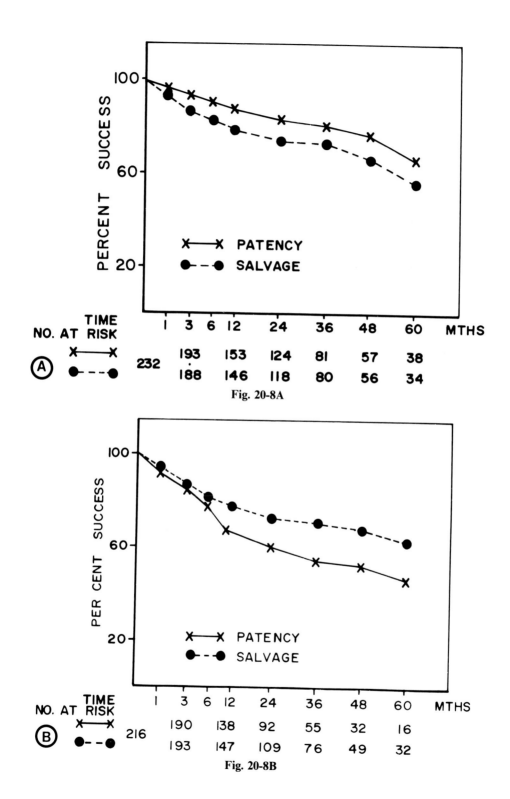

Fig. 20-8A

Fig. 20-8B

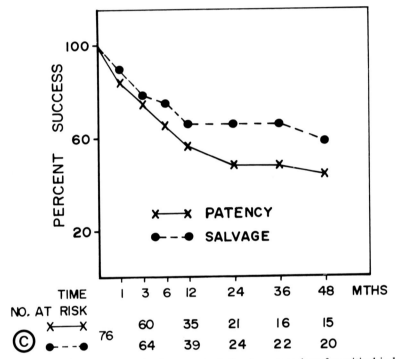

Fig. 20-8. Cumulative patency and salvage rates following operations for critical ischaemia. (A) Aorto-femoral reconstruction—the long-term salvage rate is approximately 10% worse than the patency rate. (B) Femoro-popliteal bypass—the early patency and salvage rates are identical but the long-term salvage rate is approximately 15% better than the patency rates. (C) Femoro-tibial bypass—the early patency and salvage rates are similar but the long-term salvage rate is approximately 20% better than the patency rate.

is not severely diseased and that it is technically impossible to limit proximal recon-struction to one side, this should more realistically allow simultaneous femoro-popliteal bypass. However, even if an aorto-bifemoral graft is required, failure to adequately increase flow should lead to early femoro-popliteal bypass before the chance to save the leg is lost.

It is in these patients that any arteriographic study is difficult to evaluate. Flow can be so slow that a patent profunda femoris artery may not be seen—it can be detected with the Doppler probe, perhaps by a Duplex scan, or occasionally by surgical exploration and operative arteriography. As yet, there is little information to show whether intra-arterial pressure studies or Doppler pulse wave analyses predict that proximal reconstruction alone is likely to be sufficient to heal a conser-vative distal amputation or whether combined proximal and distal reconstruction are required to avoid major amputation.

Superficial Femoral Artery Occlusion with Distal Disease

The popliteal artery distal to a superficial femoral occlusion may be patent, occluded, or left as an "isolated segment," and occlusions may extend into the tibial arteries for variable lengths. Whether the pedal arch is patent affects long-term graft patency.[23]

In contrast to proximal aorto-iliac reconstructions, a technically successful femoro-distal bypass usually leads to tissue healing unless the defect is too large to allow reasonable skin apposition. Resting APrI increased by more than 0.15 after technically successful femoro-distal bypass in most legs studied (Fig. 20-9). The more common reason for early failure in the study was graft thrombosis due to a poor runoff and this usually led to major amputation. We performed 216 femoro-popliteal bypass grafts and 76 femoro-tibial grafts for critical ischaemia; 15% and 25% respectively blocked within the first 3 months, usually with the need for ampu-

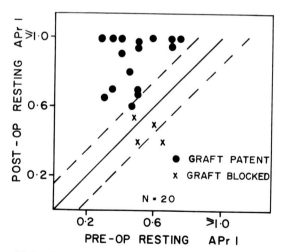

Fig. 20-9. Comparison of pre- and early postoperative resting ankle pressure indices in patients with critical isch-aemia treated by femoro-distal bypass. Most patients showed improved APrI by more than an arbitrary level of 0.15 if the bypass was technically successful.

tation (Figs 20-8B and 20-8C). However, once tissues healed, many patients were then left with an adequate circulation even if the graft then thrombosed and some 20–25% of these bypass grafts that blocked beyond 3 months did not lead to major amputation.

Thus, the best way to improve early patency and long-term salvage is to identify the most suitable arteries for distal anastomoses and this requires good arteriography. Conventional preoperative arteriography is often unsatisfactory, even if perfusion is increased by intra-arterial vasodilators or reactive hyperaemia. Preoperative IA DSA[19] or intraoperative femoral or popliteal arteriography[21,22] demonstrate the tibial arteries far better than blind surgical exploration. If these techniques are not used to supplement or even replace conventional arteriography, then many needless amputations will be performed.

One study showed that when conventional arteriography failed to reveal a patent tibial artery beyond an occlusion, IA DSA nevertheless revealed an artery suitable for femoro-tibial bypass in about one-third of legs; if no patent artery was shown by IA DSA, none was found at surgical exploration.[19] In another study, 40% of over 100 patients had been rejected for reconstruction on the basis of the preoperative arteriogram, with the likely need for major amputation, yet intraoperative femoral arteriography showed that all but one had an artery suitable for reconstruction, with early success in each case and with long-term success equal to other patients treated by femoro-tibial bypass.[21] It would not be our experience to find such a high proportion of patients with an artery suitable for bypass; an appreciable number of diabetics had no suitable artery displayed by any technique. In another study of over 50 patients, intraoperative popliteal arteriography showed the site for distal anastomosis better in 75%.[24] It also demonstrated opportunities for a double or triple graft, helped predict the likely outcome, and indicated whether further surgery was worthwhile if the graft failed.

The Doppler probe can be used to detect patent tibial and peroneal arteries distal to a femoro-popliteal occlusion. If it is possible to obtain APrI, then one or the other artery must be patent. Often there are poor anastomoses between the tibial arteries so that the artery that provides the higher APrI should be the best for a bypass. The Doppler probe can demonstrate whether the pedal arch is patent and which is the dominant artery supplying it, and thus the one best suited to receive a bypass graft. The arch is patent if there is a signal over the first metatarsal space. Each tibial artery is compressed in turn, just as with Allen's test for the hand, to determine which is the dominant feeding artery.

Sympathectomy

Experience from 231 surgical sympathectomies until 1978 and 290 chemical sympathectomies since, persuades us that either method can relieve mild to moderate rest pain or assist healing of small ulcers or conservative amputation for limited gangrene in some 60% of patients.[54] There is a mean doubling of total blood flow, shown by plethysmography, and capillary blood flow, shown by isotope clearance studies, after sympathectomy.[46]

A reliable technique to confirm sympathetic denervation is the skin potential response or psychogalvanic reflex.[55] However, it is more difficult confidently to predict that sympathectomy will increase blood flow. Two approaches have been used. The first is to identify those patients whose ischaemia is so severe that this indirect procedure could not possibly be effective. An APrI higher than 0.35[28] or ankle systolic pressure above 30 mm Hg[56] may predict success, but it is more difficult to define levels that predict failure. The other approach is to measure whether blood flow is increased by manouevres that simulate sympathectomy, such as spinal, sympathetic, or peripheral nerve blockade, or alternatively by reflex or local heating and reactive hyperaemia; in practice, these methods are either just as traumatic as chemical sympathectomy itself or not sufficiently accurate to help make the clinical decisions.[46]

ACKNOWLEDGMENTS

I appreciate the assistance from my colleagues, Prof. D. F. Scott, Mr. T. J. Devine, Mr. A. H. Johnston, and Mr. M. J. Denton of the Department of Vascular Surgery, Prince Henry's Hospital, Melbourne, and to Mr. R. B. King. We are most grateful to the Windemere Foundation for generous financial support. My thanks are due to Mrs. Ann Tremayne and Miss Kim Myers for the computer analyses and Miss Marion Cook for the secretarial assistance.

REFERENCES

1. Patton DD: Introduction to clinical decision making. Semin Nucl Med 8:273, 1978
2. Metz CE: Basic principles of ROC analysis. Semin Nucl Med 8:283, 1978
3. Junger M, Chapman BLW, Underwood CJ, et al: A comparison between two types of waveform analysis in patients with multisegmental arterial disease. Br J Surg 71:345, 1984
4. Johnston KW, Kassam M, Cobbold RSC: Relationship between Doppler pulsatility index and direct femoral pressure measurements in the diagnosis of aortoiliac occlusive disease. Ultrasound Med Biol 9:271, 1983
6. Flanigan DP, Collins JT, Schwartz JA, et al: Hemodynamic and arteriographic evaluation of femoral pulsatility index. J Surg Res 32:234, 1982
6. Baird RN, Bird DR, Clifford PC, et al: Upstream stenosis. Its diagnosis by Doppler signals from the femoral artery. Arch Surg 115:1316, 1980
7. Thiele BL, Bandyk DF, Zierler RE, et al: A systemic approach to the assessment of aortoiliac disease. Arch Surg 118:477, 1983
8. Flanigan DP, Williams LR, Schwartz JA, et al: Hemodynamic evaluation of the aorto-iliac system based on pharmacologic vasodilation. Surgery 93:709, 1983
9. MacPherson DS, Evans DH, Bell PRF: Common femoral artery Doppler wave-forms: A comparison of three methods of objective analysis with direct pressure measurements. Br J Surg 71:46, 1984
10. Sumner DS, Strandness DE: Aortoiliac reconstruction in patients with combined iliac and superficial femoral arterial occlusion. Surgery 84:348, 1978
11. Marinelli MR, Beach KW, Glass MJ, et al: Noninvasive testing vs clinical evaluation of arterial disease. JAMA 241:2031, 1979
12. Laing S, Greenhalgh RM: The detection and progression of asymptomatic peripheral arterial disease. Br J Surg 70:628, 1983
13. Brewster DC, Perler BA, Robison JG, et al: Aortofemoral graft for multilevel occlusive disease. Arch Surg 117:1593, 1983

14. Bell PRF, Charlesworth D, DePalma RG, et al: The definition of critical ischaemia of a limb. Br J Surg 69 (suppl):S2, 1982

15. Gilfillan I, Myers KA, Scott DF, et al: Inter-observer variability for assessment of femoral and popliteal pulses. Submitted for publication.

16. Carter SA: Arterial ausculation in peripheral vascular disease. JAMA 246:1682, 1981

17. Slot HB, Strijbosch L, Greep JM: Interobserver variability in single-plane aortography. Surgery 90:497, 1981

18. Thiele BL, Strandness DE: Accuracy of angiographic quantification of peripheral atherosclerosis. Prog Cardiovasc Dis 26:223, 1983

19. Kubal WS, Crummy AB, Tunipseed WD: The utility of digital arteriography in peripheral vascular disease. Cardiovasc Intervent Radiol 6:241, 1983

20. Karlsson S, Jonsson K, Aspelin P, et al: Intravenous arteriography in the preoperative evaluation of advanced atherosclerosis. Acta Radio Scand (Diagn) 23:193, 1982

21. Ricco J, Pearce WH, Yao JST, et al: The use of operative prebypass arteriography and Doppler ultrasound recording to select patients for extended femoro-distal bypass. Ann Surg 198:646, 1983

22. Scarpato R, Gembarowicz R, Farber S, et al: Intraoperative prereconstruction arteriography. Arch Surg 116:1053, 1981

23. O'Mara CS, Flinn WR, Neiman HL, et al: Correlation of foot arterial anatomy with early tibial bypass patency. Surgery 89:743, 1981

24. Roedersheimer LR, Feins R, Green RM: Doppler evaluation of the pedal arch. Am J Surg 142:601, 1981

25. Evans DH, Quin RO, Bell PRF: The significance of blood pressure measurements in patients with peripheral vascular disease. Br J Surg 67:238, 1980

26. Brewster DC, Waltman AC, O'Hara PJ, et al: Femoral artery pressure measurement during aortography. Circulation 60 (Suppl 1):120, 1979

27. Verhagen PF, van Vroonhoven TJMV: Criteria from intra-arterial femoral artery pressure measurements combined with reactive hyperaemia to assess the aorto-iliac segment; a prospective study. Br J Surg 71:707, 1984

28. Pearce WH, Yao JST, Bergan JJ: Noninvasive vascular diagnostic testing. Curr Probl Surg 20:461, 1983

29. Carter SA: The definition of critical ischaemia of the lower limb and distal systolic pressures. Br J Surg 70:188, 1983

30. Keagy BA, Pharr WF, Thomas D, et al: Comparison of reactive hyperemia and treadmill tests in the evaluation of peripheral vascular disease. Am J Surg 142:158, 1981

31. Quin RO, Evans DH, Fyfe T, et al: Evaluation of indirect blood pressure measurement as a method of assessment of peripheral vascular disease. J Cardiovasc Surg 18:109, 1977

32. Vincent DG, Salles-Cunha SX, Bernhard VM, et al: Noninvasive assessment of toe systolic pressures with special reference to diabetes mellitus. J Cardiovasc Surg 24:22, 1983

33. Nicholas GG, Myers JL, De Muth WE: The role of vascular laboratory criteria in the selection of patients for lower extremity amputation. Ann Surg 195:469, 1982

34. Barnes RW, Thornhill B, Rittgers SE, et al: Prediction of amputation wound healing. Arch Surg 116:80, 1981

35. Baker JD, Dix D: Variability of Doppler ankle pressures with arterial occlusive disease: An evaluation of ankle index and brachial-ankle pressure gradient. Surgery 89:134, 1981

36. Ouriel K, McDonnell AE, Metz CE, et al: A critical evaluation of stress testing in the diagnosis of peripheral vascular disease. Surgery 91:686, 1982

37. Berkowitz HD, Hobbs CL, Roberts B, et al: Value of routine vascular laboratory studies to identify vein graft stenosis. Surgery 90:971, 1981

38. Ramsey DE, Manke DA, Sumner DS: Toe blood pressure: A valuable adjunct to ankle pressure measurement for assessing peripheral arterial disease. J Cardiovasc Surg 24:43, 1983

39. Relf IRN: The detection of peripheral arterial disease using Doppler ultrasound, and its association with risk factors. MSc. Thesis Monash University, 1983

40. Lo CS, Myers KA, Wahlqvist ML, et al; Relation between Laplace damping factor and risk factors for atherosclerosis. Submitted for publication.

41. Baker JD, Machleder HI, Skidmore R: Analysis of femoral artery Doppler signals by Laplace transform damping method. J Vasc Surg 1:520, 1984

42. Wyss CR, Matsen FA, Simmons CW, et al: Transcutaneous oxygen tension measurements on limbs of diabetic and nondiabetic patients with peripheral vascular disease. Surgery 95:339, 1984

43. Burgess EM, Matsen FA, Wyss CR, et al: Segmental transcutaneous measurements of Po_2 in patients requiring below-the-knee amputation for peripheral vascular insufficiency. J Bone Jt Surg 64-A:378, 1982

44. Silberstein EB, Thomas S, Cline J, et al: Predictive value of intracutaneous Xenon clearance for healing of amputation and cutaneous ulcer sites. Radiology 147:227, 1983

45. Holstein P: Level selection in leg amputation for arterial occlusive disease: A comparison of clinical evaluation and skin perfusion pressure. Acta Orthop Scand 53:821, 1982

46. Myers KA: Haemodynamic studies in peripheral vascular disease. MS thesis University of Melbourne, 1968

47. Doubilet P, Abrams HL: The cost of underutilization. N Eng J Med 310:95, 1984

48. Gunn IG, Cowie TN, Forrest H, et al. Haemodynamic assessment following iliac artery dilatation. Br J Surg 68:858, 1981

49. Johnston KW, Colapinto RF, Baird RJ: Transluminal Dilatation: An alternative? Arch Surg 117:1604, 1982

50. O'Mara CS, Neiman HL, Flinn WR, et al. Haemodynamic assessment of transluminal angioplasty for lower extremity ischaemia. Surgery 89:106, 1981

51. King RB, Myers KA, Scott DF, et al: Aorto-iliac reconstructions for intermittent claudication. Br J Surg 69:169, 1982

52. Archie JP, Feldtman RW: Intraoperative assessment of the haemodynamic significance of iliac and profunda femoris artery stenosis. Surgery 90:876; 1981

53. Flanigan DP, Gray B, Schuler JJ, et al: Utility of wide and narrow blood pressure cuffs in the hemodynamic assessment of aortoiliac occlusive disease. Surgery 92:16, 1982

54. Myers KA, King RB, Scott DF, et al: Surgical treatment of the severely ischaemic leg: Salvage rates. Br J Surg 65:779, 1978

55. Cronin KD, Kursner RLG: Assessment of sympathectomy—the skin potential response. Anaesth Intenc Care 7:353, 1979

56. Walker PM, Johnston KW: Predicting the success of a sympathectomy: A prospective study using discriminant function and multiple regression analysis. Surgery 87:216, 1980

Ian L. Green
and Roger M. Greenhalgh

21

Objective Evaluation of the Femoral Pulse

Accurate assessment of the aorto-iliac segment is of considerable importance when deciding on the management of patients with symptoms of peripheral arterial disease. For many, the standard method of assessment for peripheral disease is by history, examination, and angiography. Attempts to improve on this led to the use of direct intraarterial pressure measurements either at the time of arteriography or operation.

Noninvasive tests are used in an attempt to discover at the outset whether the aorto-iliac segment is diseased or not as this affects the management. Most tests relate to the velocity of blood. Many efforts have been made to improve these non-invasive techniques for aorto-iliac disease, and most have employed computer assessment of Doppler blood velocity waveforms including pulsatility index,[1,2] Laplace transform damping,[3,4] and the principal component method.[5]

When assessing any of these techniques, the main question to be asked is whether they are significantly better than what the clinician can achieve by using his fingers to palpate the femoral pulse. Recently, Campbell[6] suggested that clinical assessment is better than any one of these sophisticated tests for diagnosing marked aorto-iliac stenoses of $>50\%$. This suggests that the movement of the artery wall may provide more useful information than the velocity of blood.

Consequently, a method for assessing the femoral pulse more objectively than palpation is desirable. Ideally, a hand-held device to be placed over the femoral artery to detect movement of the arterial wall with more precision than the fingers is what could prove more useful than all of the sophisticated tests relating in some way to velocity profile.

METHODS

A Siemens variable capacitance transducer (Fig. 21-1) was placed over the common femoral artery at the mid-inguinal point after the artery had been located by palpation. If the pulse was clinically absent, the position of the artery was found using a simple Doppler ultrasound probe and the position marked. In nearly all

DIAGNOSTIC TECHNIQUES AND ASSESSMENT
PROCEDURES IN VASCULAR SURGERY

© 1985 Grune & Stratton
ISBN 0-8089-1721-8 All rights reserved

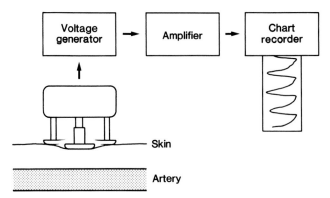

Fig. 21-1. The variable capacitance pressure transducer is held over the common femoral artery by hand. The changes in capacitance caused by movement of the arterial wall are converted into changes in voltage which are amplified and fed to a rapid pen chart recorder.

cases satisfactory signals were obtained holding the transducer by hand with light pressure over the artery. Small side-to-side movements were used to centralize the artery under the transducer and maximize the amplitude of the signal.

The movement of the arterial wall with each pulse caused movement of the plates in the transducer altering the capacitance. The changes in capacitance were converted into a voltage which was amplified and sent to a rapid pen-chart recorder.

Figure 21-2 illustrates the sort of waveforms obtained. The top tracing shows the waveform shape obtained from a common femoral artery with a relatively disease-free aorto-iliac segment. The lower tracing represents a waveform from a common femoral artery with a markedly stenosed aorto-iliac segment. The reduction in amplitude can be seen, as well as a loss of the dicrotic notch. In addi-

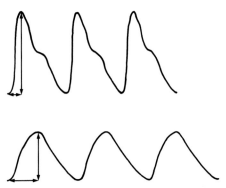

Fig. 21-2. Pulse rise time. Diagram of waveforms representing lateral movement of the common femoral artery wall with each pulse. The upper waveform is from a common femoral artery with a normal aorto-iliac segment. The lower waveform is from a common femoral artery where there is a marked stenosis in the aorto-iliac segment. Note the reduction in amplitude and increase in 'rise time.'

tion, the time taken from the lowest point of the waveform to its peak, which has been termed the "rise time," increases with disease. It was this rise time that we investigated further.

The common femoral pulse rise time was calculated simply from the chart recordings using a ruler to measure the rise time from 10 consecutive waveforms and averaging the results. The mean rise time was calculated in milliseconds after allowance for the speed of the recording.

Of the 59 patients studied, 46 were male and 13 were female (age, 38–80 years). All were being considered for arterial reconstruction of the lower limb.

Presenting symptoms are given in Table 21-1. All of the 59 patients were examined clinically by a consultant or senior registrar. The results of palpation of the femoral pulse were graded into three categories: normal, reduced, and absent.

Table 21-1
Presenting Symptoms of
Patients Considered for
Arterial Reconstruction

Symptom or Procedure	No.
Intermittent claudication	21
Ischaemic rest pain	29
Ulceration/gangrene	9
Total	59
Clinical examination	59
Aorto-iliac segments investigated	118

Note. Clinical examination included palpation of the common femoral pulse on both sides.

Examination of both sides gave 118 aorto-iliac segments for further study. There is no perfect test or standard for assessing aorto-iliac disease, so clinical examination of the pulse and the pulse rise time was compared with both angiographic assessment and direct pressure measurement, even though there are limitations of accuracy for both of these techniques.

Angiography was performed on 51 of the patients. The roentgenogram films of the aorto-iliac segments were assessed by direct measurement (Fig. 21-3). The minimum diameter of the most severe stenosis in the segment was measured and compared with the nearest distal artery which appeared free from disease, taking care to avoid any post-stenotic dilatation.

Direct pressure studies were carried out on those patients who were operated on. In 80 instances in which the common femoral artery was exposed, a 21-gauge needle was used to puncture the artery (Fig. 21-4) which was connected via manometer tubing and a three-way tap to a Gould-Statham pressure transducer. A 20-gauge cannula inserted into the radial artery was also connected to the same transducer. The three-way tap allowed rapid switching between the two sites of measurement. The common femoral systolic pressure and the radial systolic pressure were measured and used to calculate the common femoral/radial systolic pressure ratio. In 36 patients, 40 mg of papaverine was injected intraarterially to enhance flow and simulate the effect of exercise.

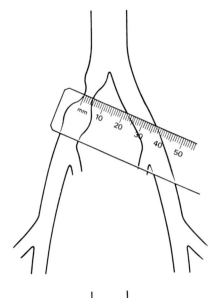

Fig. 21-3. Direct measurement of the angiogram of 102 aorto-iliac segments. The narrowest part of the most severe stenosis is measured and compared with the diameter of the nearest distal artery which appeared disease free and avoiding any post stenotic dilatation (in this case corresponding to the lower edge of the ruler).

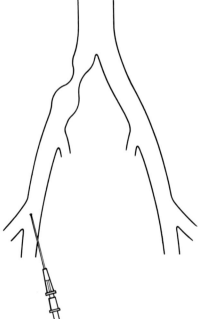

Fig. 21-4. Intraoperative direct pressure measurements from the common femoral artery. These are compared with direct measurements from the radial artery. The common femoral systolic pressure divided by the radial systolic pressure gives the common femoral/radial systolic pressure ratio.

RESULTS

We compared the established methods of angiographic assessment and direct pressure ratios. Figure 21-5 shows the pressure ratios on the vertical axis decreasing as the disease increases. The angiographic degrees of stenosis are shown on the horizontal axis with complete occlusion on the right. It will be seen that there is very little change in pressure ratio up to approximately 50% stenosis. A marked

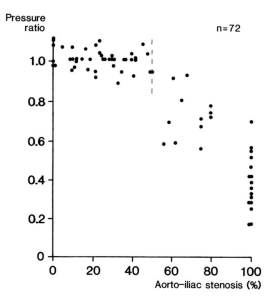

Fig. 21-5. Comparison of pressure ratios with angiographic degrees of stenosis. The pressure ratios change little up to approximately 50% stenosis.

reduction in ratio then occurs. The pressure ratios therefore give very little information about disease that causes only minor degrees of stenosis.

The pulse rise time was compared against both the angiographic stenoses and the pressure ratios. Figure 21-6 shows the pulse rise time on the vertical axis and angiographic degrees of stenosis on the horizontal axis. At the top of the graph are those points where the waveform was so flat that accurate assessment of the pulse rise time was not possible ($= \infty$). All but three of these points were associated with completely occluded aorto-iliac segments and all cases were found to show >50% stenosis on the arteriogram.

With all other readings, pulse rise time and degrees of stenosis were compared by linear regression. There was a highly significant correlation coefficient of 0.80 ($P < .001$). Stenoses >50% were generally associated with rise times of >200 ms.

Figure 21-7 shows the pulse rise time compared with the direct pressure ratios. Again the pulse rise time is plotted vertically against pressure ratios on the horizontal axis. Here the correlation coefficient is -0.82 ($P < .001$). Again, almost all of the reduced pressure ratios occur with pulse rise times of >200 ms.

Clinical palpation of the pulse is then compared with both the angiographic degree of stenosis and with the direct pressure ratio. Figure 21-8 shows the common femoral pulses graded as normal = 2, reduced = 1, and absent = 0 on the vertical axis and the angiographic degree of stenosis on the horizontal axis. When the pulse was absent, 18 of 22 of the limbs had occluded aorto-iliac segments and all were graded as >50% stenosis.

The finding of a clinically normal pulse was generally a reliable indicator that aorto-iliac stenosis was <50%. However, in seven of 61 cases the angiogram suggested a severe stenosis, up to 80%.

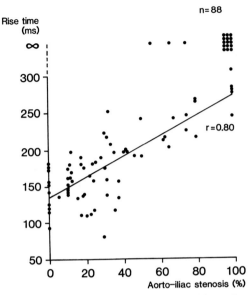

Fig. 21-6. Comparison of pulse rise time with angiographic degrees of stenosis. At the top are 18 instances where the waveform is too flat to assess the pulse rise time (∞). Highly significant correlation coefficient of 0.80 ($P < .001$) between pulse rise time and angiographic degree of stenosis.

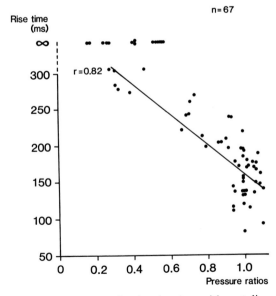

Fig. 21-7. Comparison of pulse rise time with systolic pressure ratios. Highly significant correlation coefficient -0.82.

246

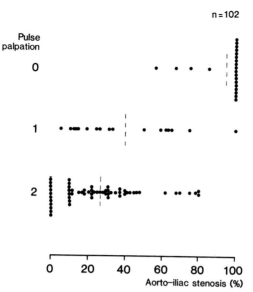

Fig. 21-8. Comparison of clinical pulse examination with angiographic degree of stenosis. Top, absent pulse grade 0; middle, diminished pulse grade 1; lower, normal pulse grade 2.

The finding of a clinically reduced pulse proved to be a very unreliable guide to the degree of stenosis with a scatter from almost complete normality to complete occlusion.

When the clinical examination was compared with the direct pressure ratio, the overall trend was similar (Fig. 21-9). Absent pulses were all associated with reduced pressure ratios of <0.7. Normal pulses generally indicated pressure ratios of >0.9, but again in four out of 40 cases marked disease was suggested by pressure ratios of <0.8. For the reduced pulse there was again a wide scatter. The results have been analysed in terms of sensitivity, specificity, and overall accuracy.

Although the clinician is mainly concerned with stenoses of >50%, it is important to see if any of the tests reliably detect minor angiographic disease of 25%–50% (Table 21-2). The overall accuracy of clinical examination was 58%. It must be remembered that since we are dealing with two groups (0–24% and

Table 21-2
Sensitivity, Specificity, and Accuracy for Minor Degrees of Angiographic Stenosis

Parameter	Sensitivity	Specificity	Accuracy
Clinical examination (reduced pulse) $N = 67$	16	81	58
Pulse rise time (170 ms) $N = 56$	70	72	71
Direct pressure ratios (0.97) $N = 45$	29	79	56
Ratios after papaverine (0.87) $N = 31$	40	88	65

Note. Data are expressed as percent. Accuracy was for distinguishing 25%–50% stenosis from <25% stenosis. Only the pulse rise time was a significant improvement over chance (50%).

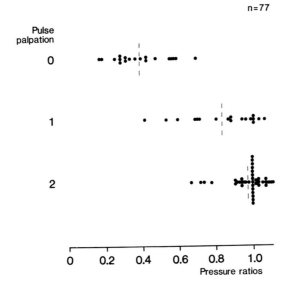

Fig. 21-9. Comparison of clinical pulse examination with systolic pressure ratio. Top, absent pulse grade 0; middle, diminished pulse grade 1; lower, normal pulse grade 2.

25%–50% stenosis) an accuracy of around 50% might be achieved by random allocation. Clinical examination is thus very poor for the assessment of these degrees of stenosis.

Pulse rise time gave an overall accuracy of 71%, direct pressure measurements were 56% accurate, and direct pressure ratios after papaverine were 65% accurate.

Only the result of the pulse rise time was significantly different from chance using the chi-squared test ($\chi^2 = 5.39$; $P < .05$).

Table 21-3 shows the accuracy results for >50% stenosis. Now the sensitivity for clinical examination is greatly improved giving an accuracy of 83% overall in this study. However, using pulse rise time, the sensitivity and specificity were both higher, giving an accuracy of 94%, significantly better than clinical examination ($\chi^2 = 5.57$; $P < .02$). The accuracy using this noninvasive technique was similar to that obtained by direct pressure measurement after exposure of the artery at operation.

Table 21-3
Accuracy for Detecting >50% Angiographic Aorto-Iliac Stenosis

Parameter	Sensitivity	Specificity	Accuracy
Clinical examination, $N = 102$	81	85	83
Pulse rise time (200 ms), $N = 88$	97	93	94
Direct pressure ratios (0.92), $N = 72$	93	94	94

Note. Data are expressed as a percent. The pulse rise time was significantly better than clinical examination ($P < .02$).

DISCUSSION

In 1978 Levenson et al[7] used direct needle puncture of the common femoral artery to obtain pressure waveforms. They found that the rate of rise of the pressure wave (dP/dt) was reduced in aorto-iliac disease. This femoral systolic slope (as they referred to it) when compared with the aortic systolic slope was thought to be more sensitive than the femoral/aortic systolic pressure index for diagnosing aorto-iliac disease. The decrease in the rate of rise of the pulse was, they felt, due to the attenuation of the higher frequencies present in the femoral waveform. All of these rates of rise were calculated from the pressure trace after direct needle puncture.

Bird[8] found that the upstroke time from thigh pulse volume recordings was a sensitive indicator for aorto-iliac disease. This was confirmed more recently by Campbell.[6] However, it is known that thigh pulse volume recordings are affected by proximal superficial femoral and profunda femoral disease. The pulse volume recorder is a noninvasive segmental plethysmograph but its trace relates to the movement of the artery wall with the pulse. The simple pressure transducer used here is simply held over the common femoral artery to record its movements. It can be performed at the patient's bedside and in the clinic on the first occasion a patient is seen so that the clinician knows instantly how to advise the patient. The equipment is less complex and vastly less expensive compared with pulse volume recording. Unlike sophisticated tests to analyse the blood velocity profile such as pulsatility index, Laplace transform damping, and the principal components method, no on-line computer is required for analysis.

CONCLUSIONS

Palpation of the femoral pulse is 83% accurate in the assessment of $>50\%$ stenoses of the aorto-iliac segment, but hopeless for $<50\%$ stenoses. Pulse rise time is better (71% accurate) for $<50\%$ stenosis and better for $>50\%$ stenosis (94% accurate). The test is simple and inexpensive.

However, the absence of a clinically palpable femoral pulse has, so far, proved to be absolutely specific for aorto-iliac disease of $>50\%$ stenosis. In this case there is no need for further noninvasive testing. The pulse rise time is of value when the pulse is either apparently normal or reduced. This simple hand-held pressure transducer assesses aorto-iliac disease better than the fingers alone which is more than can be said for other more sophisticated noninvasive tests. It is also just as good as direct invasive pressure measurement, which is far more inconvenient, painful, and not available in the clinic when the patient is first seen.

REFERENCES

1. Gosling RG, Dunbar G, King DH, et al: The quantitative analysis of occlusive peripheral arterial disease by a non intrusive ultrasonic technique. Angiology 22:52–55, 1971
2. Gosling RG, Key DH: Arterial assessment by Doppler shift ultrasound. Proc Roy Soc Med 67:447, 1974
3. Baird RN, et al: Upstream stenosis: Its diagnosis by Doppler signals from the femoral artery. Arch Surg 115:1316–1322, 1980

4. Clifford PC, Skidmore R, Bird D, et al: Femoral artery Doppler signal analysis in lower limb ischaemia. J Cardiovasc Surg 23:69–74, 1982
5. Macpherson DS, Evans DH, Bell PRF: Common femoral artery Doppler waveforms: A comparison of three methods of objective analysis with direct pressure measurements. Br J Surg 71:46–49, 1984
6. Campbell WB: MS Thesis London: Laplace Transform Analysis of Doppler Waveforms in Lower Limb Ischaemia. 1984, pp 130–136
7. Levenson SH, Guillou PH, Terry HJ, et al: Pulse pressure wave analysis in the diagnosis of aorto-iliac disease. Ann Surg 2:161–165, 1978
8. Bird DR: Non-invasive investigation in lower limb ischaemia. MChir Thesis, University of Cambridge, 1980

David Charlesworth

22

Measurement of Hydraulic Impedance: Ideal But Impractical

In an ideal world, given time, space, and sufficient funds to command the services of a multi-disciplinary team and all the equipment they needed, one could generate data that would allow a surgeon to calculate, with some degree of certainty, the probability of failure for a particular reconstruction. In practice surgeons lean heavily on their 'experience' and rule of thumb in reaching such decisions. To eliminate the element of chance they need information at two stages in the management of their patients. They need information that will help them choose the most appropriate operation in any given set of circumstances, and they need information that will tell them whether the operation they have just completed is working satisfactorily.

To illustrate this proposition we can use femoro-popliteal bypass as an example. To make the first decision the surgeon needs to know something (preferably quantitative rather than qualitative information) about the 'run-in' 'run-off' and the properties of the conduit he proposes to use to construct his bypass.

RUN-IN

An estimate of whether atherosclerosis in the aorta and iliac vessels has compromised flow in the common femoral artery can be arrived at by measurement of how pressure and flow are altered by passage through the iliac vessels. Mean pressure and flow are relatively insensitive to minor changes in the calibre of an artery and a very tight stenosis (> 75%) is required before they are affected.[1] Measurement of how pulsatile pressure and flow waves are damped by transmission through an artery is more sensitive to minor stenoses, but estimates of impedance and energy loss are the most sensitive indices of how discontinuities in the wall of an artery affect the flow through it (Fig. 22-1).[2–4]

In practice, information about run-in is obtained either by waveform analysis of ultrasound signals obtained by insonnating the common femoral artery or by differ-

DIAGNOSTIC TECHNIQUES AND ASSESSMENT
PROCEDURES IN VASCULAR SURGERY
© 1985 Grune & Stratton
ISBN 0-8089-1721-8 All rights reserved

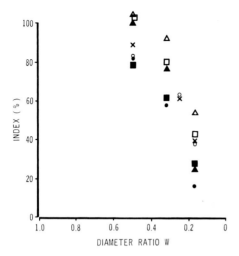

INDEX (%)

DIAMETER RATIO W

Fig. 22-1. A graph illustrating how several indices are affected by increasing stenosis. The Y axis shows the change in an index reducing from 100% (unaffected) to 0. The X axis shows the degree of stenosis as the diameter ratio W, the ratio of the diameter of the stenosis to the diameter of the tube. ($\triangle$), mean flow; ($\bigcirc$), mean pressure; ($\square$), 1/resistance (= conductance); ($\blacktriangle$), reduction in amplitude of flow wave; ($\bullet$), reduction in amplitude of pressure wave; ($\blacksquare$), 1/impedance (= admittance); and ($\times$) energy.

ential pressure studies.[5–10] Both tests can be carried out at operation but it is usually more convenient to insonnate the artery and carry out the waveform analysis before operation.

THE MECHANICAL PROPERTIES OF THE BYPASS

Choice of conduit for a femoro-popliteal bypass is not difficult, one has a choice either of autologous vein or of a prosthesis. The results obtainable when vein is used are better than for prostheses, but the choice of which prosthesis is more difficult. The mechanical properties of the saphenous vein, when used as a bypass, are affected by the diameter of the vein and the method of its preparation. It seems likely that there will be considerable variation between individual veins. Arteries (and veins) are compliant, that is to say the radius, and hence the cross sectional area, varies directly with pressure and the walls are said to be visco elastic. Arteries are a mixture of different tissues that make them visco elastic and there is a slight delay in the response to stress. This behaviour can be represented by: (1) Edyn and η if stress varies cyclically the oscillation is strain is

$$\frac{S}{\sqrt{\text{Edyn} + \eta^2 w^2}}$$

where S = strain, Edyn = dynamic modulus of elasticity, η = coefficient of viscosity of the wall, and w = circular frequency ($2\Pi f$); and (2) the elastic behaviour can be calculated in terms of wave speed and Poissons ratio

$$\text{Wave speed} = \sqrt{\frac{Eh}{2rp(1 - \sigma^2)}}$$

where E = Young's elastic modulus, h = wall thickness, r = radius, p = density of the fluid, and σ = Poisson ratio.

Prostheses are incompliant (apart from those of biologic origin) but they are of uniform construction and the problem of quantitating their mechanical behaviour is simpler; it is very unlikely that there is any individual variation amongst prostheses of the same make. But in the case of prostheses of biologic origin there may well be variations with time. This means that only one set of measurements for each type of prostheses need to be taken and the results can be freely applied to prostheses that are similar in both manufacture and dimensions. To ascertain whether the properties of a prosthesis change with time requires further measurement.

When one considers a particular prosthesis or vein it would be helpful to know its resistance in comparison to that of the collateral circulation. If it is higher than that of the collaterals then the majority of blood will continue to follow collaterals and only a little will go down the prosthesis, circumstances that would predispose to early thrombosis. There is, however, a conflict of interests in that prostheses are less likely to occlude if the velocity of flow through them is high. Hence a narrow tube with a low resistance is ideal (Fig. 22-2).

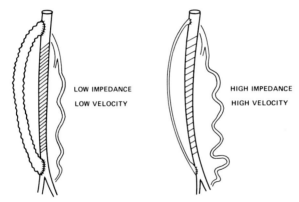

LOW IMPEDANCE

LOW VELOCITY

HIGH IMPEDANCE

HIGH VELOCITY

Fig. 22-2. The ideal prosthesis is a narrow tube with low resistance, i.e. high impedance and high velocity.

In this context it is much more appropriate to measure the impedance of the prosthesis rather than resistance because flow is pulsatile and in diastole may be reversed. The relationship between oscillatory pressure and oscillatory flow at a point in the circulation is termed the 'input impedance' of the system distal to the point of measurement. It is defined for sinusoidal waves and can only be computed for a sinusoidal pressure and flow of the same frequency. The relationship consists of two terms, the ratio of the peak amplitudes (moduli) of the two waves and the time relationship between oscillations, phase (Fig. 22-3). If $|P|$ is the modulus of pressure and $|Q|$ the modulus of the flow, the sinusoidal pressure wave is described by

Fig. 22-3. Representation of a pressure wave which varies sinusoidally with time: frequency, $f = 1/T$; modulus of $P = |P|$; and phase of $P = 2\pi tp/T$.

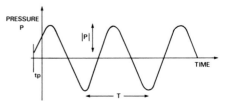

$|P| \cos (2\pi ft + \theta)$ and flow by $|Q| \cos (2\pi ft + \phi)$, where if f is frequency, t is time, and θ and ϕ are the phase of pressure and flow relative to the time origin, then at frequency f the modulus of impedance $|Z| = |P|/|Q|$ and the phase of impedance $\psi = \theta - \phi$. Input impedance is the impedance at the origin of an arterial network, modified by reflections. Impedance is usually represented by a spectrum of modulus against frequency. Pressure and flow waves can be broken down mathematically into a series of sinusoidal waves by Fourier analysis and waves of similar frequency used to derive the impedance spectrum. The properties of a prosthesis which affect its impedance are the characteristic impedance at the point of measurement $Z\delta$ and the propagation constant γ. The characteristic impedance is that which would be obtained if there were no reflections in the system. The propagation constant is a complex number which describes wave transmission in the conduit of interest. Complex numbers consist of a real and an imaginary part, the real part of γ describes how the amplitude of a wave is attenuated and the imaginary part, the delay imposed on a wave, called the phase shift (Fig. 22-4). We have used measure-

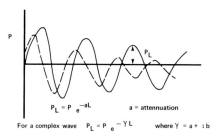

Fig. 22-4. Two waves at different frequencies and attenuated with time. The propagation constant

$$\gamma = i2\pi f \frac{(1 - \sigma^2)^{1/2}}{\delta} \frac{1}{(1 - F_{10})^{1/2}}$$

where $i = \sqrt{-1}$, $\delta =$ wave speed, and $\sigma =$ Poisson ratio.

ment of both impedance and propagation constant to characterise various prostheses and to compare them with vein.

We found that prostheses fabricated from man-made materials behaved in a similar way. Their longitudinal impedance was far in excess of that of vein of similar dimensions and there was a direct relationship between impedance and frequency, the higher the frequency the higher the impedance (Fig. 22-5).

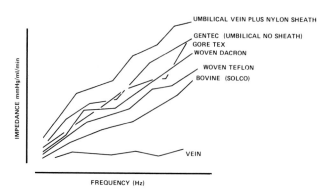

Fig. 22-5. The impedance of various prostheses varies with frequency. From Taylor S (ed): Recent Advances in Surgery. London, Butterworth, 1980. With permission.

Prostheses of biologic origin have an impedance and propagation constant comparable to autologous vein and we have some evidence to support the view that the mechanical properties of bypasses, particularly prostheses of biologic origin, change with time.[11,12] The elastic behaviour of the wall of a prosthesis can be described quantitatively from measurements of pulse wave transit time and calculation of a propagation constant. If two ultrasound probes are used to insonnate simultaneously the opposite ends of a bypass, one can measure the pulse wave transit time and calculate the wave speed and propagation constant at intervals in time. The information is useful in that it allows one to confirm that the conduit is patent and it allows an estimate of how the function of the wall is affected by time (fibrosis).

Autologous vein has a low impedance that is not related to frequency (ie, impedance is constant over a range of frequencies), and impedance fell when flow through the vein increased, implying some form of 'relaxation' in the wall in response to the increased flow, a property unique to veins and one assumes also to arteries.[13] Over a small range (4–6 mm), the longitudinal impedance of autologous vein bypasses varied only slightly in contrast to prostheses where the impedance varies inversely with diameter (Fig. 22-6).

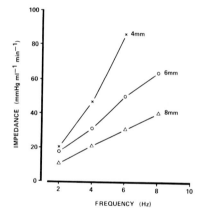

Fig. 22-6. A graph illustrating how the characteristic impedance of a prosthesis is related to its diameter. Y axis impedance mmHg mL^{-1} min^{-1}, X axis frequency. Three diameters of the same type of prosthesis were measured.

RUN-OFF

Of the three variables said to influence the success of bypass operations, the least is known about run-off. Data about the clinical success of femoro-popliteal bypass are usually presented in such a way that claudicants can be separated from patients with critical ischaemia. Ischaemia usually occurs when the run-off is poor, due to the effect of disease in the tibial arteries, but run-off is difficult to quantitate. One method is to count how many of the terminal branches of the popliteal artery are seen to be patent on an angiogram. This method takes no account of how 'diseased' individual branches are, and methods which try to incorporate this information to weight the overall estimate are imprecise. It is usual to separate patients into one of two groups, good run-off (two or three patent branches) or poor run-off (one or less) accepting that the method is imperfect. In the circumstances it is not surprising that surgeons cannot agree on what influence run-off plays on the success of a bypass. Measurement of the input impedance at the popliteal artery (site of distal anastomosis) may help to solve this problem, but there are practical difficulties that have yet to be overcome.

We have used measurement of impedance to check the function of femoro-popliteal bypass at the end of operation. We measured imput impedance in the common femoral artery before the bypass was inserted and after the bypass had been completed. Comparison of the two allowed us to identify those bypasses that failed early.[13] The input impedance in the common femoral artery is affected by (1) the impedance of the bypass, (2) the impedance of the collateral circulation, and (3) the impedance of the 'run-off' below the knee; however, the method cannot be used to measure the impedance of the run-off independent of the constraints imposed by bypass.

In summary hydraulic impedance is sensitive to small changes in the calibre of blood vessels, more so than waveform damping, but to calculate it in real time requires a considerable amount of support in the form of both men and material. It seems to be the most promising way of quantitating run-off, but its value in this context is as yet unknown.

REFERENCES

1. Weale FE: Haemodynamics of incomplete arterial obstruction. Brit J Surg 51:9, 689–693, 1984
2. Cave FD: Hydraulic impedance in occlusive arterial disease of the leg. Ph.D Thesis, University of Manchester, 1977
3. Cave FD and Charlesworth D: Arterial stenosis: an experiment to determine how best to quantify the hydraulic effects of a stenosis. Phys Med Biol 26:6, 1087–1097, 1981
4. Berguer R and Hwang NHC: Critical Stenosis. Surgery, 180:39–50, 1974
5. Harris PL, Taylor LA, Cave FD et al: The relationship between Doppler ultrasound assessment and angiography in occlusive disease of the lower limbs. Surg Gyn Obst 138:911–914, 1974
6. Charlesworth D, Harris PL, Cave FD and Taylor LA: Undetected aorto-iliac insufficiency. A reason for failure of saphenous bypass grafts for obstruction of the superficial femoral artery. Brit J Surg 62:567–570, 1975
7. Dr Morais D and Johnston KW: Assessment of aorto-iliac disease by non-invasive quantitative Doppler waveform analysis. Brit J Surg 68:789–792, 1981
8. Aukland A and Hurlow RA: Spectral analysis of Doppler ultrasound: its clinical application in lower limb ischaemia. Brit J Surg 69:539–542, 1982
9. Junger M, Chapman BLW, Underwood CJ and Charlesworth D: A comparison between two types of waveform analysis in patients with multisegmental arterial disease. Brit J Surg 71:345–348, 1984
10. Moore WS and Hall AD: Unrecognised aorto-iliac stenosis. Arch Surg 103:633–638, 1971
11. Chapman BLW and Charlesworth D: An in-vivo method of measurement of the mechanical properties of vascular prostheses: the mechanical properties of saphenous vein bypass grafts. Phys Med Biol 28:9, 1067–1074, 1983
12. Chapman BLW and Charlesworth D: Mechanical properties of gluteraldehyde stabilized human umbilical vein measured in vivo. Brit J Surg 70:530–532, 1983
13. Cave FD, Walker A, Naylor GP and Charlesworth D: The hydraulic impedance of the lower limb. Brit J Surg 63:408–412, 1976

Simon D. Parvin
and Peter R. F. Bell

23

Peripheral Resistance: Assessment by Infusing Blood at a Series of Constant Flow Rates

As surgeons have become more aggressive in their approach to the management of peripheral vascular disease, femorodistal reconstruction to vessels beyond the popliteal trifurcation has been more commonly performed. In this group of patients the results achieved are inferior to those possible when grafting to the supragenicular or immediately infragenicular popliteal artery. The severity of the disease present in many of these latter cases is such that it has been difficult deciding whether it is correct to proceed to reconstructive surgery, reconstruction with some adjunctive procedure such as arteriovenous fistula formation, or directly to primary amputation. One of the main problems has been that the preoperative arteriograms have been inadequate to visualise and define the pedal vessels or even on occasions the tibial vessels in the calf. When seen, the calf vessels often have multiple stenoses present and may not properly connect with the vessels of the foot. We felt that an objective measurement of peripheral resistance within the vessel under reconstruction would be more useful in this severe disease group since it may provide an accurate measure of the entire runoff including collaterals. Resistance was therefore measured in a series of dogs to establish the method, and subsequently in humans to test the hypothesis.

ARTERIOGRAPHY

In proximal reconstructive procedures the use of preoperative arteriography is often sufficient to allow a decision regarding operability, the site of distal anastomosis, and the likely outcome. This is because the vessels are of larger diameter and the flow in the more proximal procedures is therefore much greater. As distal procedures become more common, greater attention is paid to vessel calibre and the significance of the presence of the pedal arch has been stressed. Despite this graft patency does not correlate well with arteriography. Imparato[1] showed that if the

DIAGNOSTIC TECHNIQUES AND ASSESSMENT
PROCEDURES IN VASCULAR SURGERY

© 1985 Grune & Stratton
ISBN 0-8089-1721-8 All rights reserved

artery under reconstruction communicated with the pedal arch the two year patency rate was 39.5%. All his early failures were in patients without a pedal arch or in those where the artery failed to communicate with it. More recently Dardik[2] emphasised the importance of the pedal arch and showed that when it was patent there was a 75% graft patency compared to a 47% patency rate when the arch was absent. In patients without a patent arch, the "reasonably good" graft survival was attributed to the presence of "extensive arborization around the ankle." The assessment of arteriograms of the pedal vessels is necessarily highly subjective particularly when there are multiple stenoses in an already narrow vessel and the foot may depend almost entirely upon a flimsy collateral circulation to maintain it. In the same paper Dardik was able to adequately visualise runoff into the pedal vessels in only 64 of 290 cases. Various methods of enhancing the quality of the arteriogram have been suggested. Kahn and colleagues[3] suggested that reactive hyperaemia induced by the application of a tourniquet to the limb under study might improve the film quality by increasing blood flow. They showed that contrast transit time to the popliteal artery was halved and that contrast concentration was improved. However, the seven minutes of arterial occlusion recommended to induce hyperaemia would not be possible in the majority of patients with severe ischaemia. Feins[4] also used reactive hyperaemia but showed that a delay of up to seven minutes after release of the cuff was common before achieving a maximal increase in flow. Routine use of intraoperative arteriography can easily overcome most of the limitations of preoperative studies. In 1983 Dardik[5] suggested that the "feel" of the plunger in the syringe when injecting for the arteriogram was a useful way of assessing runoff, and in a subjective way he was assessing peripheral resistance by this manoeuvre. Harris and Campbell[6] have suggested that in severe peripheral vascular disease arteriography is inadequate and that measurement of peripheral resistance or impedance might be a more useful test of runoff.

PERIPHERAL RESISTANCE

The use of peripheral resistance measurement has not been described in a prospective way as an adjunct or alternative to arteriography to define prognosis or operability. Bliss[7] in his thesis measured resistance after reconstruction in patients undergoing femoropopliteal bypass. He concentrated on the different types of relationship between pressure and flow and stressed that it was important to measure resistance at maximal flow. This point had previously been emphasised by Wheale.[8] Conrad[9] showed that in healthy medical students resting toe flow measured plethysmographically varied 27-fold, while after maximal vasodilatation it still varied by 6-fold even under exactly similar conditions. She also showed that resistance was higher in those with vasospastic disease than normal and higher still in those with occlusive disease. Folse[10] showed that resistance in the superficial femoral artery decreased with increasing muscular activity. Delin and Ekestrom[11] suggested that pressure or flow measurement alone were insufficient to define prognosis in reconstructive surgery, but were able to show how resistance fell after a successful reconstruction. Mundth[12] could find no correlation between outcome or arteriographic assessment and resistance but stressed the inadequacy of the arteriograms. Sonnenfeld[13] measured peripheral resistance at rest and under maximal flow conditions before and after blood transfusion in patients undergoing reconstructive surgery. He confirmed the reduction in resistance with increasing flow but did not correlate these findings with outcome in terms of graft survival. Barner[14] looked at resistance in relation to graft survival but was unable to show any differences between patent and occluded grafts, either as a whole or when considered in relation to the number of vessels available for runoff.

Poiseuille, a physicist as well as a physician, intended to study the flow properties of blood, but was unable to anticoagulate it and therefore turned to study the flow of pure liquids in rigid glass tubes. His equation relates the flow and pressure of a Newtonian fluid in a cylindrical tube (Equation 1). In the case of human blood vessels the tubes are not cylindrical and the fluid is nonNewtonian. Despite these drawbacks the Poiseuille formula is regularly used to describe the haemodynamics of distal arteries.

Equation 1 $\quad Q = \dfrac{K \cdot P \cdot D^4}{L}$

Q = volume flow
P = pressure drop
D = diameter of the tube
L = length of the tube
K = constant

The Poiseuille formula can be simplified to Equation 2, which is analogous to Ohm's law where the constant K is the fluid resistance.

Equation 2 $\quad P1 - P2 = KQ$

$P1$ = arterial pressure
$P2$ = venous pressure
K = constant

The resistance is defined by Equation 3, and is inversely proportional to the fourth power of the radius and proportional to the viscosity. Clearly as the vessel gets smaller or becomes more narrow as a result of atheroma the resistance increases precipitously.

Equation 3 $\quad K = \dfrac{8\mu L}{\pi R^4}$

μ = viscosity
R = radius

For practical purposes resistance has been calculated using the following equation.

$$\text{Resistance} = \frac{\text{Arteriovenous pressure gradient}}{\text{Flow}}$$

$$= \frac{1 \text{ mmHg pressure drop}}{1 \text{ ml/min blood flow}} = 1 \text{ PRU (mmHg/ml/min)}$$

$$1 \text{ PRU (Peripheral resistance unit)} = 1000 \text{ mPRU}$$

All results presented have been measured in mPRU.

METHOD OF MEASUREMENT

The artery to be reconstructed is first exposed by an appropriate incision. After exposure the artery is mobilised and controlled over a sufficient length to permit cannulation and subsequent graft anastomosis. An arteriogram is then performed by hand injection of contrast medium via a manometer line connected to a size 16 gauge intravenous cannula. This cannula is subsequently used to infuse blood during resistance measurement. Blood is withdrawn from the femoral artery into four 100 ml glass syringes each containing 1000 IU of Heparin. The syringes are then mounted on a Harvard pump and connected together by a series of manometer tubes and three way taps and to the vessel under study via a further manometer line connected to the previously placed intravenous cannula. A size 22 gauge needle is then inserted into the femoral vein and attached to a pressure transducer by a manometer line. Arterial pressure generated by the infusion is measured by direct cannulation of the artery under study with a 27 gauge needle connected to a pressure transducer in the same way as the venous line. The cannula itself is inserted into the artery at least 1 cm distal to the tip of the infusing cannula, with the tip pointing distally and the bevel on the needle at right angles to the direction of flow. Before the infusion is started, existing arterial collateral pressure is measured together with the corresponding venous pressure. The blood is pumped into the artery at a series of flow rates (9, 38, 76, 117, and 153 ml/min), allowing a graph of pressure against flow to be drawn for each study. The infusion starts at the highest flow rate and is maintained until constant. The Harvard pump has a continuously variable gear ratio so that the rate of infusion can be reduced without stopping the infusion. Once the pressure generated by any one flow rate is constant the flow is reduced to the next flow rate. At the end of the first complete set of flows, Papaverine 15 mg is introduced into the infusing line by means of a three way tap next to the cannula. The measurements are then repeated but only at the higher flow rates (76, 117, and 153 ml/min). The apparatus is shown diagrammatically in Figure 23-1.

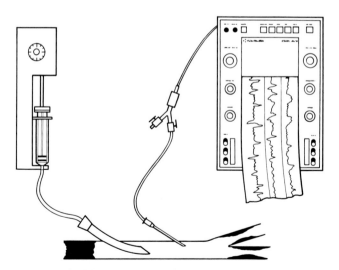

Fig. 23-1.   Diagram of the Harvard pump.

In our early experiments the pressure was measured via a pressure transducer connected by a manometer line to a three way tap immediately adjacent to the infusing cannula. The resistance of the three way tap and cannula itself resulted in a falsely high pressure recording some 200 mmHg higher than that made through the direct needle puncture. Since three way taps and cannulae vary from batch to batch it was decided that this variable but potentially considerable error was best avoided by the direct needling method.

Blood has been used to measure resistance in all cases. This obviated the need to make a correction for viscosity and haematocrit induced by using saline or some other infusion fluid. We have experienced no adverse effects from this policy in over 60 examinations.

We have infused at known flow rates and measured the pressure generated rather than the other way round because the measurement of pressure can be performed more accurately and more cheaply than flow. In addition it is technically very difficult to get a good fit of the flow probe around small and diseased vessels.

All measurements have been recorded on a chart recorder which has allowed subsequent analysis of results with computer storage.

ANIMAL EXPERIMENTS

Before being used in humans the above method was tested in a series of ten dogs in order to check the method and the reproducibility of the results. Each dog was given a general anaesthetic. Anaesthesia was induced with thiopentone and maintained with oxygen, nitrous oxide, and Hypnorm. The animals were intubated and ventilated, and pulse, blood pressure, urine output, and CVP were recorded continuously with intermittent recording of blood gases. In each case the technique described above has been used but in order to simulate the human ischaemic limb, the hindlimb was first rendered ischaemic by the technique described by Johansen and Bernstein.[15] The terminal aorta, last ipsilateral lumbar artery, both internal iliac arteries, and all branches of the iliac and femoral artery from the aorta above to the stifle below were ligated together with the main trunk of the external iliac artery itself.

Bernstein found that, using this technique, all of the animals developed irreversible gangrene of the limb and none survived. Pressure was measured in the femoral vein via a cannula sutured into a side branch of the femoral vein with its tip within the lumen. Similarly arterial pressure was measured by a cannula placed distal to the infusing cannula in a branch of the main artery with the tip of the cannula just emerging into the main artery.

Results

A typical trace produced on the chart recorder is reproduced in Figure 23-2. In this figure arteriovenous pressure difference has been plotted against flow. In this instance slightly different flow rates were in operation. As the flow increased the arteriovenous pressure difference also increased, but not in linear proportion. The rise in pressure difference was proportionately less than the rise in flow and thus the resistance was seen to fall as the flow increased.

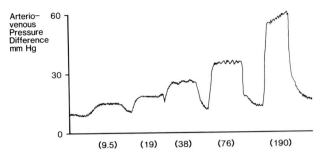

Fig. 23-2. Typical trace produced on chart recorder.

Figure 23-3 illustrates the combined results for all ten dogs and plots mean pressure (closed dots) with standard error and resistance (open dots) against flow. Resistance falls throughout the range as flow increases but at flow rates in excess of 80 ml/minute the relationship is approximately linear. The marked fall in resistance at low flow rates is probably partly due to the anomalous behaviour of blood viscosity at low shear rates and partly due to the peripheral vasodilatation occurring in the ischaemic limb. It seems likely from this that to be useful in a predictive way resistance would need to be measured in the linear part of the curve at higher flow rates, and that in this series of dogs the test was quite reproducible.

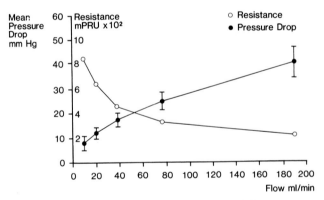

Fig. 23-3. Combined results for all ten dogs. Mean pressure (closed dots) plotted with standard error and resistance (open dots) against flow.

HUMAN STUDIES

In the light of the reproducibility of the animal experiments, it was decided that the same principle should be applied to patients to measure peripheral resistance. The long term aim of these experiments was to determine whether it might be possible to define a resistance, above which the chances of a successful graft would be so small that amputation or some other procedure should be used as the primary form of treatment. In order to provide information in as many different runoff situations as possible three groups of patients have been studied. Seven patients undergoing below knee amputation had resistance measured in the best vessel available at ankle level prior to amputation. Fifteen patients undergoing femorodistal reconstruction with adjunctive arteriovenous fistula had resistance measured at ankle level in the vessel to be used for the reconstruction. Thirty-seven patients undergoing femoropopliteal reconstruction, the majority to the infragenicular popliteal artery, had resistance measured in the popliteal artery at the site of graft anastomosis before grafting was performed. It was hoped that these three groups with a wide range of disease severity would provide a good range of resistances. In each case the preoperative arteriogram was independently assessed by a Consultant Radiologist without knowledge of the clinical details. All cases underwent intraoperative arteriography prior to resistance measurement including the amputees. The results were not made available to the Surgeon performing the operation, the actual procedure performed being based entirely on the preoperative or intraoperative arteriograms.

Results

Not all patients had pressure measured at all of the available flows, and, therefore, the numers available for analysis in each group are given. Where numbers were small, results have been omitted. All results have been analysed using the single tailed Mann-Whitney U Test.

Resistance and Operation

Figure 23-4 shows the mean resistance with standard error of all cases in each of the operation groups at three of the flow rates. In each case resistance falls as the flow increases, and in each case the resistance in the amputation group is greater than that in the femorodistal group (except at 153 ml/min), which is in turn higher than the femoropopliteal group. These findings reflect what one would expect to find given the relative severities of the disease processes present. Differences between the amputation and femoropopliteal group were significant ($p < 0.009$ at 38 ml/min and $p < 0.03$ at 76 ml/min) though there was no significant difference at 153 ml/minute. Similarly the differences between the femoropopliteal and femorodistal groups were significant at all flow rates ($p < 0.0008$ at 38 ml/min, $p < 0.0005$ at 76 ml/min, and $p < 0.01$ at 153 ml/min). There were no significant differences between the femorodistal group and the amputees. This suggested that the disease in the former group was severe enough to warrant amputation. In fact all the patients in the femorodistal group were consented for amputation at the time of reconstruction

RESISTANCE AND OPERATION

	38ml/min			76ml/min			153ml/min		
	No.	Res	S.E	No.	Res	S.E	No.	Res	S.E
Amputation	10	3707	1083	9	2060	628	6	870	279
Femorodistal	15	3174	648	15	1923	258	8	1071	235
Femoropopliteal	32	1417	103	32	986	79	26	662	72

Fig. 23-4. Mean resistance with standard error of all cases in each of the operation groups at three of the flow rates.

on the understanding that this would be performed if nothing else was possible. All those patients whose femorodistal grafts have failed have required amputation shortly afterwards for severe rest pain confirming that as a group they are very similar to those undergoing primary amputation.

Resistance and Runoff

Figure 23-5 shows the relationship between resistance and runoff. In the femorodistal group there were only small numbers for analysis and no significant differences. At 76 ml/minute the resistance of the two vessel runoff group was actually higher than the single runoff group. This finding is not surprising considering the severity of the disease present. In those with two vessels in the calf there was often no visible collateral connection between them, and the connection through into the foot was often tenuous. The two vessels were therefore in effect totally separate and of no greater advantage to the patient in terms of usable runoff than those with single vessel runoff. In the femoropopliteal group there were no significant differences between the single and two vessel runoff groups presumably as in the femorodistal group reflecting the poor collateral connection between the two vessels. However, both of these groups had significantly higher resistance than the three vessel runoff group ($p < 0.01$ at 38 ml/min, $p < 0.001$ at 76 ml/min and $p < 0.01$ at 153 ml/min for the two vessel runoff, and $p < 0.025$ at 38 ml/min, $p < 0.01$ at 76 ml/min and $p < 0.01$ at 153 ml/min for the one vessel group). Technically, satisfactory mea-

RESISTANCE AND RUNOFF

Femorodistal grafts

	38ml/min			76ml/min		
	No.	Res	S.E	No.	Res	S.E
One vessel	9	3467	1071	9	1817	389
Two vessel	4	1264	785	4	2361	470

Femoropopliteal grafts

	38ml/min			76ml/min			153ml/min		
	No.	Res	S.E	No.	Res	S.E	No.	Res	S.E
One vessel	6	1568	155	6	1121	89	5	720	83
Two vessel	9	1876	263	9	1357	204	7	1001	203
Three vessel	16	1192	121	18	734	53	14	471	45

Femoropopliteal grafts after papaverine

	117ml/min			153ml/min		
	No.	Res	S.E	No.	Res	S.E
One vessel	4	566	159	2	366	-
Two vessel	4	392	90	4	458	92
Three vessel	12	290	30	5	255	58

Fig. 23-5.   Relationship between resistance and runoff.

surement of resistance after the administration of papaverine was limited to small numbers of cases, and was performed at higher flow rates. The absolute values of resistance were considerably lower after papaverine as would be expected but the differences were only significant at 117 ml/minute between the single and three vessel runoff groups. The difficulty with measuring resistance after papaverine is due to the transient effect of the drug. There is no significant plateau of its effect before the pressure once again starts to rise. If only one measurement of resistance was being made, the postpapaverine level would be easy to measure as the lowest resistance recorded. But in these experiments resistance was being measured at several flow rates and consistent results were therefore impossible.

Resistance and Graft Survival

Figure 23-6 shows that at six months the resistance in the patent grafts is in each case lower than in the occluded grafts but the differences are not significant. However, at four months when there are more grafts available for review the differences are significant ($p < 0.007$ at 38 ml/min, $p < 0.006$ at 76 ml/min, and $p < 0.01$ at 153 ml/min). In the femorodistal group no significant differences could be demonstrated but this may have been due to the small numbers of cases available for analysis. Twelve of the femoropopliteal grafts have failed, and using the Kendall test of correlation there was found to be a significant negative correlation between survival time and resistance (tau $= -0.6$, $p < 0.003$). Of the flow rates tested in our series, resistance measured at 76 ml/minute seemed best at separating the various groups overall. No graft with a resistance greater than 1500 mPRU at 76 ml/min survived more than 1.5 months. Conversely, of 16 grafts performed with a resistance less than 1500 mPRU, 8 were still patent at the time of analysis and the mean graft survival time including both successful and failed grafts was 7.7 months. This difference was highly significant ($p < 0.001$). One of 6 grafts with a resistance greater than 1200 mPRU was still patent at the time of analysis, and the mean graft survival time was 3.35 months. Of the 11 grafts with a resistance less than 1200 mPRU, 5 were still patent at the time of analysis. The mean survival time in this group was 7.9 months. This difference was also significant ($p < 0.05$).

RESISTANCE AND GRAFT SURVIVAL - FEMOROPOPLITEAL GRAFTS

Grafts patent at 6/12 vs. grafts thrombosed at 6/12

	38ml/min			76ml/min			153ml/min		
	No.	Res	S.E	No.	Res	S.E	No.	Res	S.E
Patent	11	1206	154	11	874	83	11	488	95
Not patent	6	1491	455	11	1041	311	6	745	207

Grafts patent at 4/12 vs. grafts thrombosed at 4/12

	38ml/min			76ml/min			153ml/min		
	No.	Res	S.E	No.	Res	S.E	No.	Res	S.E
Patent	21	1236	82	21	847	60	15	516	49
Non patent	6	2225	383	6	1621	305	6	1166	244

Fig. 23-6. Resistance in the patent grafts at six months is lower than in the occluded grafts, but the differences are not significant.

CLINICAL APPLICATION

The difficulty experienced in assessing runoff is well illustrated by the two arteriograms (Figs. 23-7 and 23-8). In the first there is two vessel runoff and in the second single vessel runoff into the peroneal artery only. The resistance of both of these runoff situations was the same at 550 and 580 mPRU. Our experience thus far suggests that both of these grafts have a good chance of success. It is unlikely that on purely radiological grounds these two arteriograms would have been assessed to have the same resistance. With our limited experience of looking at graft survival time so far it would seem that there is a reasonable correlation between resistance and outcome and that resistance measurement may prove useful prognostically. It should be possible to measure resistance at a single flow rate probably in the range 75 to 125 ml/minute and use a cutoff of between 1000 mPRU and 1500 mPRU. Patients with a resistance above this level should be treated by either primary amputation, which may not be appropriate in many cases, or by the addition of an adjunctive arteriovenous fistula. Patients with a resistance below 1000 mPRU have a good chance of prolonged graft survival. The X-rays shown above indicate that one cannot make this decision on radiological grounds alone. The place of papaverine is not clear. In our experiments so far it has not proved helpful, but the

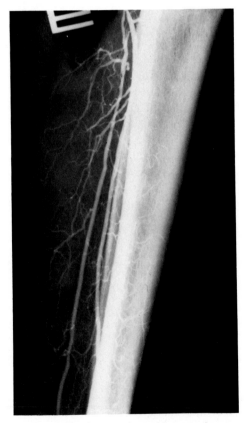

Fig. 23-7.   Difficulty experienced in assessing runoff.

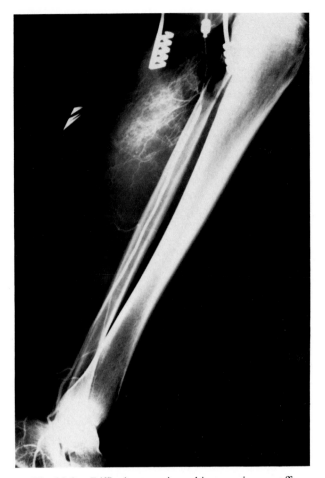

Fig. 23-8.   Difficulty experienced in assessing runoff.

situation would be different if resistance was only being measured at a single flow rate. The cutoff level of resistance has also to be determined more accurately, but this can only be achieved if more cases are studied. In our own centre we have now abandoned measurement of resistance at multiple flow rates and are attempting to simplify the technique so that it can be performed at a single flow rate without the need for special equipment or technical help.

   Ultimately it would be more sensible to perform comparisons of graft survival in relation to an objective measure of runoff rather than to an arbitrary and subjective assessment of arteriograms. This would permit meaningful comparisons of series from different centres and must surely be the goal of this type of research.

REFERENCES

1.   Imparato AM, Kim GE, Madayag M, et al: Angiographic criteria for successful tibial arterial reconstructions. Surgery 74:830–838, 1973
2.   Dardik H, Ibrahim IM, Sussman B, et al: Morphologic structure of the pedal arch and

its relationship to patency of crural vascular reconstruction. Surg Gynaecol Obstet 152:645–648, 1981

3. Khan PC, Boyer DN, Moran JM, et al: Reactive hyperaemia in lower extremity arteriography: An evaluation. Radiology 90:975–980, 1968

4. Feins RH, Roedersheimer LR, Baumstark AE, et al: Predicted hyperaemic angiography: A technique of distal arteriography in the severely ischaemic leg. Surgery 89:202–205, 1981

5. Dardik H, Sussman B, Ibrahim IM, et al: Distal arteriovenous fistula as an adjunct to maintaining arterial and graft patency for limb salvage. Surgery 94:478–486, 1983

6. Harris PL, Campbell H: Adjuvant distal arteriovenous shunt with femorotibial bypass for critical ischaemia. Br J Surg 70:377–380, 1983

7. Bliss BP: Thesis for Master of Surgery. University of London, 1968

8. Wheale SRF, Taylor GW, Rothwell-Jackson RL: Measurement of regional vascular resistance at operation. Br J Surg 52:627–630, 1964

9. Conrad MC, Green HD: Hemodynamics of large and small vessels in peripheral vacular disease. Circulation 29:847–853, 1964

10. Folse R: Alterations in femoral blood flow and resistance during rhythmic exercise and sustained muscular contractions in patients with arteriosclerosis. Surg Gynaecol Obstet 121:767–776, 1965

11. Delin A, Ekestrom S: Evaluation of reconstructive surgery for arterial stenoses from intraoperative determinations of flow, pressure and resistance. Acta Chir Scand 130:35–41, 1965

12. Mundth ED, Darling RC, Moran JM, et al: Quantitative correlation of distal arterial outflow and patency of femoropopliteal reversed saphenous vein grafts with intraoperative flow and pressure measurements. Surgery 65:197–206, 1969

13. Sonnenfeld T, Cronenstrand R, Nowak J: Leg haemodynamics during reconstructive vascular surgery. Br J Surg 66:586–589, 1979

14. Barner HB, Kaminski DL, Codd JE, et al: Haemodynamics of autogenous femoropopliteal bypass. Arch Surg 109:291–293, 1974

15. Johansen K, Bernstein EF: Revascularisation of the ischaemic canine hindlimb by arteriovenous reversal. Ann Surg 190:243–253, 1979

Enrico Ascer
and Frank J. Veith

24

Outflow Resistance Measurements in Infrainguinal Bypass Operations By Injecting Saline and Measuring the Integral of Pressure

It is well known that infrainguinal arterial reconstructions are less successful when more distal arteries are utilized. Infrapopliteal bypasses have consistently yielded lower patency rates than femoropopliteal bypasses.[1] The relatively high incidence of early failure after infrapopliteal bypasses has stimulated the search for a reliable predictor of graft success or failure. Various preoperative criteria, including arteriographic evaluation of the run-off bed and hemodynamic and clinical assessment of the degree of ischemia have proven to be unreliable prognostic indices of graft outcome.[2-4] These factors have not provided criteria whereby graft patency rates can be improved without excluding a substantial number of patients from successful limb salvage. Furthermore, intraoperative measurement of femoropopliteal bypass graft flow rates and outflow tract resistance have proven to be inconsistent predictors of graft patency.[5-9] These inconsistencies may relate either to the use of inaccurate methodology or to the fact that these studies only evaluated femoropopliteal bypasses in which the outflow resistance was not high enough to cause early graft failure.

The use of standard electromagnetic flow meters for evaluating bypass flows and outflow resistance presents several inaccuracies. In vivo calibration of these instruments is frequently difficult. Reliable quantitation of flow rates often cannot be obtained, especially when low-flow, small vessel bypasses are being evaluated. These arteries may be of very small caliber, calcified, and thick walled. Although the flow probes can be applied to a vein graft, they cannot be used directly on polytetrafluoroethylene (PTFE) grafts.

We attempted to calculate outflow resistance with a constant-infusion pump and a pressure transducer. This method was time-consuming and cumbersome. Another major disadvantage was related to the possible generation of dangerously high pressures within the system, placing the distal anastomosis at risk of rupture.

DIAGNOSTIC TECHNIQUES AND ASSESSMENT
PROCEDURES IN VASCULAR SURGERY

© 1985 Grune & Stratton
ISBN 0-8089-1721-8 All rights reserved

Furthermore, this method increased the risk of contamination. Accordingly, we have developed a new method for measuring outflow resistance for all infrainguinal arterial reconstructions.[10,11] Our new method overcomes the aforementioned disadvantages and is simple, accurate, and reproducible. Measurements can be obtained in less than 10 minutes.

This chapter has four purposes: (1) to report our results with measurement of outflow resistance as a predictive factor for graft outcome; (2) to report on the evaluation of the vasospastic component of outflow resistance (i.e., that portion that can be eliminated by papaverine injection) and the determination of its role in graft patency; (3) to show that critically high outflow resistance values can be used as a guide to modify the surgical procedure to obtain graft patency under otherwise unfavorable circumstances, and (4) to compare outflow resistance values to preoperative factors that could possibly predict graft success or failure.

METHODS

Patients

Intraoperative outflow resistance measurements were obtained during 104 infrainguinal arterial reconstructions for limb salvage in 96 patients at Montefiore Medical Center from July 1982 to December 1983. There were 56 men and 40 women (age, 51–88 years; mean, 68 years). Cardiovascular risk factors were frequent and often multiple (Table 24-1). The indications for surgery were rest pain in 19 patients (18%), nonhealing ischemic ulcer in 37 (36%), and gangrene in 48 (46%). There were 46 femoropopliteal (FP) bypasses and 58 bypasses to infrapopliteal arteries (FD). Expanded PTFE (WL Gore & Associates, Flagstaff, Ariz) grafts were used in 57 instances (35 FP, 22 FD), autogenous saphenous vein grafts were used in 44 (11 FP, 33 FD), and the remaining three operations (all FD) were performed with composite grafts. No veins smaller than 3.0 and 4.0 mm in diameter were used for FD and FP bypasses, respectively. Six-millimeter PTFE grafts were used for FP bypasses and tapered 6.5 to 4.5 mm for FD bypasses.

Of the 46 FP bypasses, 19 were to the below-knee popliteal artery, whereas 27 were inserted above the knee. Nineteen of the FP bypasses were inserted into an isolated popliteal artery segment. Of the 58 FD bypasses, 16 were to the anterior tibial artery, 10 to the posterior tibial, 18 to the peroneal, and 14 to the dorsalis

Table 24-1
Cardiovascular Risk Factors (96 Patients)

Risk Factor	Number of Patients	Percent
Age > 65 years	70	73
Previous myocardial infarction/congestive heart failure	43	45
Diabetes	59	61
Hypertension	63	66
Smoker/chronic obstructive pulmonary disease	46	48
Stroke	12	13

pedis. Twenty-three of the FD bypasses were performed with an intact pedal arch and 35 were performed when the pedal arch was either incomplete or absent.

Angiographic visualization of the inflow and outflow tracts was obtained preoperatively in all cases. In addition, completion arteriograms were routinely performed intraoperatively to verify the adequacy of the surgical technique and, in some instances, to define more clearly the morphologic characteristics of the outflow bed.

Noninvasive hemodynamic evaluation of the lower extremity, including segmental blood pressures and pulse volume recording tracings, were obtained before and after operation in many of these cases.

Our criteria and techniques for infrainguinal limb salvage bypass operations, patient follow-up, and determination of graft patency have been described in detail elsewhere.[12] All operations were performed under general anesthesia with isoflurane in conjunction with nitrous oxide, oxygen, and muscle relaxants. Systemic blood pressure was continuously monitored via a radial artery catheter. For high-risk patients, a central venous line was inserted, and whenever indicated, a balloon-tipped catheter was placed in the pulmonary artery for measurement of left ventricular function. In addition, core temperature was monitored throughout the procedure.

Method for Measurement of Outflow

After completion of the distal anastomosis of the bypass, 20–50 ml of normal saline solution was injected with a syringe into the fluid-filled graft and allowed to flow into the bypass outflow bed. During injection, the pressure generated in the graft was measured and electrically integrated. This pressure integral was a function of the outflow bed resistance that could be quantitated by the application of the hydraulic analog of Ohm's law to the arterial system, $R = P/F$, where R = resistance (mmHg/ml/min), P = pressure (mmHg), and F = flow (ml/min).

Assuming the resistance to be constant during the fluid injection, the numerator and denominator of this equation can be integrated, according to L'Hôspital's rule:

$$R = \frac{\int_0^t P \, dt}{\int_0^t F \, dt}$$

Since, by definition, the integral of flow ($\int_0^t F \, dt$) is the volume (V) injected, we can solve for resistance:

$$R = \frac{\int_0^t P \, dt}{V}$$

Thus, this equation permits the determination of resistance by measuring the integral of pressure and the volume of fluid injected.

To integrate the pressure generated during injection, we built an analog computer using 741 type operational amplifiers. This instrument is connected to an arterial pressure monitoring system that is available in every operating room. In our studies we used a standard Statham transducer and datascope (870 model) equipped with a P3 pressure module to display the digital readout. The graft is occluded proximally and a 21-gauge butterfly needle is inserted into the lumen of the graft and connected to the transducer by polyethylene tubing (Fig. 24-1). To avoid the resistance effect of the arterial back pressure generated through collateral flow into the recipient arterial segment, the measured back pressure in this segment is electrically zeroed before starting to integrate the pressure by the saline injection through the graft. If the back pressure is pulsatile, the mean pressure is electrically zeroed. To minimize the arterial and graft compliance variables, the pressure integration is started only after 5–15 ml of saline solution has been injected. By this time a pressure plateau has been reached and can be seen on the datascope. This plateau represents the injection pressure, which should be kept between 30 and 50 mmHg for femoropopliteal bypasses and between 40 and 60 mmHg for infrapopliteal bypasses. The amount of leakage from the distal anastomosis, if any, is measured by injecting 20 ml of saline solution into the graft and collecting the leakage in a small container placed under the distal incision. The percentage of leakage is used to accurately estimate the actual volume injected for use in calculating outflow resistance.

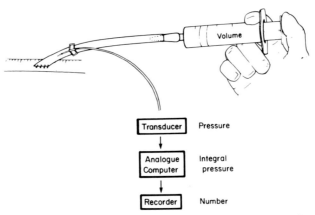

Fig. 24-1. Diagram illustrating method for measuring outflow resistance during bypass operation. After completion of distal anastomosis, graft is filled with saline solution and a syringe is attached to proximal end. A 21-gauge butterfly needle is inserted near distal anastomosis and connected to pressure transducer by polyethylene tubing. Analog computer, situated between transducer and recorder, displays electrically integrated pressure as a number.

Measurements by this technique have been performed with proximal and distal segments of the recipient artery unclamped (total outflow resistance), with the distal segment gently occluded (proximal outflow resistance), and finally, with the proximal segment gently occluded (distal outflow resistance) (Fig. 24-2).

To offset the possible occurrence of intraoperative arterial vasoconstriction and its effects on the measurement of outflow resistance, we repeated these measurements after local intraarterial injection of a standard dose of 60 mg papaverine hydrochloride in 60 patients (29 FP, 31 FD).

This entire investigation was carried out in accordance with the requirements of our Institutional Review Board for Human Research.

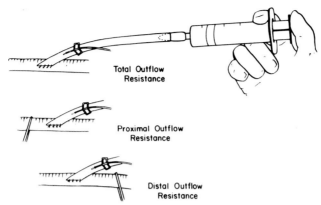

Fig. 24-2. Diagram shows how different components of outflow resistance were measured. Total outflow resistance is obtained when both proximal and distal segments of recipient artery are unclamped; proximal outflow resistance is obtained by gently occluding distal segment of recipient artery; and finally, distal outflow resistance is obtained by gently occluding proximal segment of recipient artery and allowing fluid to flow only into distal portion of artery.

Definition of Graft Patency and Exclusions

Three study patients died within the first three months after operation. These patients were excluded from the analysis. For the purpose of this study, early graft patency was considered to be up to three months.

Statistical Analyses

To correlate outflow resistance measurements with graft outcome and the type of bypass performed, a two-way analysis of variance was used. Since the probability distributions for vascular resistance changes in resistance, and related measurements appeared to be positively skewed and nonnormal, logarithmic transformations were applied to all of these measurements. Such transformation of the data resulted in homoscedasticity and distributions that appeared normal. Although the analyses were carried out using the transformed data, all summarizations of the data are presented using means and standard deviations of the untransformed resistance measurements along with medians and their respective upper (75%) and lower (25%) quartiles. Two-dimensional contingency tables were analyzed using the chi-square of Fisher exact tests, as appropriate.

RESULTS

Total Outflow Resistance and Overall Early Patency

A significant relationship was found when the total outflow resistance measurements (both segments of the recipient artery unclamped) were correlated with graft patency. The mean resistances for patent and occluded grafts were 0.39 ± 0.26 and

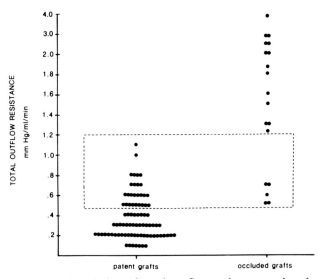

Fig. 24-3. Correlation of total outflow resistance and early graft patency in 101 infrainguinal arterial reconstructions. Although this method was valuable as predictor of graft patency, the area of overlap between 0.5 and 1.2 mmHg/ml/min prevented measurements from being perfect predictors in some cases.

1.62 ± 0.83 mmHg/ml/min, respectively ($P < .0001$) (Fig. 24-3). All grafts with a total outflow resistance >1.1 mmHg/ml/min occluded with the first three postoperative months and all grafts with a total outflow resistance <0.5 mmHg/ml/min remained patent. However, when the measured resistance was between these two values, three-month graft patency could not be predicted.

Distal Outflow Resistance and Overall Early Patency

Distal outflow resistance measurements (proximal segment of the recipient artery occluded) were also found to be a good predictor of graft outcome. The mean distal outflow resistance values for patent and occluded grafts were 0.46 ± 0.28 and 2.15 ± 1.07 mmHg/ml/min, respectively ($P < .0001$). Moreover, this technique provided values that were even better predictors of graft patency than the total outflow resistance values. A critical level of 1.2 mmHg/ml/min was identified. All bypasses with outflow resistance ≥ 1.2 mmHg/ml/min occluded within three months, whereas all bypasses with values below this level remained patent (Fig. 24-4).

Distal Outflow Resistance and Type of Bypass

As expected, distal outflow resistance measurements obtained during FP bypasses were found to be significantly lower than those obtained from FD bypasses, 0.33 ± 0.24 and 1.17 ± 0.99 mmHg/ml/min, respectively ($P < .001$) (Fig. 24-5). Interestingly, only one FP graft had an outflow resistance >1.2 mmHg/ml/min, although 19 (41%) were inserted into an isolated popliteal artery segment. This was the only FP graft that failed.

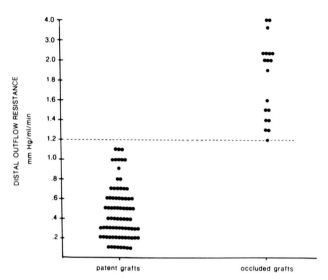

Fig. 24-4. Correlation of distal outflow resistances and early graft patency in 97 infrainguinal arterial reconstructions. A critical level of 1.2 mmHg/ml/min was identified.

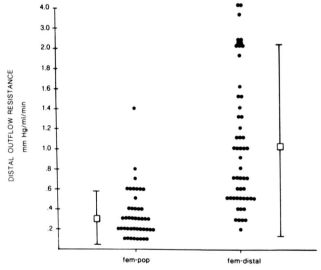

Fig. 24-5. Correlation of distal outflow resistances and type of bypass. There was significant difference between mean and standard deviations for both groups. Note that only one graft in femoropopliteal group had outflow resistance >1.2 mmHg/ml/min.

Changes After Papaverine Injection

In 60 grafts (28 FP, 32 FD) the median total outflow resistance before papaverine was 0.32 mmHg/ml/min (lower quartile 0.22 mmHg/ml/min; upper quartile 0.6 mmHg/ml/min), and after papaverine it was 0.25 mmHg/ml/min (lower quartile 0.15 mmHg/ml/min; upper quartile 0.42 mmHg/ml/min). This difference was statistically significant ($P < .001$). The same trend was observed in 53 grafts (24 FP, 29 FD) in which the median distal outflow resistance before papaverine was 0.57 mmHg/ml/min (lower quartile 0.24 mmHg/ml/min; upper quartile 1.02 mmHg/ml/min), and after papaverine it was 0.36 mmHg/ml/min (lower quartile 0.17 mmHg/ml/min; upper quartile 0.72 mmHg/ml/min) ($P < .01$), as shown in Fig. 24-6.

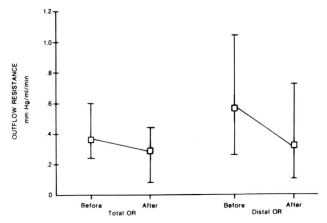

Fig. 24-6. Comparison of outflow resistances before and after local injection of papaverine in 60 bypasses. Both total and distal outflow resistances was significantly lowered by papaverine. Data are represented as medians and quartiles.

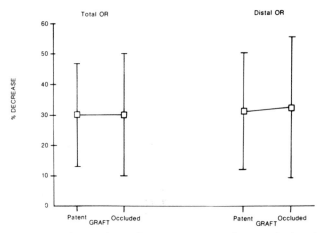

Fig. 24-7. Comparison of mean percentage decrease (induced by papaverine) in total and distal outflow resistances for patent and occluded grafts. No statistically significant difference was noted between the two groups.

Table 24-2
Degree of Papaverine Response (% Decrease)
and Possible Risk Factors

Factors	% Resistance Decrease	P value*
Diabetes		
Diabetic	29	
Non-diabetic	36	NS
Arterial calcification		
Calcified	32	
Non-calcified	23	NS
Distal anastomosis		
Popliteal	31	
Infrapopliteal	27	NS

* Fisher's exact test.

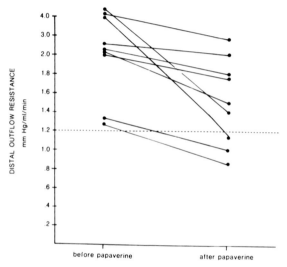

Fig. 24-8. Comparison of distal outflow resistance measurements before and after papaverine for nine failed bypasses. Note that in three cases (33%) distal outflow resistance was lowered to below the critical value of 1.2 mmHg/ml/min.

The effect of papaverine on outflow resistance measurements was not predictive of bypass success or failure. The mean percentage decrease in total outflow resistance for the nine FD bypasses that failed within three months was 30 ± 20.3%, and for the 51 bypasses (28 FP, 23 FD) that remained patent it was 30 ± 17.1%. Similarly, the mean percentage decrease in distal outflow resistance of bypasses (nine FD) that failed was 32 ± 22.8% and for the 44 bypasses (24 FP, 20 FD) that remained patent it was 31 ± 18.7% (Fig. 24-7). Further analysis showed that factors believed to influence the degree of the vasodilating response to papaverine, such as diabetic status, presence or absence of arterial calcification, and insertion of the graft into the popliteal or infrapopliteal arteries, failed to do so (Table 24-2).

Interestingly, when the distal outflow resistance measurements obtained before and after papaverine were plotted for the bypasses that occluded, a decrease in three of these to a value <1.2 mmHg/ml/min was observed (Fig. 24-8).

Outflow Resistance and Angiographic Criteria

In our earlier experience with 64 infrainguinal bypasses, a significant relationship ($r = .6$; $P < .0001$) was found when the four angiographic groups (isolated, nonisolated, with intact pedal arch, without intact pedal arch) were correlated with outflow resistance measurements (Fig. 24-9). However, when the means of the outflow resistance values were compared individually, the nonisolated group was not significantly different from the isolated group, nor was the intact pedal arch group significantly different from the absent pedal arch group.

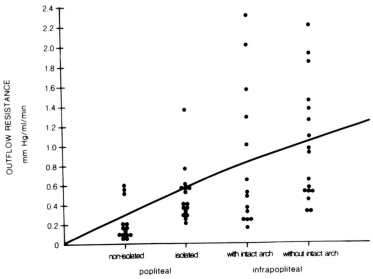

Fig. 24-9. Correlation of distal outflow resistance and angiographic pattern in 64 infrainguinal reconstructions (31 FP; 33 femorodistal).

Outflow Resistance and Overall Noninvasive Hemodynamic Measurements

Poor correlation was found between outflow resistance and ABPI ($r = 0.12$; $P = NS$), as shown in Figure 24-10. Ankle brachial pressure indices results were also found to be unreliable predictors of graft patency by the Fisher's exact test. Correlation of outflow resistance and PVR amplitudes at the ankle level is shown in Figure 24-11 ($r = 0.1$; $P = NS$). These amplitude results were found not to be significant predictors of graft patency by the Fisher's exact test.

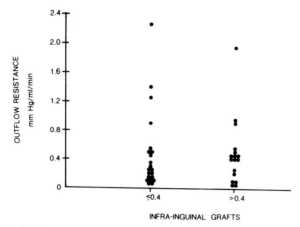

Fig. 24-10. Correlation of distal outflow resistance and ankle brachial pressure indices (ABPI) for infrainguinal reconstructions ($r = 0.12$; $P = $ NS).

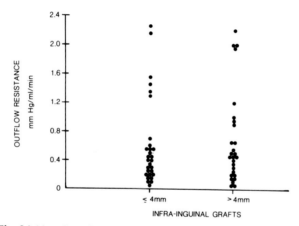

Fig. 24-11. Correlation of distal outflow resistance and PVR ankle amplitude tracings in 33 infrainguinal reconstructions ($P = $ NS).

Outflow Resistance and Other Variables in Femorodistal Bypasses

Because of the high occlusion rate in FD bypasses (19 of 55; 33%) (Fig. 24.5), an analysis of several variables that may predict graft failure was possible. These included diabetes, the presence of extensive arterial calcification as noted by the operating surgeon, use of PTFE graft material, and the absence of an intact pedal arch. None of these variables alone was found to be a significant predictor of early graft failure. However, total or distal outflow resistance measurements ≥ 1.2 mmHg/ml/min, regardless of the use of papaverine, were invariably associated with bypass failure within three months (Table 24-3).

Table 24-3
Comparison of Risk Factors and Graft Outcome in
55 Infrapopliteal Reconstructions (%)

Variable	Diabetes	Arterial Calcification	PTFE Graft Material	No Pedal Arch	Total or Distal Outflow Resistance >1.2 mmHg/ml/min
Patent	59	64	57	65	0
Occluded	41	36	43	35	100
P value*	NS	NS	NS	NS	<.001

* Fisher's exact test.

Outflow Resistance and Selection of Cases for Sequential Bypass

Three FD bypasses in which the distal outflow resistance measurement was >1.2 mmHg/ml/min occluded intraoperatively. During the same operation, a thrombectomy of the graft was performed in conjunction with an extension to a second distal artery. More recently, when the distal outflow resistance was >1.2 mmHg/ml/min, we performed primary sequential bypasses. All six sequential grafts have remained patent for over three months (Table 24-4). It is interesting to note in retrospect that of the 18 FD grafts that occluded, 12 patients (67%) were suitable for a sequential bypass to a different leg artery.

Table 24-4
Application of Resistance Measurements to Improve Patency
(>1.2 mmHg/ml/min) to Improve Patency

Primary Bypass (OR >1.2 mmHg/ml/min)	Outcome	Extension	Outcome
Posterior tibial	Occluded	Anterior tibial	Patent
Posterior tibial	Occluded	Peroneal	Patent
Dorsalis pedis	Occluded	Peroneal	Patent
Posterior tibial	. . .	Dorsalis pedis	Patent
Dorsalis pedis	. . .	Posterior tibial	Patent
Popliteal	. . .	Peroneal	Patent

DISCUSSION

It is generally believed by vascular surgeons that poor graft outflow with high outflow resistance is an important cause of early graft failure. The present investigation provides a simple, rapid, and reproducible intraoperative method for quantitating the outflow resistance of a bypass. Because of the rarity of early failures in femoropopliteal bypasses, even with bypass insertions into isolated popliteal artery segments, this outflow resistance measurement is of no discriminate value in predicting early failure of this operation. However, in bypasses to infrapopliteal arteries, high outflow resistance is not a rare finding and is a major cause of early graft occlusion. When the total outflow resistance measurement was modified by occluding the proximal outflow from the graft so that only the distal outflow resistance was measured, our method provided a highly accurate index of failure and success. All infrapopliteal bypasses with distal outflow resistances of 1.2 units or more thrombosed in the early postoperative period while all bypasses with lower resistances remained patent at least three months.

It is of interest that our measurements of bypass outflow resistance have failed to correlate with other preoperative hemodynamic and angiographic parameters, some of which have been thought to indicate a "poor" or "high" resistance outflow bed and to contraindicate attempts at arterial revascularization.[6,13] The poor correlation of measured outflow resistance with these parameters may explain why they have been disappointing predictors of bypass outcome.

It is well known that vasoconstriction can occur during infrainguinal arterial reconstructions and that it can be reversed with papaverine. These findings were confirmed by our study. A significant decrease in outflow resistance was observed in both FP and FD bypasses after local injection of papaverine, even in the presence of arterial calcification and diabetes. However, the degree of this vasodilatory response did not segregate bypasses destined to fail from those that would function three months or more. Thus, the concept of the so-called fixed resistance as a cause of early graft failure was not confirmed by our data.

However, elimination of the vasospastic component of the outflow resistance identified a subgroup of patients (33%) in whom a distal outflow resistance of more than 1.2 mmHg/ml/min were lowered to below the critical value. Although these grafts eventually occluded, it is interesting to speculate that perhaps long-term vasodilating therapy might improve patency rates in this setting.

The occurrence of intraoperative bypass failure in the presence of an outflow resistance >1.2 mmHg/ml/min prompted us to perform an immediate graft thrombectomy with extension of the graft as a sequential bypass to a second artery in three cases.[14] Figure 24-12 (A, B, and C) illustrates one such case. The successful outcome of these bypasses has encouraged us to perform primary sequential bypasses in three other situations that also appeared hopeless because of critically high outflow resistances. All six grafts have remained patent. This finding prompts us to raise two speculative possibilities. First, the additional outflow tract provided by the sequential limb may have increased flow through the proximal portion of the sequential graft. This increased flow through the long part of the graft may have been the decisive factor in improving patency. Second, although both distal limbs of the sequential grafts had low flow rates they remained patent. This suggests that short grafts may tolerate higher outflow resistances and lower flow rates than longer grafts.[15]

The described method for measuring outflow resistance may be beneficial for identifying some technical defects, particularly those at or distal to the distal anastomosis. A high outflow resistance in a femoropopliteal bypass should alert the surgeon to this possibility. However, not all technical defects will be identified and our method should not obviate the need for completion angiograms.

At present, high outflow resistance should not be used as the sole criterion for performing a major primary amputation. Some bypasses with high distal and total outflow resistances have succeeded long enough to permit foot lesions to heal and remain healed after graft closure has occurred. Perhaps increased experience with resistance measurements and other factors will allow criteria to be established for excluding the possibility of a successful bypass and limb salvage. However, this is not yet the case.

Moreover, the uniform accuracy of distal outflow resistance as a predictor of

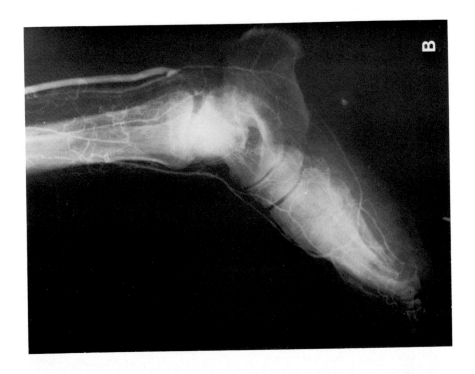

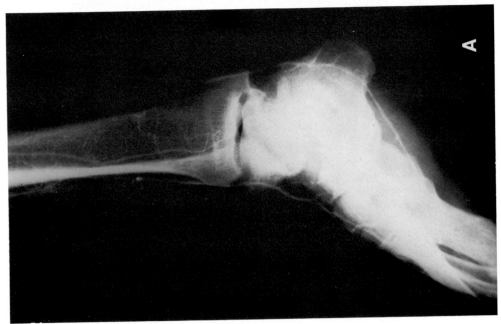

282

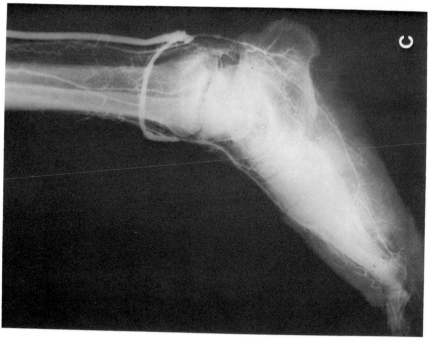

Fig. 24-12. (A) Preoperative arteriogram demonstrates patent dorsalis pedis and posterior tibial arteries. (B) since posterior tibial artery appeared to be of superior quality, femoroposterior tibial bypass was performed. Distal outflow resistance was >1.2 mmHg/ml/min. The graft occluded in the operating room. (C) Thrombectomy of femoroposterior tibial bypass graft and extension to dorsalis pedis artery were performed. Graft remains patent over four months.

bypass success and failure cannot persist. False-positive and false-negative determinations are expected to occur. Low resistance arterial reconstructions may fail because of a problem in the graft or its inflow tract. Both these areas are not assessed at all by our method. Similarly, a distal intimal flap that is nonobstructive but becomes so with time may cause a bypass with low outflow resistance to fail. This underscores the need not to substitute resistance measurements for completion angiography.

Finally, improvements in arterial prostheses, bypass techniques, or pharmacologic manipulation of platelet/coagulation systems may enable bypasses to be performed successfully although the distal outflow resistance exceeds 1.2 mmHg/ml/min. This possibility points up the importance of using our resistance measuring method to standardize cases used in the evaluation of different graft materials, new surgical techniques, and adjunctive drug therapies.

REFERENCES

1. Bergan JJ, Veith FJ, Bernhard VM, et al: Randomization of autogenous vein and poly-tetrafluoroethylene grafts in femoral-distal reconstruction. Surgery 92:921, 1982

2. Koontz, TJ, Stansel HC Jr: Factors influencing patency of the autogenous vein-femoropopliteal bypass graft: An analysis of 74 cases. Surgery 71:753, 1972

3. Miller VM: Femoropopliteal bypass graft patency: An analysis of 156 cases. Ann Surg 180:35, 1974

4. Ricco JB, Flinn WR, McDaniel MD, et al: Objective analysis of factors contributing to failure of tibial bypass grafts. World J Surg 7:347, 1983

5. Barner HB, Kaminski DL, Codd E, et al: Hemodynamics of autogenous femoropopliteal bypass. Arch Surg 109:291, 1974

6. Dean RH, Yao JST, Stanton PE, et al: Prognostic indicators in femoropopliteal reconstructions. Arch Surg 110:1287, 1975

7. Mannick JA, Jackson BT, Coffman JD, et al: Success of bypass vein grafts in patients with isolated popliteal artery segments. Surgery 61:17, 1967

8. Mundth ED, Darling RC, Moran JM, et al: Quantitative correlation of distal arterial outflow and patency of femoropopliteal reversed saphenous vein grafts with intraoperative flow and pressure measurements. Surgery 65:197, 1969

9. Terry HJ, Allan JS, Taylor GW: The relationship between blood-flow and failure of femoropopliteal reconstructive arterial surgery. Br J Surg 59:549, 1972

10. Ascer E, Veith FJ, Morin L, et al: Quantitative assessment of outflow resistance in lower extremity arterial reconstructions. J Surg Res 37:8, 1984

11. Ascer E, Veith FJ, Morin L, et al: Components of outflow resistance and their correlation with graft patency in lower extremity arterial reconstructions. J Vasc Surg 1985 (in press)

12. Veith FJ, Gupta SK, Samson RH, et al: Progress in limb salvage by reconstructive arterial surgery combined with new or improved adjunctive procedures. Ann Surg 194:386, 1981

13. Imparato AM, Kim GE, Madayag M, et al: Angiographic criteria for successful tibial arterial reconstructions. Surgery 74:830, 1973

14. Edwards WS, Gerety E, Larkin J, et al: Multiple sequential femoral tibial grafting for severe ischemia. Surgery 80:722, 1976

15. Veith FJ, Gupta SK, Weiser RK, et al: Short vein grafts in limb salvage arterial reconstructions, In Bergan JJ, Yao JST (eds) Evaluation and Treatment of Upper and Lower Extremity Circulatory Disorders. Orlando, Fla, Grune & Stratton, 309:17, 1984

D. Preston Flanigan

25

Peroperative Doppler Testing and Imaging in Patients with Lower-Limb Ischemia

The purpose of preoperative Doppler testing and imaging is to determine if lower extremity symptoms suggestive of ischemia are truly of ischemic origin and, if so, to determine the severity and location of the arterial occlusive process. Additionally, intraoperative techniques can be used to assess even better the location of the occlusive process and to determine the technical adequacy of the vascular procedure, thus avoiding the need for reoperation by allowing repair of technical errors at the time of the primary operation.[1]

Peroperative imaging includes the use of both intraoperative arteriographic and ultrasonic imaging. Preoperative arteriography and intraoperation completion arteriography are covered elsewhere in the volume. The imaging part of this chapter will be limited to intraoperative prebypass arteriography and intraoperative imaging ultrasound.

PREOPERATIVE DOPPLER TESTING

The principles of Doppler ultrasound are not repeated here. Suffice it to say that the Doppler shift caused by moving blood cells can be converted to an audible frequency range and/or can be charted against time to produce a Doppler analog waveform.

The normal Doppler analog waveform obtained from the axial arteries of the lower extremity are triphasic in nature (Fig. 25-1A). The first component is representative of forward flow during systole, the second component is a result of reversed flow during diastole, and the third component is representative of forward flow in late diastole. Disease that narrows the lumen of an artery being tested can cause changes in the waveform in proportion to the degree of narrowing. With mild disease, the third component disappears rendering the waveform biphasic and causing a possible irregularity of the waveform secondary to turbulence (Fig. 25-1B). As greater stenoses are encountered or the artery becomes occluded the component of reverse flow disappears and the waveform becomes monophasic (Fig. 25-1C). In

DIAGNOSTIC TECHNIQUES AND ASSESSMENT
PROCEDURES IN VASCULAR SURGERY

© 1985 Grune & Stratton
ISBN 0-8089-1721-8 All rights reserved

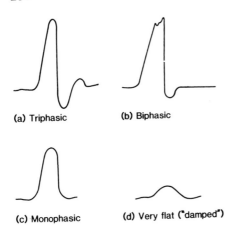

(a) Triphasic   (b) Biphasic

(c) Monophasic   (d) Very flat ("damped")

Fig. 25-1. Doppler analog waveform tracings in various stages of arterial occlusive disease. (A) Normal triphasic waveform. (B) Biphasic waveform with mild turbulence as seen with mild arterial disease. (C) Monophasic waveform as seen with severe stenoses or occlusion. (D) Low amplitude monophasic waveform as seen with total arterial occlusion with poor collateralization.

situations of good collateral flow around arterial occlusions, the waveform amplitude remains normal or only slightly depressed. With poor collateral, the amplitude decreases and the waveform may be nearly flat (Fig. 25-1D).[2]

INTRAOPERATIVE DOPPLER TESTING

Doppler examinations can be carried out under sterile conditions in the operating room to assess the results of lower extremity revascularization.[3] The test consists of performing segmental pressure measurements using a sterile Doppler probe and blood pressure cuffs. The sphygmomanometer and main Doppler unit are not sterile and are positioned adjacent to the operating table (Fig. 25-2). Measurements are made following revascularization but prior to wound closure. Pressures are usually taken at the ankle and, occasionally, at the thigh level.

In the situation of bypassing single segment disease, the ankle index should become normal following bypass. If this does not occur several factors may be at cause. There may be inadequate inflow to the graft: this situation can be evaluated by the intraoperative measurement of intraarterial pressure in the donor artery. Alternatively, there could be a technical problem at the proximal or distal anastomosis. This possibility can be assessed in infrainguinal reconstruction by measure-

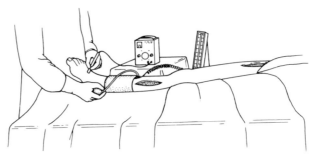

Fig. 25-2. Method of measuring Doppler-derived segmental pressures on the operating table. From Williams LR, et al. Am J Surg 144:578, 1982. With permission.

ment of segmental Doppler-derived pressures over the graft. If the pressure index over the mid portion of the vein graft is normal, then the problem is not at the proximal anastomosis and is either at the distal anastomosis, the distal segmental of the graft, or in the runoff vessels. These possibilities can be assessed by the use of completion intraoperative arteriography or by intraoperative ultrasonic imaging. Situations unique to in-situ saphenous vein bypass procedures are uncut venous valves and unligated arterio-venous fistulae. Both of these factors can prevent the ankle pressure index from becoming normal. Intraoperative arteriography can usually detect these problems and localize them for correction. The incompressible nature of polytetrafluoroethylene grafts precludes segmental pressure measurements over the graft. In this situation, intragraft pressures may be obtained by needle punctures of the graft.

When patients have multisegment disease, only part of which is bypassed leaving disease between the distal anastomosis and the ankle, the ankle index will usually not increase to normal. In this situation, it would be helpful to know what degree of increase should occur following bypass. This ability to predict the increase in ankle pressure following bypass would also be helpful preoperatively in patients with multisegment disease to determine the extent of revascularization required. Practically, this usually means determining whether an inflow procedure, an outflow procedure, or both will be required in a given patient.

To predict the pressure index at a given level following bypass, one needs to know the preoperative pressure index at that level and the preoperative pressure index at the proposed site of the distal anastomosis (Fig. 25-3).[4] This information can be obtained with segmental Doppler-derived pressures except in the case where the distal anastomosis is to be in the common femoral artery. In these patients, common femoral artery pressure must be obtained preoperatively by arterial puncture. The premise supporting this approach is that the pressure index at the level of the distal anastomosis will be normal following a technically adequate bypass performed in a situation of normal inflow. The percent increase between the preoperative and postbypass pressure at the level of the distal anastomosis should be the same percent increase seen at any site distal to the distal anastomosis.

We studied correlations between the predicted pressure index and the actual postoperative pressure index attained for both suprainguinal ($N = 49$) and infrainguinal ($N = 134$) bypasses (Fig. 25-4). The correlation was excellent for both suprainguinal and infrainguinal revascularizations. In the suprainguinal group only 4% of pressure indices failed to increase to within 0.1 of the predicted value and in the infrainguinal group only 9% failed to achieve this level.[4]

$$\text{Predicted Pressure Index} = \frac{\text{Preoperative Pressure Index}}{\text{Preoperative Pressure Index}}$$

Predicted Pressure Index
(level of interest)

= Preoperative Pressure Index
(level of interest)

—————————————————————

Preoperative Pressure Index
(site of proposed distal anastomosis)

Fig. 25-3. Formula for the prediction of pressure index at any level following arterial bypass. From Flanigan DP, Williams LR, Schuler JJ: Perioperative and intraoperative assessment in limb revascularization, In Bergan JJ, Yao JST (eds): Evaluation and Treatment of Upper Limb Extremity Circulatory Disorders. Orlando, Fla, Grune & Stratton, 1984, pp 135. With permission.

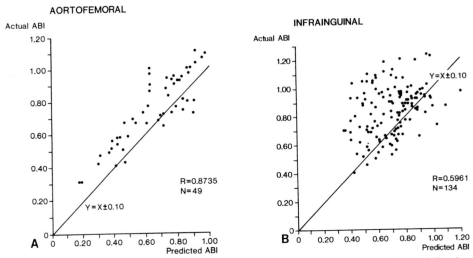

Fig. 25-4. Correlation between predicted and actual ankle/brachial pressure index following suprainguinal (A) and infrainguinal (B) revascularization.

POSTOPERATIVE DOPPLER TESTING

The purpose of early postoperative Doppler testing is to assess graft function during a period when failure is most likely. Many patients may not have adequate palpable pulses postoperatively to allow for accurate detection of graft failure or impending failure. Yao and Bergan have described the use of hourly Doppler-derived ankle pressure measurements postoperatively for this purpose (Fig. 25-5).[5] A return of the ankle index to the preoperative level indicates graft thrombosis and allows for timely remedial therapy. A declining ankle pressure index indicates impending failure and may indicate the need for intervention to avoid graft thrombosis and possible limb loss.

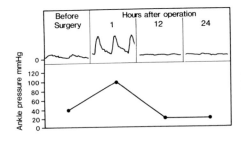

Fig. 25-5. Postoperative monitoring of bypass graft patency using Doppler measurements. From Yao, JST and Bergan JJ, Surg Clin North Am 54:23, 1974. With permission.

PEROPERATIVE IMAGING

Prebypass Operative Arteriography

The need for accurate and complete preoperative arteriography cannot be over-emphasized. Disastrous consequences can result from bypass to an inappropriate vessel or even worse from not performing a bypass procedure in a patient with

Fig. 25-6. Technique of prebypass operative arteriography. From Flanigan DP, Williams LR, Keifer TJ, et al: Prebypass operative arteriography. Surgery 92:627, 1982. With permission.

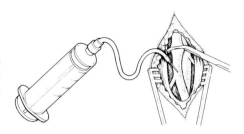

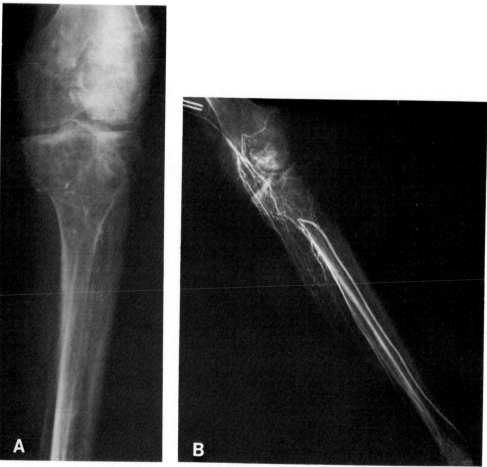

Fig. 25-7. (A) Preoperative arteriogram showing no patent axial vessels. (B) Prebypass operative arteriogram demonstrating patent axial calf arteries acceptable for bypass. From Flanigan DP, Williams LR, Keifer TJ, et al: Prebypass operative arteriography. Surgery 92:627, 1982. With permission.

critical ischemia because arteriography incorrectly demonstrated no recipient vessel. Prebypass operative arteriography is useful in avoiding such errors by providing a complete view of the more distal lower extremity arterial anatomy when pre-operative studies appear inadequate or because amputation is being entertained because of the preoperative arteriographic demonstration of no recipient vessel.

The technique may be performed at any level but most commonly the common femoral or popliteal arteries are used. When preoperative arteriography demon-strates a patent popliteal artery it is used preferentially as the injection site since the technique is more reliable at this location. When the popliteal artery is not visual-ized on preoperative arteriography or it is felt to be unwise to dissect the popliteal vessels, the common femoral artery is used.

The technique is the same for both sites except for the amount of contrast injected and the delay prior to exposure of the film.[6] Dissection of the artery is performed and a proximal inflow occlusion clamp is applied (Fig. 25-6). The film is placed in a sterile cassette cover and placed under the part of the leg (not under the

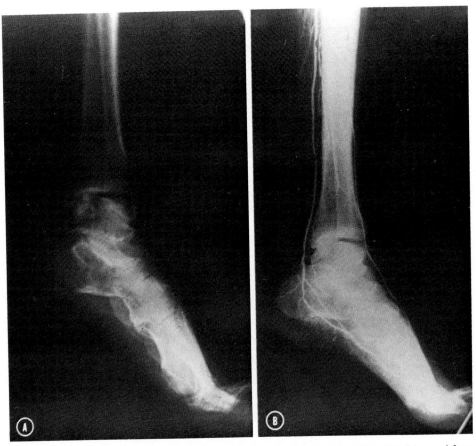

Fig. 25-8. (A) Preoperative arteriogram showing poor visualization of the distal leg and foot arteries. (B) Prebypass operative arteriogram showing the dorsalis pedis, posterior tibial, and pedal arch arteries. From Flanigan DP, Williams LR, Keifer TJ, et al: Prebypass operative arteriography. Surgery 92:627, 1982. With permission.

operating table) to be visualized. In the femoral artery, 60 cc of full-strength contrast is injected via a 19-gauge needle and exposure of the film is accomplished at seven seconds following injection. In the popliteal artery 15 cc of contrast is injected using a 23-gauge needle and exposure is made immediately following injection.

The utility of the technique in a given practice will depend on the quality of the preoperative arteriography available. In our experience, prebypass operative arteriography was of benefit 91% of the time it was used.[6] In 66% of the patients, bypasses were performed to vessels that were not visualized on preoperative arteriograms (Fig. 25-7) and in 25% of the patients the technique changed the proposed site of the distal anastomosis by providing improved visualization of vessels that were poorly visualized on preoperative studies (Fig. 25-8). In 93% of our patients in whom amputation was thought necessary because of critical ischemia and preoperative nonvisualization of recipient vessels, limb salvage was obtained as a result of employing prebypass operative arteriography and appropriate bypass.

INTRAOPERATIVE ULTRASONIC IMAGING

The main advantage of ultrasound over arteriography for intraoperative assessment of the technical adequacy of revascularization is that it is noninvasive. It avoids the use of contrast agents and the associated complications of nephrotoxicity and volume overload. Additionally, it allows visualization in multiple planes at multiple angles in real-time as contrasted to the single-plane static views provided by arteriography. The disadvantage of ultrasound is that examination is somewhat limited to the operative wound, thus limiting the proper visualization of the runoff vessels. Additionally, current ultrasound probe design is such that some sites are technically difficult to visualize.[7]

Intraoperative imaging ultrasound is made possible through the advent of real-time, B-mode, high-resolution small parts scanners. The technique employs 7.5–12 MHz B-mode ultrasound using either mechanical sector or linear array technology. The test is performed using a hand-held ultrasound probe that is either gas sterilized or enclosed in a sterile plastic sleeve for operative use. Acoustic coupling gel is placed between the sleeve and probe. The operative wound is filled with sterile saline for further acoustic coupling and the probe is manipulated over the vascular site providing a real-time image (Fig. 25-9). The image resolution is <1 mm. The image is projected on a black and white monitor adjacent to the operating table. The main ultrasound unit, also adjacent to the operating table, is operated by an ultrasound technician. Interpretations are made in real-time by the operating surgeon. Hard copy is available on polaroid film, video tape, or roentgenogram film.

Prior to clinical use, the accuracy of the technique was determined in the animal laboratory. Defects consisting of 1–5 mm intimal flaps, subintimal hema-

Fig. 25-9. Illustration of longitudinal (A) and transverse (B) intraoperative ultrasound scanning of an end-to-side arterial anastomosis. From Sigel B, Flanigan DP, Schuler JJ, et al: Detection of vascular defects during operation by imaging ultrasound. Ann Surg 196:473, 1982. With permission.

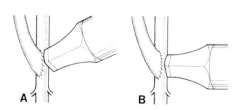

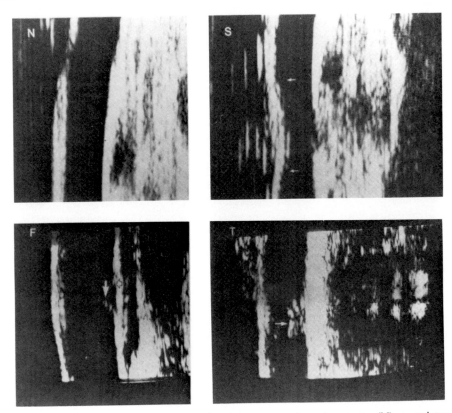

Fig. 25-10. Operative ultrasonograms showing a normal canine aorta (N), a strictured canine aorta (S), a canine aorta with an intimal flap (F), and a canine aorta with intraluminal thrombus (T). From Coelho JCU, Sigel B, Flanigan DP, et al: Detection of arterial defects by real-time ultrasound scanning during vascular surgery: An experimental study. J Surg Res 30:535, 1981. With permission.

tomas, thrombi, and strictures were created in canine aortas (Fig. 25-10).[8] Ultrasound correctly identified 100% of all lesions except for 1-mm flaps which were identified 67% of the time. Ultrasound was further evaluated in this model and was found to be superior to both single-plane portable and serial biplane arteriography in the detection of these defects (Table 25-1).[9] The technique likewise was evaluated clinically in comparison to arteriography.[7] The main difference in this setting was a greatly superior positive predictive value for ultrasound (Table 25-2).

The appearance of defects created in the canine aorta as seen on ultrasound are shown in Figure 25-10. Intimal flaps, in addition to being echogenic, can be seen to move toward and away from the arterial wall with arterial pulsation. Thrombi remain fixed and strictures are evidenced by a decrease in the size of the arterial lumen. Figure 25-11 shows an example of actual clinical operative sonograms obtained in a patient undergoing femoral popliteal bypass.

Of 841 vascular sites examined, 21% showed ultrasonic defects.[7] The percent distribution of these defects is shown in Table 25-3. All of these defects were not considered significant as only 32% were repaired for an overall repair rate of 7%. The decision to repair a defect is difficult and depends on the size, location, and type

Table 25-1

Percent Accuracy of Ultrasound *V* Portable and Serial
Biplane Arteriography

Defects	Portable Arteriography	Serial Biplane Arteriography	Ultrasonography
2 × 5 mm flaps	59%	75%	95%
5 × 5 mm flaps	61%	73%	96%
Thrombi	67%	84%	100%
Strictures	73%	79%	85%

Table 25-2

Clinical Comparison of Operative Ultrasonography
and Arteriography

Test	Ultrasonography	Arteriography
Sensitivity	92.3%	92.3%
Specificity	97.5%	93.8%
Accuracy	96.8%	93.5%
Positive predictive value	85.7%	70.6%
Negative predictive value	98.7%	98.7%

Table 25-3

Relative Frequency of Defects

Defect	Percent Frequency
Intimal flaps	44%
Thrombi	23%
Strictures	30%
Other	3%

Table 25-4

Repaired Ultrasound Defects

Defect	Size	Number	Location
Intimal flap	1 mm	1	T
	2 mm	2	P, T
	3 mm	3	2P, T
	4 mm	1	T
	5 mm	6	IC, 2F, 3P
	7 mm	2	A, CC
Thrombus	Total	4	P, 2T, Splenorenal
	4 × 5 mm	1	IC
	5 × 5 mm	1	Portacaval
Stricture	30%	2	2T
	40%	4	IC, F, vein graft, portacaval
	50%	3	2F, T
Inverted graft	⋯	1	P-T graft

Note. IC = internal carotid, CC = common carotid, F = femoral, P = popliteal,
T = tibial, and A = aorta. There were 31 defects in 26 patients.

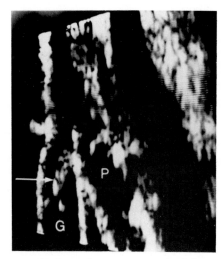 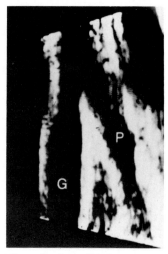

Fig. 25-11. (A) Operative sonogram of a vein graft (G) to distal popliteal artery (P) anastomosis showing intraluminal graft thrombus and a popliteal artery intimal flap. (B) Appearance of the same anastomosis after correction of the defects.

of defect encountered. Additionally, the type of operation being performed and the condition of the patient must be considered in the decision to reopen a vessel to effect repair. Tables 25-4 and 25-5 show defects repaired and not repaired respectively at a time when we had scanned 411 sites. The current approach is not different after scanning 841 sites.

Indications for vessel reentry have been subjective and empiric. It is difficult to know if the indications are appropriate since it can only be assumed that complications would have followed nonrepair of those defects actually repaired. The validity of the subjective criteria are supported by our experience with 174 infrainguinal bypass procedures in which the one-month patency rate was not sta-

Table 25-5
Unrepaired Ultrasound Defects

Defect	Size	Number	Location
Intimal flap	1 mm	6	IC, 3F, P, T
	2 mm	44	6CC, IC, 3IC, 26F, 6P, T, SUBCL
	3 mm	15	3A, 3CC, 2EC, 6F, P
	4 mm	6	A, CC, 2F, 2P
	5 mm	2	A, EC
	6 mm	1	A
Thrombus	2 × 2 mm	1	Splenorenal
	3 × 3 mm	1	Splenorenal
	3 × 5 mm	1	F
Stricture	28%	6	2F, P, vein graft, portacaval, splenorenal
	40%	1	P

Note. IC = internal carotid, EC = external carotid, CC = common carotid, F = femoral, P = popliteal, T = tibial, SUBCL = subclavian, and A = aorta. There were 84 defects in 65 patients.

Table 25-6
One-Month Patency of Lower Extremity Bypass
Grafts According to Operative Ultrasound
Findings

Patient Group	One-Month Patency
No ultrasound defect	90%
Unrepaired ultrasound defects	98%
Repaired ultrasound defects	88%

Note.   There was a total of 174 grafts.

tistically different for those with no defects, those with no defects that were repaired, and those with defects judged to be insignificant and, therefore, left unrepaired (Table 25-6).

REFERENCES

1. Flanigan DP, Williams LR, Schuler JJ: Perioperative and intraoperative assessment in limb revascularization, In Bergan JJ, Yao JST (eds): Evaluation and Treatment of Upper Limb Extremity Circulatory Disorders. Orlando, Fla, Grune & Stratton, 1984, pp 135
2. Nichalaides AN, Gordon-Smith IC, Dayandas J, et al: The value of Doppler blood velocity tracings in detection of aortoiliac disease in patients with intermittent claudication. Surgery 80:774, 1976
3. Williams LR, Flanigan DP, Schuler JJ, et al: Intraoperative assessment of limb revascularization by Doppler-derived segmental blood pressures. Am J Surg 144:578, 1982
4. Williams LR, Flanigan DP, Schuler JJ, et al: Prediction of improvement in ankle blood pressure following arterial bypass. J Surg Res 1985 (in press)
5. Yao JST, Bergan JJ: Application of ultrasound to arterial and venous diagnosis. Surg Clin North Am 54:23, 1974
6. Flanigan DP, Williams LR, Keifer TJ, et al: Prebypass operative arteriography. Surgery 92:627, 1982
7. Flanigan DP: Intraoperative Vascular Ultrasound. Presented at the Meeting of the Society for Clinical Vascular Surgery, Palm Spring, Calif, 1984
8. Coelho JCU, Sigel B, Flanigan DP, et al: Detection of arterial defects by real-time ultrasound scanning during vascular surgery: An experimental study. J Surg Res 30:535, 1981
9. Coelho JCU, Sigel B, Flanigan DP, et al: An experimental evaluation of arteriography and imaging ultrasonography in detecting arterial defects at operation. J Surg Res 32:1982

Brian P. Heather, Ian L. Green,
Charles N. McCollum, and Roger M. Greenhalgh

26

Intraoperative Detection of Arterio-Venous Fistulae After In-Situ Vein Bypass

After all valves have been rendered incompetent and proximal and distal anastomoses are completed, the final important stage of in-situ vein bypass is the detection and ligation of residual branches of the long saphenous vein that may act as arterio-venous fistulae. The method chosen to detect such potential fistulae will be influenced to the same extent by the technique used for valve disruption.

If valves in the thigh portion of the vein are cut with either a modified Hall stripper or the floating intraluminal valve cutter described by Leather et al,[1] significant lengths of vein may remain unexposed. On the other hand, if the Leather valvulotome is used to cut valves along the whole vein, as is our usual practice, it is essential that the entire length of vein is exposed along its outer surface to enable use of the instrument under direct vision. Such long continuous incisions are easily closed with a continuous subcuticular polypropylene suture and, in our experience, have caused no problems with postoperative wound healing.

Obvious branches of the vein are dealt with by division and ligation, by application of a silver clip, or by ligation in continuity by oversewing with a fine non-absorbable suture. Excessive circumferential mobilisation of the vein in search of branches is, however, probably best avoided since one of the claimed advantages of the in-situ technique is improved nutrition of the vein by leaving it undisturbed in its bed.

Lengths of vein that have not been exposed are best examined by on-table angiography using a marking grid of subcutaneous needles. This technique, as described by Karmody et al,[2] not only demonstrates arterio-venous fistulae, which can be located and ligated through small separate incisions, but also reveals potential areas of narrowing or kinking in the vein (Fig. 26-1). With the full length of vein exposed, it is possible to use either a sterile Doppler probe or an electromagnetic flow meter to detect residual arterio-venous fistulae.

Figures 26-2 to 26-7 illustrate our own current technique using a Gould Stathom SP2204 self-zeroing electromagnetic flow meter. The probe is placed proxi-

DIAGNOSTIC TECHNIQUES AND ASSESSMENT
PROCEDURES IN VASCULAR SURGERY

© 1985 Grune & Stratton
ISBN 0-8089-1721-8 All rights reserved

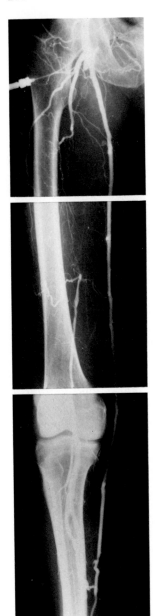

Fig. 26-1. Arteriogram demonstrating an in situ vein graft with a large arterio-venous fistula filling the deep veins. Some stenosis of the vein is also noted just above the fistula.

mally on the vein and initially records combined graft and fistula flow. The vein is then temporarily occluded by finger and thumb just distal to the probe to check the accuracy of the meter's zero reading. The point of occlusion by a compressing digit is gradually moved distally along the vein until the appearance of a wave form and a positive flow reading suggests that a vein branch has just been passed. The vein is carefully explored at the indicated site, the branch is ligated in continuity, and ligation is confirmed by return of the flow reading to zero. Sequential occlusion of the vein is continued in this fashion down to the distal anastomosis at which time the

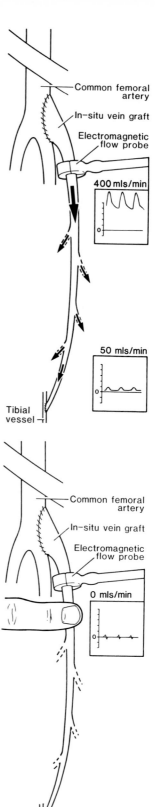

Fig. 26-2. Diagram of an in-situ vein graft with several hidden branches present. The electromagnetic flow probe placed just past the proximal anastomosis shows a very high flow. However, flow measurements at the distal end of the graft would show that only a small proportion of the flow is reaching the distal artery.

Fig. 26-3. Occlusion of the graft just distal of the probe stops all flow and the flow meter should register zero.

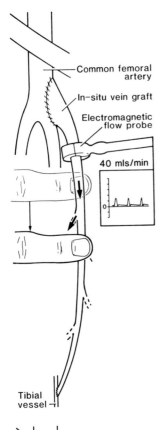

Fig. 26-4. As the finger occluding the graft is moved distally, the flow should remain at zero. The presence of flow indicates a patent vein branch proximal to the point of occlusion. This allows localisation of the branch so that it can be tied with only minimal mobilisation of the vein.

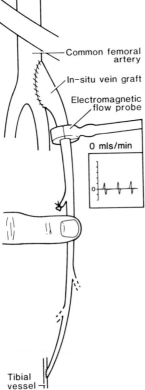

Fig. 26-5. After tying the branch, flow should return to zero when the vein is occluded just distal to this point. The flow waveform may indicate some forward flow but with an equal reversal. This is due to some expansion of the compliant vein walls with each pulse and the effect increases as the graft is occluded more distally.

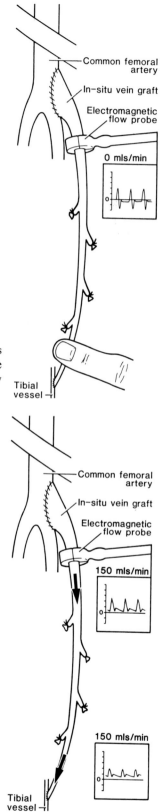

Fig. 26-6. The graft is occluded more distally and branches are tied if any flow occurs in the graft. Finally, the graft can be occluded next to the distal anastomosis and the graft flow should be zero.

Fig. 26-7. The graft is released and all flow will now be reaching the distal artery. Flow measurements made distally should confirm this if the correct size flow probes are used, but this should not be necessary. Although the flow at the top and the bottom of the graft is equal, the shape of the velocity profile alters down the graft. This is again largely due to the compliance of the vein walls.

final flow in the vein bypass itself is recorded. Using this technique, we have not found it necessary to perform additional on-table angiography to detect arterio-venous fistulae. However, if the final flow in the in situ bypass is inadequate, an operative arteriogram is performed to investigate the distal vessels and appearance of the distal anastomosis.

REFERENCES

1. Leather RP, Corson JD, Karmody AM: Instrument evaluation of the valve incision method of in-situ saphenous vein bypass. J Vasc Surg (in press)
2. Karmody AM, Leather RP, Corson JD, et al: The in-situ saphenous vein arterial bypass by valve incision, In Greenhalgh RM (ed): Vascular Surgical Techniques. London, Butter-worths, 1984, pp 191–198

H. Loeprecht
H. Weber
and J. Monnig

27

Vascular Endoscopy

For more than six decades intraluminal inspection of blood vessels and cardiac chambers has constituted a challenge for both physicians and surgeons.[1] But its problems were many: (1) Blood in the vessel segment of interest had to be replaced by a suitable transparent medium; (2) Suitable instruments with an excellent optical system were needed.

Advances in reconstructive vascular surgery provided new impetus for research in vascular endoscopy. In the late 1960s, J. Vollmar introduced the techniques as a routine procedure after vessel repair. The instruments available at that time were either rigid with excellent lens systems or flexible (fiber bronchoscopes).[2,3] However, their use was confined to vessels of large caliber, e.g., the iliac arteries and veins. Not before the advent of fiberscopes with a small diameter did the technique find further applications.

Once the requisite instruments had become available for a widespread use of arterioscopy and venoscopy, it was of interest to see whether vascular endoscopy could replace other intraoperative quality control procedures in clinical routine, particularly intraoperative angiography, flow measurements, or simple exploration of the reconstructed vessel segments.

ENDOSCOPIC INSTRUMENTS AND ACCESSORIES

While the early rigid scopes (Storz Comp.) with Hopkins lens systems offered images of excellent quality, their ridigity made them unsuited for routine intraoperative use. Therefore we have come to replace them by fiberscopes of Olympus (BF-6C, PF-27L) with a diameter of 6 mm and 2 mm. These scopes are sterilizable in ethylene oxide and can be stored under sterile conditions. Ringer's solution in plastic bags with clip-on pressure cuffs is used for flushing. A cold light source, Olympus CLE-F, provides light for both direct inspection and photographic documentation. Photographs are taken with a detachable OM-1 camera with a magnifying tube and a built-in flash with synchronizer. Most important among the accessories is the angioscopy catheter, which is critical for the success of endoscopy

DIAGNOSTIC TECHNIQUES AND ASSESSMENT
PROCEDURES IN VASCULAR SURGERY

© 1985 Grune & Stratton
ISBN 0-8089-1721-8 All rights reserved

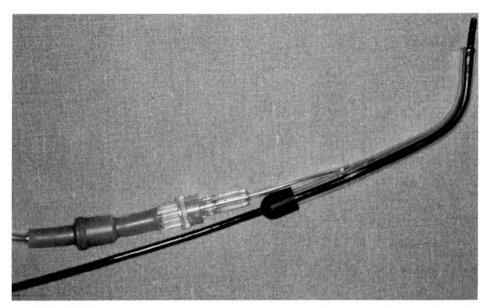

Fig. 27-1.   The angioscopy-cannula for the 2 mm endoscope with separate flushing channel.

in the periphery (Fig. 27-1). This doublelumen catheter was expressly designed by us for visualizing small-caliber vessels. It accommodates the scope, which is introduced through a rubber cap, and has an integrated perfusion channel for injecting the perfusion medium (manufactured by Rüsch Comp., FRG).

TECHNIQUE

Arterioscopy

It is done after vessel repair, i.e., after thrombendarterectomy, bypass implantation, or disobliteration of occluded graft limbs. Intraoperative quality control after embolectomies has recently been added to its applications.

Retrograde arterioscopy towards proximal requires prior proximal blockade with an occluding balloon (5-F Fogarty catheter) (Fig. 27-2). Large caliber arteries are then examined with the 6 mm scope. This is introduced with the built-in flushing channel, and the blood is flushed out of the vessel segment of interest. The scope is then advanced to the level of the balloon. While pulling it back the vessel can be meticulously inspected step by step. The quality of surgery can be evaluated from a three-dimensional image and the condition of the vessel lumen can be documented.

Orthograde arterioscopy does not require distal balloon blockade, but the flow should be interrupted cranial to the point of access. It should preferentially be done with the 2 mm scope.

This is introduced towards the extremity together with the angioscopy catheter through which some Ringer's solution (about 30 to 40 ml) is first infused under pressure (Fig. 27-3). Then the scope is advanced. Normally it can be brought down to the mid-calf level, i.e., to a point where it completely occludes the artery exam-

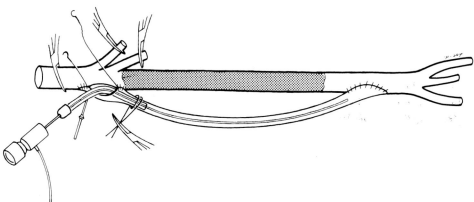

Fig. 27-3. Control endoscopy after reconstructive procedure of lower limb arteries in an orthograde way using a 2 mm endoscope.

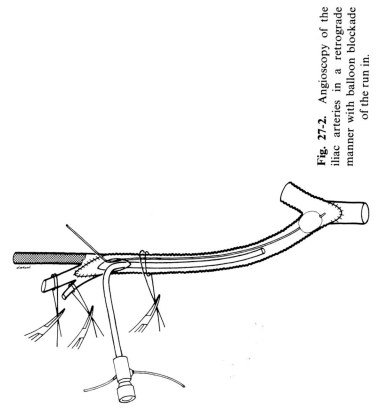

Fig. 27-2. Angioscopy of the iliac arteries in a retrograde manner with balloon blockade of the run in.

305

ined. This procedure provides for adequate flushing of the vessel and offers a clear view of the vessel segments passed by the instrument. Major inflow from a collateral can easily be handled by pulling the scope back, injecting some more perfusion medium, and readvancing the instrument. This maneuver can be repeated as often as desired with minimal perfusion volumes. It provides the examiner with a three-dimensional view of intraluminal details after thrombendarterectomy, of the condition of the valves after homologous vein grafting, both in situ and reversed, and of the distal anastomosis after bypass surgery. Photographic documentation can easily be obtained with the equipment described.

Venoscopy

Endoscopy of the deep veins predominantly serves the purpose of intraoperative quality control during venous thrombectomy so that the scope can be introduced through the access of choice, i.e., the groin or the adductor channel. Unlike arterioscopy, venoscopy requires appreciably larger flushing volumes.

Technique of Iliac Venoscopy

After disobliteration has been completed, an occluding balloon is introduced proximally through the venotomy in the groin (Fig. 27-4). Inflation at the common iliac junction provides for adequate blockade. The 6 mm scope is then advanced to the level of the balloon and flushing is instituted through the flushing channel. This will readily visualize the segment between the balloon and the iliac bifurcation so that the vessel wall can be inspected for mural clots or a venous spur that is present

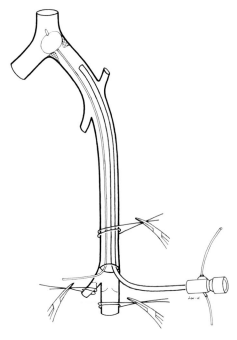

Fig. 27-4. Method of endoscopy of the pelvic veins after venous thrombectomy using 6 mm endoscope with the built-in flushing channel.

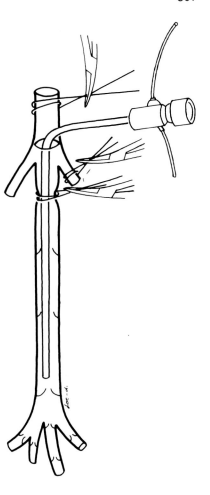

Fig. 27-5. Angioscopic techniques for the examination of the femoral vein after thrombectomy.

at the left iliac vein junction in 10–20% of patients.[4] The profuse inflow from the
internal iliac vein can normally not be adequately coped with by flushing through
the flushing channel. Pulling the balloon back to the level of the iliac bifurcation
and subsequently flushing the external iliac vein again has been found to be quite
useful. This can normally be done without any problems. Even the ascending
lumbar vein can readily be entered and inspected with the 6 mm scope. For iliac
venoscopy as described, about 500–1000 ml of Ringer's solution are required. The
flushing volume should be brought to the anesthetist's knowledge so that he can
account for it in the fluid balance.

   Femoral venoscopy (Fig. 27-5) including the popliteal vein can be done with
both 6 mm scope of the 2 mm instrument with the angioscopy catheter. Both of
them can readily be maneuvered past the valves by careful manipulation and
advanced down to the popliteal vein. While the larger scope will be trapped at this
level, the 2 mm instrument can be forwarded even further distal. Flushing at this
level requires much smaller flushing volumes, because the only major inflow is likely
to be contributed by the deep femoral vein. Photographic documentation can be
obtained with the OM-1 camera.

CLINICAL APPLICATIONS AND RESULTS

Thrombendarterectomy

Semiclosed disobliteration of long occluded segments in the arterial system is an attractive procedure, because the occluded interbifurcational segment can be cleared through two small arteriotomies at the bifurcations with suitable instruments, e.g., the ring stripper. But thrombendarterectomies of such extended segments should invariably be associated with an intraoperative quality control procedure which, together with the inspection of the occluding cylinder, should enable the surgeon to see whether or not medial sleeves or intimal tags have been left behind. These may, after all, be responsible for subsequent reocclusion or restenosis. Vascular endoscopy is helpful in this respect, because it offers a three-dimensional view of the disobliterated vessel segment; residual material can be removed by instrumentation; and the completeness of the procedure can be documented.

The angiogram in Fig. 27-6, which was taken a few months after semiclosed disobliteration of the superficial femoral artery, shows evidence of early high-grade restenosis. Intraoperative quality control by angiography or endoscopy was omitted in this case. Incomplete disobliteration is likely to be responsible for restenosis or failure of thrombendarterectomy in the majority of cases.

Thrombendarterectomy should always be considered for restoring flow in long occluded segments. Whenever vein grafts of adequate length are not available

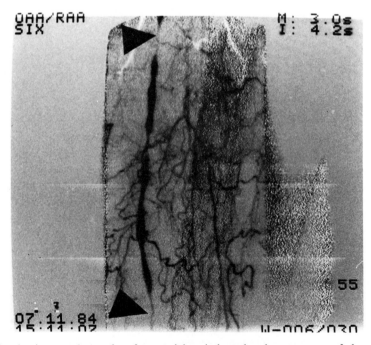

Fig. 27-6. Angiogram 6 months after semiclosed thrombendarterectomy of the superficial femoral artery: Severe restenosis as no intraoperative control method was applied during the primary operation.

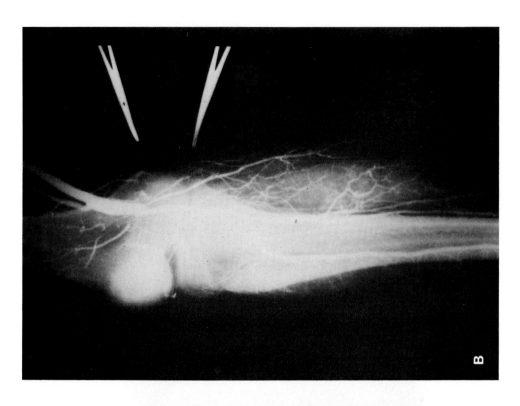

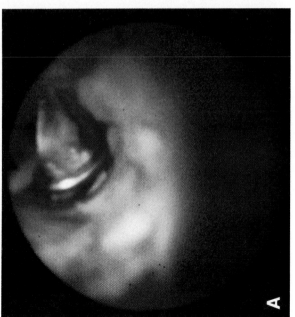

Fig. 27-7. (A) Attempted TEA of the popliteal artery with unsuperable calcified stenosis: Note the stripper with the TEA-cylinder. (B) Control X-ray after reconstruction with a femoro-popliteal below knee bypass graft.

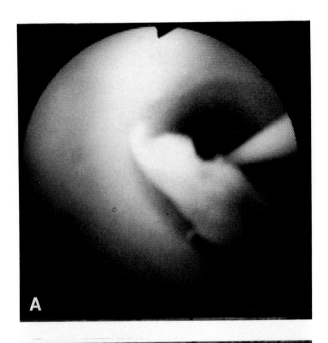

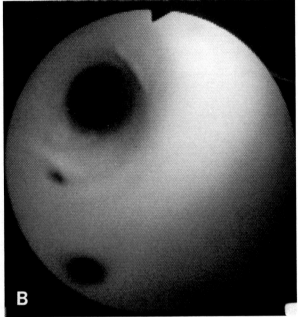

Fig. 27-8. (A) Semiclosed retrograde TEA of the external iliac artery. Remaining internal tag at the vessel wall. (B) Control angioscopy after removal of the intimal tag with the ring stripper: smooth arterial wall.

because of caliber mismatch or anatomical variants, as happens often enough. The use of synthetic graft material with its attendant disadvantages can be avoided by disobliterating the superficial femoral artery and bypassing the occluded segment across the knee joint with homologous vein (Fig. 27-7).

The external iliac artery can equally be disobliterated by retrograde thromb-endarterectomy. In this procedure, inflow is blocked from proximal by balloon inflation of cross-clamping through an extraperitoneal approach and the scope is introduced proximally from below to inspect the disobliterated segment (Fig. 27-8). Normally the occluding material at the iliac bifurcation will come off smoothly without any major floating intimal tags.

Bypass Implantation

Intraoperative quality control of both autologous vein grafts or Dacron and PTFE grafts is mainly directed towards the distal anastomosis and the junction with the downstream vessels. If autologous vein grafts are used, the graft lumen is another point of interest because venous valves may cause septation or stenosis.

For evaluation, the 2 mm scope with the angioscopy catheter is introduced at the level of the proximal anastomosis after the distal anastomosis has been completed and advanced towards distal. In the direction of flow the entire bypass and, particularly, the distal anastomosis can thus be viewed to see whether the junction between the graft and the native artery is smooth and regular or whether the suture line is irregular and whether intimal tags have been left behind along an extended segment. The scope can then be advanced beyond the anastomosis to the point at which the artery examined will no longer accept it.

Even in long femoro-tibial bypasses the distal anastomosis can normally be well seen on endoscopy, because the graft usually has a larger caliber than the recipient vessel. The scope will easily duplicate the curvature of the graft or of an extraanatomical bypass, e.g., to the anterior tibial artery. The detailed information obtainable by vascular endoscopy is best illustrated by comparison with intraoperative angiography, which has so far been the most reliable intraoperative quality control procedure (Fig. 27-9). Intraoperative angiography shows the junction with the anterior tibial artery to be smoooth. On simultaneous endoscopy the walls are seen to be smooth with only some minor blood deposits in the graft. It should be stressed that interrupted sutures were used at the tip of the anastomosis in this case. In the case of a bypass anastomosed to the tibio-peroneal trunk intraoperative angiography failed to show any definite stenosing material at the level of the anastomosis (Fig. 27-10). On endoscopy, by contrast, the suture line was found to bulge and a major intimal tag was seen to project into the lumen. Based on the angiographic evidence, a redo was omitted in this case. No more than six months later the graft had occluded, but as there was adequate compensatory flow the patient could be spared an amputation.

Disobliteration of Graft Limbs

After graft limb disobliteration with a ring stripper or a balloon it is imperative to know whether poor technique at the proximal or distal anastomosis or simply intimal hyperplasia at the suture line were responsible for graft failure. Retrograde

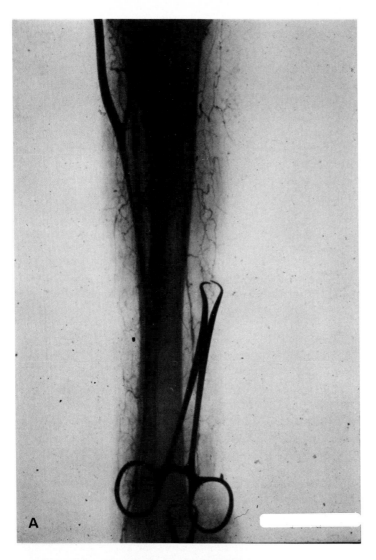

A

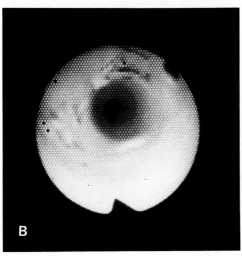

B

Fig. 27-9. Femoro-tibio anterior bypass graft using Gore-Tex-Prosthesis (ring inforced). (A) Control by intraoperative angiography. (B) Endoscopic finding of a very smooth suture line and no alteration of the vessel wall (2 mm endoscope).

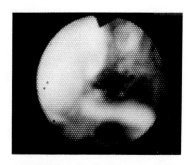

Fig. 27-10. Endoscopic control after femoro-popliteal below knee graft (Gore-Tex), very rough suture line and flotating intimal tag. Reocclusion of the graft 6 months later (2 mm endoscope).

endoscopy with prior balloon blockade will readily visualize the iliac vessels. In our material the proximal anastomosis or the graft limb itself were not found to be responsible for reocclusion. We rather consistently found intimal hyperplasia at the tip of the anastomosis to have caused stenosis with subsequent reocclusion, particularly in 2-level procedures in which a tapering graft limb was sutured into the profunda femoris artery in terms of profundal revascularization. With the help of the 2 mm scope even the distal profunda femoris artery can be inspected. The concept is illustrated by the case of a female with reocclusion after iliofemoral bypass surgery. Postprocedural endoscopy showed pronounced endothelial changes (Fig. 27-11) around the anastomosis attributable to manipulation. The distal artery was normal and delicate.

Endoscopy thus serves a dual purpose: The quality of disobliteration can be established beyond doubt and, more important still, the causes of failure can be identified. A simple maneuver will show whether reocclusion is attributable to kinking of the graft limb or merely to outflow obstruction by intimal hyperplasia. This is important because proximal inflow obstruction due to kinking or malposition of the graft limb will necessitate additional proximal replacement. It goes without saying that this also applies to disobliteration of occluded femoro-popliteal or femoro-tibial bypasses. In these, instrumentation is usually confined to the syn-

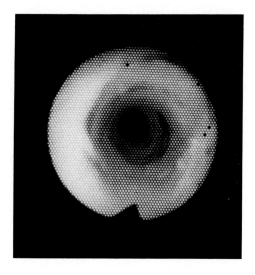

Fig. 27-11. View on the profunda femoris artery after disobliteration of the occluded graft and removal of thrombi in the deep femoral artery. Endothelial damage after Fogarty maneuver a potential starting point for secondary reocclusion.

thetic graft component. For illustration a combined graft consisting of a double-helix PTFE graft proximally and a homologous saphenous vein graft across the knee down to the anterior tibial artery is shown. Neither the vein graft nor the PTFE graft showed any surgery-related damage. But a slender crescent-shaped valvular ridge (Fig. 27-12) was found to project into the venous lumen. As there was no intraluminal obstruction proximally and distally, external compression presumably of the synthetic graft is likely to have been responsible for graft failure.

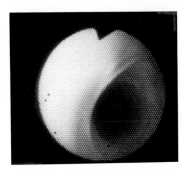

Fig. 27-12.   Valvular edge in a v. saphena graft to the anterior tibial artery.

Intraluminal Quality Control after Embolectomy

Intraoperative postembolectomy quality control procedures are designed to rule out residual clots in the periphery or in the profunda femoris artery. In the past, intraoperative angiography was found to be the most helpful technique for this purpose. We ran a small parallel group of patients who were examined by simultaneous endoscopy, using the small-size scope and found the information obtainable intraoperatively to compare favorably with that of intraoperative angiography. However, intraluminal postembolectomy quality control of peripheral vessels by endoscopy is limited by the diameter of currently available scopes. Developments in the future will show whether more, and more peripheral, information can be obtained with scopes of smaller diameters.

VENOSCOPY

Venoscopy is mainly done for assessing the completeness of disobliteration in patients with recent vein thrombosis. Often partially organized clots are found to be present. These can be removed with ring strippers. Repeat intraluminal inspection will then normally show smooth walls. In patients with thrombosis of more than 8 day's standing, unsuspected by clinical evidence, extensive fibrous organization from the vessel wall is usually seen and villous connective tissue projects into the lumen. This material can no longer be stripped away with the ring stripper. Outflow at the level of the left iliac vein junction is another point of interest, because May and Husny reported 10–20%[4] of patients to have a venous spur of variable size (ranging from a simple fibrous ridge to a larger mass with filiform narrowing of the lumen) in this location. Endoscopy will provide a direct view of the situation, while on blind exploration the balloon catheter may often enough inadvertently be advanced into the ascending lumbar vein, wrongly suggesting patency (Fig. 27-13). Endoscopy also has an important bearing on management, because it will indicate whether ilio-iliac bypass or resection of the venous spur with patch plasty are needed.

Femoral venoscopy through a venotomy in the groin after disobliteration of the vein in patients with recent vein thrombosis can be done with the 6 mm scope because the cross-section of the femoral vessels is large enough to admit the instrument. It is important to make sure that the scope is carefully manipulated, lest it enters the deep femoral vein. With full vision the valves can easily be negotiated and the entire popliteal vein can be examined endoscopically. Even soft recent clots are no obstacle to the scope, which can be passed alongside them to assess their size, identify older organized parts and signs of recanalization with fibrous webs crossing the lumen (Fig. 27-14). Recent mural clots can be easily stripped away with the balloon or the ring stripper with full visual control of the situation.

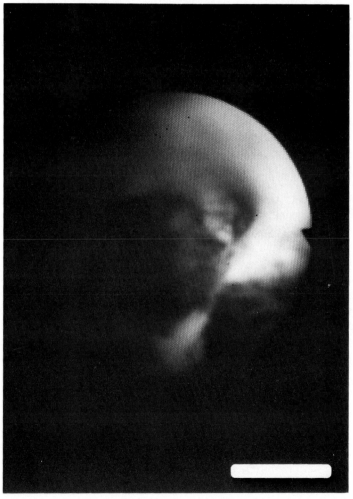

Fig. 27-13. Retrograde endoscopy of the pelvic veins. Typical venous spur at the confluens of the iliac vein as the localizatory factor for ilio-femoral venous thrombosis.

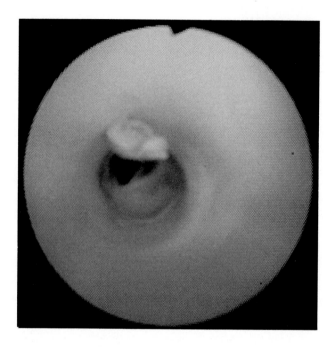

COMPLICATIONS

Vollmar reported three potential complications[5] (Table 27-1): (1) Mechanical injury to the vessel wall; (2) infection; and (3) fluid overload. Ever since we have routinely done vascular endoscopy after reconstructive vascular surgery or venous thrombectomy we have not encountered any of these complications. It is imperative, however, to manipulate and advance the scopes with utmost care. Particularly in the lower leg arteries the scope should never be forcefully advanced, because this may give rise to dissection.

As the scopes are gas-sterilizable and the procedure is done under sterile conditions, infectious complications have not been seen in our material. Even photogra-

Table 27-1
Complications of Angioscopy

1. Mechanical lesions to the vessel wall
   Perforation or dissection
   Distension damage (uncontrolled pressure perfusion!)
   Disruption of venous valves

2. Infection
   Local bacterial contamination
   Septicemia

3. "Fluid overload" by perfusion
   (Vollmar 1974)

phic documentation with the nonsterile camera attached to the scope has not caused any problems if the usual precautions are taken. Between examinations the non-sterile camera is covered with sterile drapes.

If properly done, orthograde endoscopy requires little perfusion fluid. No doubt, the volume of the flushing fluid, which may enter the circulation, is largest in iliac venoscopy. Therefore, it is important to work briskly using the technique described earlier. In more than 50 venous thrombectomies done in the past 2 years we have never seen any severe electrolyte imbalances which would have had serious consequences for the patient.

CONCLUSION

Vascular endoscopy is not only a toy for vascular surgeons, but provides a convincing view upon the reconstructed arterial or venous segment. Technical faults and remaining sclerotic plaques can be identified and also removed. In the venous field it allows us to be sure about complete disobliteration of the occluded deep femoral, pelvic veins or anatomical abnormalities (venous spur). In our hand vascular endoscopy replaces the intraoperative angiography as control-measurement of choice in peripheral arterial reconstructions as well as after arterial embolectomy. The 3-dimensional view is superior to the 2-dimensional one in angiography, which frequently misses smaller dissections. In contrast (caused by the diameter) the angiography gives better information concerning the "run-off" in the peripheral arteries.

In the future we see the possibility of interventional endoscopic maneuvers removing remaining plaques of intimal tags by Laser-Coagulation, on which field experimental work is already under progress. Vascular endoscopy in this way promises still an impetuous development for the improvement of our operative results.[5,6]

REFERENCES

1. Cutler ED, et al: The surgical treatment of mitral stenosis: Experimental and clinical studies. Arch Surg (Chicago) 9:689, 1924
2. Vollmar JF: Die Gefäßendoskopie: ein neuer Weg der intraoperativen Gefäßdiagnostik. Endoscopy 1:141, 1969
3. Vollmar JF, Junghanns K: Die Endoskopie der Arterien. In: von Otteryann R (ed.): Fortschritte der Endoskopie. New York: Schattauer-Verlag Stuttgart, 1970, pp 2–25
4. May R, Thurner J: The cause of the predominantly sinistral occurrence of thrombosis of the pelvic veins. Angiology 8:419, 1957
5. Vollmar JF, Storz LW: Vascular endoscopy. Surg Clin North Amer 54:111–122, 1974
6. Treat MR, Weld FM, White J, et al: Laser endarterectomy in vivo. Circulation 66:366, 1982
7. v. Stiegman G, Kahn D, Rose AG, et al: Laser endarterectomy. Surg Gynecol Obstet 1984 (in press)

B. M. Jones
Jeremy O. Roberts
and Roger M. Greenhalgh

28

Perioperative Assessment for Microvascular Anastomoses

Any procedure involving microvascular surgery depends for its success on the establishment and maintenance of patent arterial and/or venous anastomoses. In plastic and reconstructive surgery the frequency of vascular complications of free skin flaps has been reported as ranging from 7 to 40%.[1] Reduction in the unacceptably high figure has only been achieved by application of standards at least as demanding as those prevailing in large vessel surgery. To approach the goal of 100% success, attention must be given to selection, operative technique, and assessment of anastomoses and postoperative monitoring.

SELECTION OF VESSELS

Careful planning is essential in microvascular surgery, particularly in relation to the vascular pattern of both donor and recipient vessels. Selection of vessels anatomically suitable and free from atheroma is made before surgery, but this decision may be modified by findings at the time of operation.

Arteries

The recipient artery must be assessed for size and quality. In traumatised limbs the adequacy of the collateral circulation must be assessed. Clinical examination of the arterial pulses and circulatory status should be reinforced by objective assessment. Simple transcutaneous ultrasound Doppler flowmetry is of some value, but the information obtained is qualitative, making interpretation difficult. More sophisticated techniques go some way to providing quantitative data.[2] Arteriography has limitations when applied to very small vessels, and the timing of exposures must be planned precisely. In addition, to avoid trauma to the recipient vessel, the cannulae should be introduced via a different artery, distant to the proposed operation site. Digital subtraction angiography may well be of great value in this field, but may require intra arterial injection.

DIAGNOSTIC TECHNIQUES AND ASSESSMENT
PROCEDURES IN VASCULAR SURGERY
© 1985 Grune & Stratton
ISBN 0-8089-1721-8 All rights reserved

Veins

Assessment of the venous drainage is less satisfactory. Skin marking of the superficial veins is useful as these can be used if there are no suitable deep veins accompanying the artery. Venography is not indicated, as small vessel display is poor and the contrast medium may damage the vascular endothelium and cause clotting.

OPERATIVE TECHNIQUE

Microvascular surgery is a specialised technique requiring specific training, equipment, and facilities. Magnification is provided by binocular loupes (Fig. 28-1) and the operating microscope (Fig. 28-2).

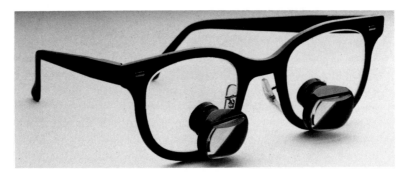

Fig. 28-1.   Binocular operating loupes, original magnification 2.5 × .

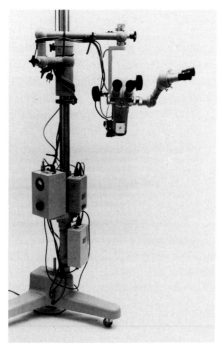

Fig. 28-2.   Zeiss operating microscope, original magnification up to 60 × .

In the process of isolating and preparing vessels for anastomosis, great care must be taken over attaining haemostasis and minimising trauma to the vessels. The recipient artery must have a strong perfusion pressure and the vein free drainage. If vein or artery is found to be damaged or diseased then it must either be resected until a healthy part is reached or an alternative recipient vessel used. This may require an interpositional reversed vein graft. The site and orientation of the anastomoses should be chosen such that the risk of tension, kinking, and excessive angulation of the vessels after skin closure is minimised. Anastomoses may be end-to-end or end-to-side. The latter is mandatory if there is marked inequality of vessel size or if the recipient vessels are required for the maintenance of distal circulation. Interrupted sutures are used for all microvascular anastomoses, the techniques having been well described.[3,4]

ASSESSMENT OF PATENCY

It has been stated that "most vascular complications (of free flap transfers) are post-operative confirmation of intra-operative suspicions—they should be recognised and corrected at the initial operation, not 6 to 12 hours later".[1] Clearly a reliable intra-operative patency test is required. Since a thrombus formed at a microanastomosis reaches its maximal size during the first 10 minutes after removal of the occluding clamps,[5] any patency test should be applied after this period has elapsed. Much can be learned by simply observing the finished anastomosis.

Arterial pulsation may be longitudinal, which may be forward or reverse, or expansile.[6] Forward longitudinal pulsation at the anastomosis indicates blockage as the column of blood is "hammering" against an obstruction, while reverse pulsation indicates anastomotic patency, but is only seen when the vessel distal to the anastomosis is quite straight. Expansile pulsation distal to the anastomosis indicates patency and may be confirmed by lifting the vessel over a blunt hook until it is almost occluded, when expansile pulsation and blood flow is seen at the point where the vessel is compressed. Wriggling is a pulsatile increase and decrease in the curvature of a length of artery and if present distal to an anastomosis demonstrates patency. This, however, will only occur if the distal artery already lies in a curve. It can be mimicked, in the presence of anastomotic occlusion, by forward longitudinal pulsation distorting the distal vessel.

A blocked venous anastomosis produces a tense, distended vessel upstream and a collapsed vessel downstream. Confirmatory tests of elevating and stroking the vein and observing the point of distension and refill on release were suggested.

A further manoeuvre known as the double forceps patency test has been described[7] and may be applied to arteries or veins. The vessel is emptied downstream of the anastomosis between two pairs of jewellers forceps and, after releasing the proximal forceps, refilling from across the looked for anastomosis.

These tests require accurate subjective interpretation. They involve manipulation of the vessel and do not provide a permanent record of the condition of the anastomosis at operation. An objective, permanent record of anastomotic patency is desirable.

Arteriography

On table arteriography is inappropriate as it requires needle puncture of the vessel and, in such small arteries, this constitutes unacceptable trauma.

Electromagnetic Flowmetry

The electromagnetic flowmeter has been used extensively for flow measurements in vascular surgery. Its principle of action is the measurement of the induced electric potential generated across a column of blood moving at 90° to the axis of an electromagnetic field. The development of measuring probes as small as 1 mm in diameter suggested it may be of benefit in microvascular surgery. It is necessary to obtain compression of the vessel under test by the probe of 10–15% to gain accurate readings and both probe and vessel must be submerged in fluid. These factors present problems when dealing with small vessels, since they vary in size markedly with physiological stimuli. An initial experimental study using the flowmeter for evaluating microvascular arterial anastomoses was encouraging.[8] The probe was used to assess microanastomoses in rabbit superficial femoral arteries (Fig. 28-3), a

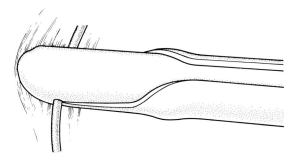

Fig. 28-3. The microelectromagnetic flow probe on the rabbit saphenous artery.

pulsatile wave form (Fig. 28-4) distal to the anastomosis correlating with patency. However, the digital read out of estimated volume flow through the anastomosis was variable and unreliable. Further investigation of the technique[9] showed an inaccurate wave form derived from the flow probe in 3 out of 21 patent anastomoses. Again, the digital read out of flow was found to be unreliable. The flowmeter has been shown to be accurate in measuring arterial flow in a 2 mm vessel supplying an island flap in the dog, over prolonged periods and under varying physiological conditions.[10] However, the conditions that must be satisfied to obtain meaningful readings are so stringent as to render it unsuitable for clinical use at present.

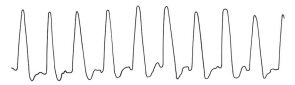

Fig. 28-4. A typical electromagnetic flow tracing obtained from a 1 mm vessel.

The Ultrasound Doppler Flowmeter

When a sound source moves relative to an observer, a frequency change can be noted consisting of an apparent shift to a higher frequency as the source approaches and to a lower frequency as it moves away. This phenomenon was described in 1842 by C. J. Doppler and has become known as the Doppler effect. The principle has been applied to biological systems, using red blood cells as the moving "object". Ultrasound waves from an external transducer are beamed onto the moving red cells, and the backscattered, shifted sound detected by a receiving transducer. The frequency shift is proportional to the relative velocity between the transducer and the red cells. A probe using this Doppler shift of sound to detect flow in blood vessels is a useful and relatively simple tool for vascular surgery.[11] Its peroperative use to assess anastomoses in peripheral vascular reconstructions reduced the number of patients requiring re-operation because of unsatisfactory flow from 30.6% to 8.6%.[12] Experimentally, directional ultrasound Doppler flowmetry has been applied peroperatively to anastomoses in 1 mm arteries and was found to assess patency with 100% accuracy.[9] The response was found to be an "all or none" phenomenon. A pulsatile noise and satisfactory wave form was obtained distal to all patent anastomoses but if the anastomosis had occluded, no Doppler noise was detectable and the tracing was flat.

It was apparent from this study that the technique was potentially valuable in predicting the fate of vascularised free tissue transfers and further work was carried out to evaluate it when applied to epigastric island flaps in rats.[13] Flaps were raised based on the femoral vessels with end-to-end microvascular anastomoses. A standard directional ultrasound Doppler flowmeter was used to insonate the inferior epigastric artery (Fig. 28-5). Of the 22 flaps raised, 18 survived; of the 4 failures, 2 were due to venous occlusion and 2 arterial. In the two venous failures a satisfactory Doppler pulse had been detected at operation and survival had been predicted. In 5 cases no Doppler pulse had been detectable at operation and failure had been anticipated; of these 2 failed and 3 survived. In all, the outcome was correctly predicted in 17 out of the 22 flaps (77%). The ability of the directional Doppler arterial pulse to discriminate between a successful and unsuccessful flap failed to reach statistical significance. An arterial Doppler signal (albeit of altered character) was detectable even with the flap's venous drainage completely occluded for one hour. This indicated the need to assess the venous anastomosis, in addition to the arterial, at the time of surgery.

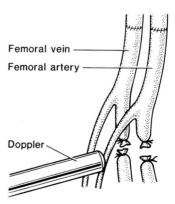

Femoral vein

Femoral artery

Doppler

Fig. 28-5. Insonation of the inferior epigastic artery.

Venous flow is difficult to detect by simple insonation, because of its low velocity. To overcome this the vein was insonated proximal to the anastomosis and gently compressed distally, producing a sudden rush of blood and an easily audible "woosh" in the presence of a patent anastomosis. This was termed the "venous flow augmentation test" (Fig. 28-6). When both arterial insonation and "venous flow augmentation test" were applied to a further 20 free flaps prediction of survival was 100% accurate. Further information as to the circulatory status of a free flap can be obtained by the use of truly directional ultrasound Doppler flowmetry with spectral analysis of the signal.[13,14] This technique gives information as to the peripheral resistance in the flap and indication of impaired venous drainage even in the presence of a patent venous anastomosis. This may be of particular value clinically, not only in the peroperative assessment of free flaps, but also in replantation surgery.

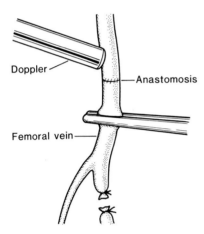

Fig. 28-6.   Venous flow augmentation test.

POST OPERATIVE MONITORING

Despite proven arterial and venous anastomosic patency at operation, blood flow in the clinical free flap may be disturbed in the post-operative period by compression of the pedicle because of oedema, constrictive dressings or postural kinking. Since the speed with which such problems are recognised and corrected determines the likelihood of flap survival,[15] post-operative monitoring of the flap circulation is essential. Most important in this surveillance is the skill and judgement of the surgeon. Clearly, however, it is impossible for him to observe the patient constantly during the post-operative period. This task, therefore, falls for much of the time upon the nursing and junior medical staff whose experience may be limited. Hence an objective mechanical monitoring technique would be of great value. The techniques that have been investigated for use on flaps with a visible surface can be categorised into clinical tests, chemical and radioisotopic methods, and instrumental methods.

Clinical Tests

Clinical tests involve observation of skin colour, the temperature of the flap, capillary refill, and bleeding characteristics.

A healthy flap has the normal colour of the donor site and is warm to the touch, with a normally delayed capillary refill after blanching of the skin by press-ure. If a small incision is made in the flap, brisk red bleeding results. Arterial insuffi-ciency is indicated by blanching, delayed capillary refill, coolness of the flap, and absence of bleeding on incision. In contrast, a congested, purple, cool flap with very rapid capillary refill and a slow purple ooze following incision indicates impaired venous drainage.

These tests suffer from many disadvantages. They all require experienced inter-pretation. Colour changes may at first be subtle and by the time they are clinically apparent, salvage of the flap may be impossible because of irreversible tissue damage. Subjective assessment of temperature change is very unreliable and incision of the flap is obviously invasive and cannot be repeated too often.

Chemical and Radioisotopic Methods

The staining of a skin flap by intravenously injected dyes, such as fluorescein, and the clearance of radioisotopes injected into a flap, are both known to give an accurate estimate of skin blood flow. However, both of these methods are obviously restricted in how often they can be repeated and so have limitations as clinical post-operative monitors of free flaps.

Instrumental Methods

Photoplethysmography,[16] interstitial fluid pressure measurement,[14,17] transcu-taneous pO_2 measurement,[18] and electromagnetic flowmetry[8,9,10] all have some value. However, they have limitations in practical application and interpretation.

Spectrophotometry

Measurement of skin colour by reflection spectrophotometry has shown poten-tial as a free flap monitor in an experimental study.[19] Indication of circulatory change was rapid, arterial and venous occlusion were distinguished, and interpreta-tion facilitated by digital display. Further clinical evaluation is awaited.

Differential Thermometry

Measurement of skin temperature is subject to many variables, not least the temperature difference found over the body in a normal subject. Any change in ambient temperature or air currents may affect a sensor on the skin surface, as will changes in thermal conductivity of the skin, or the metabolism of underlying tissues. These problems are partially overcome by measuring the temperature difference between two thermocouples, one applied to the skin of the flap and the other on adjacent nonflap skin. This monitoring technique has the advantages of simplicity and inexpensiveness. It is in wide clinical use but an experimental study[20] found its response to circulatory change to be slow and inconsistent.

Laser Doppler Flowmetry

Based on a similar system to ultrasound Doppler flowmeters, this uses a fibre-optic light guide to transmit laser light to the skin and carry backscattered, reflected light to photodetectors. Red blood cells moving within the skin cause a frequency shift of the light that is proportional to the red cell flux within a block of tissue approximately 1 mm diameter. Studies, in vitro and in vivo, have shown a rapid response in laser Doppler flowmeter output to physiological changes in skin blood flow[21] and, in a small series of clinical free flaps, it has shown potential as a post-operative monitor.[22]

Buried Flaps

As will be appreciated, all the above techniques can, at present, only be applied to flaps with a visible surface. A proportion of vascularised free tissue transfers in current use have no such visible surface, these cannot be monitored post-operatively. The use of thermocouples implanted percutaneously, and positioned in contact with the arterial wall distal to a microanastomosis, has been reported as showing promise as a post-operative monitor of buried flaps.[23,24] Limitations to the general clinical application of this technique are suggested by current experimental work by the authors and we are investigating alternative methods of anastomotic and tissue viability monitoring with implanted probes.

CONCLUSION

To achieve the aim of 100% microvascular anastomosis patency and vascularised free tissue transfer survival, scrupulous attention to detail must be paid at all stages.

An appropriate donor site and suitable recipient vessels should be chosen on clinical grounds reinforced by ultrasound Doppler flowmetry and, where indicated, arteriography. Vessel selection is then confirmed at operation.

The surgery must be carried out by a trained operator, with appropriate equipment and facilities. Anastomotic technique must be meticulous and the patency of both arterial and venous anastomoses tested by ultrasound Doppler flowmetry at least ten minutes after the release of the vessel clamps.

Post-operative monitoring should be reliable, objective, and continuous, with digital display to facilitate interpretation. Criteria not fulfilled by any current technique but with laser Doppler flowmetry showing the most potential. Finally, the surgeon must be prepared to immediately re-explore and revise any flap that develops circulatory impairment in the post-operative period.

REFERENCES

1. Daniel RK: Clinical microvascular surgery and free tissue transfers, in: Grabb WC and Smith JW (eds): Plastic Surgery. Boston, Little Brown and Company, 1979, pp 660–684
2. Gosling RG, King DH: Ultrasonic angiology, in: Harcus and Adamson (eds): Arteries and Veins. London, Churchill Livingstone, 1975, pp 61–98
3. Cobbett JR: Small vessel anastomosis. Br J Plast Surg 20:16–20, 1967
4. Greenhalgh RM, Rossi LFA, Hoare MR: The precise technique for end-to-side microvascular anastomosis with a suitable experimental model. Ann R Coll Surg Engl 63(1):28–30, 1981
5. Acland RD: Thrombus formation in microvascular surgery: An experimental study of the effects of surgical trauma. Surgery 73:766–771, 1973
6. Acland RD: Signs of patency in small vessel anastomosis. Surgery 72:744–748, 1972

7. Hayhurst JW, O'Brien BMc: An experimental study of microvascular technique, patency rates and related factors. Br J Plast Surg 28:128–132, 1975
8. Greenhalgh RM, Bourne R, Rossi LFA, et al: The value of the electromagnetic flow probe in experimental and clinical microvascular anastomosis. Ann Surg 189:311–312, 1979
9. Rossi LFA, Hoare MR, Greenhalgh RM: Peroperative proof of patency of microvascular anastomoses. Ann R Coll Surg Engl 63:189–191, 1981
10. Banis JC, Schwartz KS, Acland RD: Electromagnetic flowmetry—an experimental method for continuous blood flow measurement using a new island flap model. Plast Reconstr Surg 66:534–544, 1980
11. Yao JST, Bergan JJ: Application of ultrasound to arterial and venous diagnosis. Surg Clin North Am 54:23–38, 1974
12. Keitzer WF, Licht EL, Brossart FA, De Weese MS: Use of the Doppler ultrasonic flowmeter during arterial vascular surgery. Arch Surg 105:308–312, 1972
13. Jones BM, Greenhalgh RM: The use of the ultrasound Doppler flowmeter in reconstructive microvascular surgery. Br J Plast Surg 36:245–253, 1983
14. Jones BM: Predicting the fate of free flap tissue transfers. Master of Surgery Thesis, University of London, 1982
15. Goodstein WA, Buncke HJ Jr: Patterns of vascular anastomosis vs success of free groin flap transfers. Plast Reconstr Surg 64:37–40, 1979
16. Webster MHC, Patterson J: The photoelectric plethysmograph as a monitor of microvascular anastomoses. Br J Plast Surg 29:182–185, 1976
17. Jones BM, Sanders R, Greenhalgh RM: Interstitial fluid pressure as a circulatory monitor in skin flaps. Br J Plast Surg 36:358–362, 1983
18. Achauer BM, Black KS, Litke DK: Transcutaneous pO_2 in flaps: A new method of survival prediction. Plast Reconstr Surg 65:738–745, 1980
19. Jones BM, Sanders R, Greenhalgh RM: Monitoring skin flaps by colour measurement. Br J Plast Surg 36:88–94, 1983
20. Jones BM, Dunscombe PB, Greenhalgh RM: Differential thermometry as a monitor of blood flow in skin flaps. Br J Plast Surg 36:83–87, 1983
21. Nilsson GE, Tenland T, Oberg PA: Evaluation of a laser Doppler flowmeter for measurement of tissue blood flow. IEEE Trans Biomed Eng 27:597–604, 1980
22. Jones BM, Mayou BJ: The laser Doppler flowmeter for microvascular monitoring: A preliminary report. Br J Plast Surg 35:147–149, 1982
23. Cohn KH, May JW Jr: Thermal-energy dissipation: A laboratory study to assess patency in blood vessels. Plast Reconstr Surg 70:475–480, 1980
24. May JW Jr, Lukash FN, Gallico GG, Stirrat CR: Removable thermocouple probe microvascular patency monitor: An experimental and clinical study. Plast Reconstr Surg 72:366–379, 1983

PART V

Amputation Levels

Vance A. Spence
and Peter T. McCollum

29

Evaluation of the Ischaemic Limb by Transcutaneous Oxymetry

There has been considerable interest in the development of noninvasive methods for estimating the state of nutrition of ischaemic tissue. This interest stems from a need for objective measurements in the evaluation of the ischaemic limb particularly before and after various surgical reconstructive procedures and in the assessment of drug therapy. Perhaps the most important need for accurate assessment of ischaemia relates to the prediction of wound healing following below knee amputation, and indeed this problem has attracted considerable attention.

In recent times, the measurement of transcutaneous oxygen ($TcPO_2$) has emerged as a potentially reliable and valid method in the field of tissue viability assessment. However, the $TcPO_2$ method was developed for paediatric intensive care medicine as a noninvasive estimation of arterial oxygen partial pressure in neonates. Whether or not the same methodology is applicable to the assessment of skin perfusion in adult skin has not yet been answered, but this has not prevented an ever increasing amount of literature on $TcPO_2$ measurements in the ischaemic limb. Most of these measurements relate to the assessment of the optimum level of amputation and there appears to be a reasonable consensus concerning the range of $TcPO_2$ values that exist in the ischaemic limb. This is hardly surprising because the $TcPO_2$ gradient down the ischaemic limb is determined by a lowered oxygen delivery to the skin as a consequence of a reduced blood flow. However, a good correlation between $TcPO_2$ values and clinical findings does not mean that the transcutaneous method demonstrates the sensitivity and specificity needed to estimate tissue viability in a particular ischaemic limb. Nevertheless, there are many claims for the $TcPO_2$ method, and this review examines the evidence for such claims and assesses the potential of the method as a noninvasive test for peripheral arterial insufficiency.

DIAGNOSTIC TECHNIQUES AND ASSESSMENT
PROCEDURES IN VASCULAR SURGERY
© 1985 Grune & Stratton
ISBN 0-8089-1721-8 All rights reserved

331

THE TRANSCUTANEOUS OXYGEN METHOD

A detailed account of the principles involved in transcutaneous oxymetry, along with a description of various electrodes, is available elsewhere.[1-3] The $TcPO_2$ electrode is essentially a Clark type polarographic electrode consisting of a platinum cathode and a silver anode immersed in an electrolyte and sealed by a semipermeable membrane. If a suitable current is applied between the anode and cathode, the resulting current produced by the electrochemical reduction of oxygen in the electrolyte is proportional to the partial pressure of oxygen. The first experiments on the surfaces of the skin with a non-heated electrode produced PO_2 values ≤ 3.5 mmHg but this rose significantly to around 30 mmHg when the skin was inflamed.[4] The inflammation, or "arterialisation," of the skin produced physically or by chemical vasodilator substances allowed oxygen to diffuse from the superficial capillary layer through the skin and onto the electrode. These methods of producing vasodilation did not, however, provide a consistent standard of conditions under the electrode. This was achieved by incorporating a heating element into the electrode which created conditions of maximal hyperaemia by local heating to 43–45°C.[5] In addition to inducing hyperaemia, local heating of the skin also alters skin structure in such a way as to enhance the permeability of gases.[6] This combination of circumstances leads to a $TcPO_2$ value that approximates the oxygen partial pressure of the arterial blood (PaO_2) in normal subjects.

Despite the good correlation between the PaO_2 and $TcPO_2$ measurements, the relationship between them is complex. The PaO_2 is only one of a number of parameters that influences the $TcPO_2$ value,[2] some of which are listed in Table 29-1. In the first instance, the skin utilises oxygen as its energy source and this automatically reduces oxygen availability to the electrode that is situated directly above. The effect of this artifact will be minimised in conditions of normal blood perfusion because the increase in oxygen availability from thermal arterialisation will be relatively much greater than the increased oxygen requirements of the skin.[7] However, heating the skin has a pronounced effect on the blood oxygen tension, because the oxygen dissociation curve is shifted to the right and the PO_2 will rise approximately 20 mmHg for the 4°C increase in temperature that generally results in the dermal capillaries. The effects of these two artifacts tend to cancel each other out.

A further parameter that affects the $TcPO_2$ reading is skin thickness. This is of

Table 29-1
Physiologic and Methodologic
Parameters that Determine the
Transcutaneous PO_2 Value

Arterial PO_2 (PaO_2)
Blood perfusion
Skin metabolism
Skin thickness
Structure of the microcirculation
Electrode O_2 consumption
Electrode response time
Tissue temperature profile
Physiologic effects of hyperthermia

particular importance when measurements are being made on adult skin where considerable regional variation in thickness exists. A thick skin requires a correspondingly thick membrane to balance out the differences in diffusional resistance.[1] However, the membrane thickness is also balanced against the size of the cathode and the need for a fast response time and so it is not just a simple matter of changing membranes to suit particular thicknesses of skin. In this respect it is worth remembering that all commercially available $TcPO_2$ electrodes have their characteristics optimised for measurements on the skin of neonates and that some caution should be observed when making measurements on normal and ischaemic adult skin.

$TcPO_2$ VALUES IN NORMAL ADULT SKIN

$TcPO_2$ values obtained from the legs of young and elderly normal subjects have been extensively reported and a summary of the results is presented in Table 29-2.[8-16] In this table, the $TcPO_2$ values pertain to a particular site (ie, 10 cm below the knee (BK)) although measurements from the above knee and foot levels are also available from the same literature. There is a considerable variation in $TcPO_2$ values at the BK site ranging from 40 mmHg[11] to 100 mmHg.[8] This variation would be a little surprising if the $TcPO_2$ value was purely a reflection of the arterial oxygen tension, but, as previously discussed, there are several other parameters that determine the final result. There are also some other practical points worthy of consideration. These include preparation of the skin (shaving, stripping with sellotape, degreasing), the type of electrode used, and its temperature setting. We have recently demonstrated that two different electrodes on adjacent sites can give significantly different $TcPO_2$ readings.[16] The differences between these measurements are related to such electrode characteristics as membrane permeability and thickness and the electrode heating arrangement. These differences must be taken into account when

Table 29-2
BK $TcPO_2$ Values in Normal Subjects

Study	Equipment	Probe Temperature (°C)	No. of Subjects	Age (years)	$TcPO_2$ mmHg ± SD
Mustapha et al[8]	Radiometer	45	6	17–25	92 ± 9
Mustapha et al[8]	Radiometer	45	6	54–64	79 ± 8
Dowd et al[9]	Radiometer	45	161	?	70 ± 9
Byrne et al[10]	Kontron	45	13	30 ± 4	69 ± 8
Byrne et al[10]	Kontron	45	23	61 ± 9	60 ± 6
Franzeck et al[11]	Oxymonitor	45	24	19–75	57 ± 10
Oghi et al[12]	Oxymonitor	45	20	23–34	70 ± 10
Matsen et al[13]	Radiometer	44	13	22–35	77 ± 13
Clyne et al[14]	Kontron	44	10	51–80	63 ± 5
Wyss et al[15]	Radiometer	44	15	22–35	76 ± 11
Spence et al[16]	Radiometer	44	31	19–44	73 ± 12
Spence et al[16]	Drager	44	31	19–44	63 ± 12
Spence et al[16]	Radiometer	44	17	51–90	57 ± 11

comparing results obtained with different electrodes, or with similar electrodes used at different settings.

In an extensive study on 161 normal volunteers, Dowd et al[9] showed that the TcPO$_2$ measurements were not age dependent and that there was no gradient from proximal to distal parts of the limb. These conclusions are not supported by others, and a significant difference between BK TcPO$_2$ measurements on young and elderly normal subjects has been reported.[8,10] We have found TcPO$_2$ readings on elderly normal skin to be reduced by 5–15 mmHg, depending on the electrode used.[16] There is also a TcPO$_2$ gradient down the limb from above knee level to the foot of approximately 5–10 mmHg.[10,13,14,16]

In elderly subjects who were age-matched for vascular disease patients, a TcPO$_2$ value of 60 ± 10 mmHg is to be expected at the BK level; this should increase or decrease by a further 10 mmHg when above knee or foot sites respectively are included.

TcPO$_2$ MEASUREMENTS IN ISCHAEMIC LEGS

There are significant proximal to distal TcPO$_2$ gradients in the limbs of patients with obstructive arterial disease. These gradients may be no greater than those found in age matched control subjects when only mild vascular disease is present,[10] but the gradients become increasingly significant with progressing symptoms (Table 29-3).[10,14,16–19] Wyss et al[19] showed that limbs with low TcPO$_2$ values on the foot were more likely to have rest pain or ulcers and to eventually need amputation, but that there was a lack of perfect correlation between TcPO$_2$ measurements and clinical impression of ischaemia. Indeed, Franzeck et al[11] found extremely low TcPO$_2$ values (<10 mmHg) in several patients without ulceration or trophic skin changes but with intermittent claudication as the only complaint. Byrne et al[10] showed that claudicants had a wide range of values but that the inclusion of an excercise test improved the sensitivity of the method considerably. These results

Table 29-3
TcPO$_2$ Values in Ischaemic Legs

Study	No. of Patients	TcPO$_2$ (mmHg + SD) AK	BK	Foot	Clinical Presentation
Byrne et al[10]	17	66 ± 7	59 ± 5	56 ± 4	Mild ischaemia
Clyne et al[14]	10	67 ± 9	64 ± 9	51 ± 10	Claudicants
Wyss et al[19]	150	. . .	43 ± 17	37 ± 20	Claudicants
Byrne et al[10]	68	54 ± 7	48 ± 10	37 ± 12	Claudicants
Clyne et al[14]	9	55 ± 18	50 ± 16	36 ± 16	Severe ischaemia
Wyss et al[19]	166	. . .	36 ± 20	24 ± 22	Severe ischaemia
Ratliff et al[18]	62	52 ± 15	37 ± 17	. . .	Severe ischaemia
Burgess et al[17]	30	52 ± 3	43 ± 4	16 ± 4	Severe ischaemia
Byrne et al[10]	32	50 ± 14	29 ± 20	4 ± 4	Severe ischaemia
Spence et al[16]	21	54 ± 13	35 ± 21	17 ± 22	Severe ischaemia

Note.   AK = above knee and BK = below knee.

emphasise that the interpretation of a particular $TcPO_2$ value on an ischaemic limb is not straightforward, a finding probably due to the fact that the $TcPO_2$ is not always a good reflection of the nutritional status of the tissue beneath the electrode.

The most significant determinant of $TcPO_2$ measurements on the skin of ischaemic limbs is the local arterial perfusion pressure.[20] To achieve a normal $TcPO_2$ measurement, a several-fold increase in papillary blood flow is required, which is achieved by heating the skin beneath the electrode. Under these circumstances, there is a relaxation of resistance vessels and normal autoregulatory mechanisms that control tissue blood flow are abolished. In normal skin, the increase in tissue oxygen supply is sufficient to reduce the arterial-tissue oxygen gradient towards zero and $TcPO_2$, reflecting tissue PO_2, approaches arterial pressure.[21] In ischaemic skin, however, local perfusion pressures are reduced and this factor alone limits the degree of vasodilation induced by heating to such an extent that tissue oxygen levels fall far short of the arterial PO_2, this being reflected by a low $TcPO_2$ measurement. It is worth emphasising that the reduced $TcPO_2$ measurement results primarily from the reduced arterial blood pressure, and not, per se, a reduced tissue PO_2.[21]

Normal tissue oxygenation in the skin of patients with peripheral arterial obstructive disease is quite possible despite significantly reduced perfusion pressures.[22] This situation is possible because of the arteriolar and precapillary sphincter control mechanisms and the oxygen buffering capacity of haemoglobin which respond to a decreased oxygen delivery. The ability of these intrinsic control mechanisms to maintain tissue oxygenation has been demonstrated in an experiment on skeletal muscle in which arterial perfusion pressure was reduced from 100 mmHg to 45 mmHg.[23] At some stage, however, a state of hypoperfusion will be reached when tissue oxygen requirements simply cannot be met by autoregulatory mechanisms and critical ischaemia prevails. Whether or not $TcPO_2$ measurements can be indicative of this critical level of perfusion remains unclear, but, at present, the technique is probably not sufficiently developed.

The fact that there is a relationship between $TcPO_2$ measurements and the arterial perfusion pressures (which approximates the systolic pressure) in the ischaemic limb may, of course, be significant from a diagnostic viewpoint. There is a need for such a measurement in the assessment of the diabetic ischaemic limb, where the arteries are incompressible and normal Doppler systolic measurements are unobtainable. Indeed, $TcPO_2$ estimation has been advocated as a reasonable alternative.[19] Although Clyne et al[14] have shown a linear relationship between perfusion pressure and $TcPO_2$, it is in fact probably curvilinear,[15,19] such that the $TcPO_2$ is relatively insensitive to changes in perfusion pressure when the pressure is high but falls off steeply when there is a small but positive pressure value.[15] This means that the $TcPO_2$ method is particularly able to detect changes in perfusion pressure in the most ischaemic limbs and, indeed, such changes may be elicited by simply moving the limb from the supine to the dependent position.[10,11,24] Positional limb alterations can induce significant changes in local transmural pressure, and it is possible that the magnitude of the changes offers an added quantitative indication of the severity of ischaemia.[24] This method of classification of the adequacy of limb perfusion may significantly improve the discriminatory ability of the $TcPO_2$ method. An analysis of the wide spectrum of $TcPO_2$ values obtainable from ischaemic limbs, as listed in Table 29-3, suggests that such an improvement is necessary if the $TcPO_2$ method is to fulfill its diagnostic potential.

TcPO$_2$ MEASUREMENTS AND THE OPTIMUM AMPUTATION LEVEL

Assessment of the optimum level of amputation in an ischaemic limb can be particularly difficult in many patients. Few surgeons would dispute the desirability of retaining the knee joint, but there is a disappointing rate of BK amputations in most centres. On this basis there is a need for noninvasive methods to assist in the estimation of potential wound healing and considerable attention has focussed on the development of such methods.[25] The most recent of these to emerge is the transcutaneous oxygen method.

The success of any method to reliably predict the outcome of wound healing depends entirely on its ability to discriminate between what is to be considered potentially viable and nonviable tissue. This discrimination may never be perfect for one particular method because it may measure only one of the many nutritional variables that ultimately determines skin viability. Nevertheless, it is obviously important that the degree of overlap, constituting questionable viability, is as small as possible.

An examination of the results in Table 29-4 reveals that if the BK TcPO$_2$ value is > 35–40 mmHg a BK amputation will always heal. This finding appears important and it has been suggested that a significant number of patients could be spared

Table 29-4
Anterior BK TcPO$_2$ Values for Successful
and Unsuccessful BK Amputations

Study	Healed BK Amputations		Failed BK Amputations	
	No.	TcPO$_2$	No.	TcPO$_2$
Franzeck et al[11]	26	37 (2–62)	6	1 (0–3)
Burgess et al[17]	30	42 (26–72)	7	16 (0–36)
Dowd et al[9]	3	50 (48–53)	2	35 (34–35)
Mustapha et al[8]	9	52 ± 13	5	35 ± 8
Ratliff et al[18]	28	42 (7–72)	5	23 (5–35)
Katsamouris et al[26]	22	50 (36–66)	5	22 (3–42)

Note. Data for TcPO$_2$ are mean (range) mmHg.

above knee amputations on the basis of this criterion.[18] However, in our own laboratory, where an aggressive BK amputation policy is in operation,[27] we observed that in patients with a BK TcPO$_2$ value of ≥ 35 mmHg the selection of a BK amputation was clinically not in doubt in most patients. More importantly, there was a group of patients who had a range of clinically viable and nonviable limbs at the BK level in whom the TcPO$_2$ values varied from 0 to 35 mmHg. The problem is that healing is possible at extremely low TcPO$_2$ values,[11,18] and this fact alone suggests that the TcPO$_2$ method is a poor arbiter of tissue viability. It is clear, therefore, that TcPO$_2$ measurements can reliably predict those amputations that will heal on the basis of a value > 35 mmHg, but the technique is unable to predict those amputations that will not heal.

TcPO$_2$ MEASUREMENTS FOLLOWING OXYGEN INHALATION

One possible means of improving the discriminatory ability of the TcPO$_2$ method for assessing tissue viability might be achieved by monitoring the TcPO$_2$ changes induced by oxygen inhalation. We have previously reported on the measurement of tissue PO$_2$ transients, and demonstrated the significance of such measurements in relation to skin ischaemia.[22] Essentially, tissue PO$_2$, as measured by a needle microelectrode method was not necessarily reduced in the midcalf region of the ischaemic limb, but the response to breathing oxygen was often markedly reduced when compared to a normal skin site. In the more distal parts of the same ischaemic limb the tissue PO$_2$ was significantly reduced with no response to oxygen inhalation. The absent or reduced response to oxygen breathing is a function of local oxygen debt[27] and it is also possible to argue, theoretically, that the slope of the air to oxygen transition rate curve should be directly proportional to blood flow.[4] We have now repeated these oxygen inhalation experiments using the TcPO$_2$ method and the preliminary data are presented in Tables 29-5 and 29-6. TcPO$_2$ was measured at the AK, BK, and foot levels of 11 normal subjects (mean age, 65 $\pm$ 12 years) and 21 patients requiring amputation because of critical ischaemia. Measurements of TcPO$_2$ breathing air and oxygen and the rate of change of PO$_2$, induced by oxygen inhalation, were estimated from the TcPO$_2$ readings (Fig. 29-1). All of these parameters were significantly reduced in the ischaemic limbs at the below knee and foot levels (Table 29-5). However, an examination of the three parameter values obtained at the BK level of ischaemic subjects (Table 29-6) shows that the rate value was the best predictor of ultimate BK amputation wound healing. The TcPO$_2$ (air) values were insufficiently specific since four patients (nos. 1, 5, 7, and 13) had a TcPO$_2$ of ≤ 20 mmHg and yet achieved healing, while one patient had a TcPO$_2$ value of 32 mmHg but failed to heal. There was also some overlap for TcPO$_2$ (oxygen) values but the rate values (mmHg/min) of all four failed amputations were lower than any of those in the "healed amputation" group.

Table 29-5
TcPO$_2$ Measurements ($\pm$ SD) Breathing Air and Oxygen

Site/Subjects	No.	TcPO$_2$ (mmHg)		Rate of Change (air to oxygen) (mmHg/min)
		Air	Oxygen	
AK				
Normal subjects	11	64 $\pm$ 10	252 $\pm$ 69	66 $\pm$ 37
Ischaemic patients	21	54 $\pm$ 13	196 $\pm$ 79	48 $\pm$ 29
BK				
Normal subjects	11	59 $\pm$ 10	216 $\pm$ 64	40 $\pm$ 26
Ischaemic patients	21	35 $\pm$ 21*	115 $\pm$ 72*	21 $\pm$ 19*
Foot				
Normal subjects	11	57 $\pm$ 7	195 $\pm$ 56	49 $\pm$ 31
Ischaemic patients	21	17 $\pm$ 22*	53 $\pm$ 75*	15 $\pm$ 23*

* = significantly reduced ($P < .01$)

Table 29-6
TcPO$_2$ Values ± SD Breathing Air
and Oxygen

No.	TcPO$_2$ (mmHg)		Rate (mmHg/min)
	Air	Oxygen	
1	20	46	20
2	40	152	44
3	44	169	23
4	36	68	9
5	20	218	23
6	24	48	15
7	16	72	10
8	40	68	19
9	44	124	20
10	40	76	14
11	68	184	32
12	60	212	78
13	0	78	13
14	48	216	29
15	48	222	74
16	76	204	29
17	56	96	10
18	0	0	0
19	32	68	7
20	16	48	8
21	6	38	8

Note. The rate of change of PO$_2$ from air to oxygen breathing was measured at BK levels in 21 patients who required BK amputation. The outcome for patients no. 1–17 was success; patients 18–21 failed.

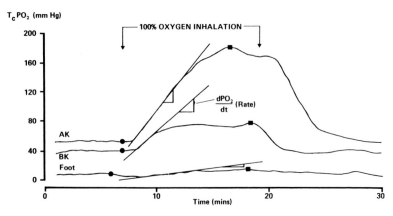

Fig. 29-1. TcPO$_2$ recordings at the AK, BK, and foot levels on an ischaemic limb. The TcPO$_2$ values breathing air (marked ●) are 52, 40, and 8 mmHg at the AK, BK, and foot levels, and the respective peak values after oxygen inhalation (marked ■) are 181, 76, and 16 mmHg. The corresponding rate values for these levels are 19, 14, and 2 mmHg/min. A BK amputation healed successfully.

As there are a small number of patients in this study the significance of the results is perhaps questionable, but the data presented in Table 29-6 confirms that healing can take place even when the $TcPO_2$ is zero at the amputation site (patient no. 13). Conversely, it is evident that a $TcPO_2$ value of 32 mmHg may not support healing when the air to oxygen transition rate is reduced (patient no. 19). In this study, a transition rate value of <9 mmHg/min denoted no healing potential.

Other attempts to measure $TcPO_2$ changes induced by oxygen inhalation have already been made. Ohgi et al[12] have shown that $TcPO_2$ measurements after oxygen inhalation were significantly reduced in ischaemic limbs, and that such measurements, in combination with exercise loading, could be used to classify the severity of ischaemia. More recently, Harward et al[28] reported on their preliminary findings in 101 patients undergoing 118 amputations and demonstrated that the initial $TcPO_2$ measurement, coupled with the response to 100% oxygen inhalation, was an excellent predictor of the outcome of lower extremity amputations. The physiologic relationship between oxygen inhalation–induced $TcPO_2$ changes, local blood flow, and the tissue oxygen exchange rate has not yet been studied. Knowledge of tissue oxygen supply, gained from oxygen-induced $TcPO_2$ rate transients, would greatly enhance the clinical application and significance of such measurements in relation to the study of tissue viability.

CONCLUSIONS

Transcutaneous oxymetry is a fairly new addition to the repertoire of the non-invasive vascular laboratory. The method is easily applied, but the interpretation of results in relation to the nutritional state of the tissues underlying the electrode is not straightforward. Considerable caution should be exercised when comparing results obtained with different electrode characteristics. In this respect, it would be useful to have some standardisation and improvements in electrode design to optimise electrode characteristics for measurements in adult skin. In severely ischaemic skin, $TcPO_2$ values to not necessarily reflect tissue PO_2 and so the relationship between low $TcPO_2$ measurements and wound healing is doubtful. However, there is sufficient evidence in support of the use of oxygen inhalation–induced $TcPO_2$ changes, along with the effects of limb dependency and exercise, to warrant further research.

REFERENCES

1. Huch R, Lubbers DW, Huch A: The transcutaneous measurement of oxygen and carbon dioxide tensions for the determination of arterial blood gas values with control of local perfusion and peripheral perfusion pressure. Theoretical analysis and practical application, in Payne JP, Hill DW (eds): Oxygen Measurements in Biology and Medicine. London, Butterworths, 1975, pp 121–138
2. Eberhard P, Mindt W, Kreuzer F: Cutaneous oxygen monitoring in the newborn. Paediatrician 5:335, 1976

3. Hebrank DR: Non-invasive transcutaneous oxygen monitoring, a review. J Clin Eng 6:41, 1981

4. Evans NTS, Naylor PFD: The systemic oxygen supply to the surface of human skin. Resp Physiol 3:21, 1967

5. Huch R, Huch A, Lubbers DW: Transcutaneous measurement of blood PO_2 ($TcPO_2$): Method and application in perinatal medicine. J Per Med 1:183, 1973

6. Van Duzee BF: Thermal analysis of human stratum corneum. J Invest Derm 64:404, 1975

7. Linhart J, Preovsky I: Oxygen consumption in the foot in man and its changes after body heating. Clin Sci 23:47, 1962

8. Mustapha NM, Redhead RG, Jain SK, et al: Transcutaneous partial oxygen pressure assessment of the ischaemic lower limb. Surg Gynaecol Obstet 156:582, 1983

9. Dowd GSE, Provan JL, Ameli FM, et al: Measurement of transcutaneous oxygen pressure in normal and ischaemic skin. J Bone Joint Surg 65:79, 1983

10. Byrne P, Provan JL, Ameli FM, et al: The use of transcutaneous oxygen tension measurements in the diagnosis of peripheral vascular insufficiency. Ann Surg 200:159, 1984

11. Franzeck UK, Talke P, Bernstein EF, et al: Transcutaneous PO_2 measurements in health and peripheral arterial occlusive disease. Surgery 91:156, 1982

12. Oghi S, Ito K, Mori T: Quantitative evaluation of skin circulation in ischaemic legs by transcutaneous measurement of oxygen tension. Angiology 32:833, 1981

13. Matsen FA, Wyss CR, Pedegana LR, et al: Transcutaneous oxygen tension measurement in peripheral vascular disease. Surg Gynaecol Obstet 150:525, 1980

14. Clyne CAC, Ryan J, Webster JHH, et al: Oxygen tension on the skin of ischaemic legs. Am J Surg 143:315, 1982

15. Wyss CR, Matsen FA, King RV, et al: Dependence of transcutaneous oxygen tension on local arteriovenous pressure gradient in normal subjects. Clin Sci 60:499, 1981

16. Spence VA, McCollum PT, McGregor IW, et al: The effect of the transcutaneous oxygen electrode on the variability of dermal oxygen tension changes. (submitted for publication).

17. Burgess EM, Matsen FA, Wyss CR, et al: Segmental transcutaneous measurements of PO_2 in patients requiring below-the-knee amputation for peripheral vascular insufficiency. J Bone Joint Surg 64(A):378, 1982

18. Ratliff DA, Clyne CAC, Chant ADB, et al: Prediction of amputation wound healing: The role of transcutaneous PO_2 assessment. Br J Surg 71:219, 1984

19. Wyss CR, Matsen FA, Simmons CW, et al: Transcutaneous oxygen tension measurements on limbs of diabetic and non-diabetic patients with peripheral vascular disease. Surgery 95:339, 1984

20. Eickoff JH, Jacobsen E: Correlation of transcutaneous oxygen to blood flow in heated skin. Scand J Clin Lab Invest 40:761, 1980

21. Eickoff JH, Engell HC: Transcutaneous oxygen tension ($TcPO_2$) measurements on the foot in normal subjects and in patients with peripheral vascular disease admitted for vascular surgery. Scand J Clin Lab Invest 41:743, 1981

22. Spence VA, Walker WF: Tissue oxygen tension in normal and ischaemic human skin. Cardiovasc Res 18:140, 1984

23. Granger HJ, Goodman AH, Granger DN: Intrinsic metabolic regulation of blood flow, O_2 extraction and tissue O_2 delivery in dog skeletal muscle, in Bicher HI, Druley DF (eds): Advances in Experimental Medicine and Biology, Vol 37A. New York, Plenum, 1973, pp 451–456

24. Hauser CJ, Appel P, Shoemaker WC: Pathophysiologic classification of peripheral vascular disease by positional changes in regional transcutaneous oxygen tension. Surgery 95:689, 1984

25. Spence VA, McCollum PT, Walker WF, et al: Assessment of tissue viability in relation to the selection of amputation level. Prosth Orthot Int 8:67, 1984
26. Katsamouris A, Brewster DC, Megerman J, et al: Transcutaneous oxygen tension in selection of amputation level. Am J Surg 147:510–517, 1984
27. Urbach F: The blood supply of tumours, in Montagna W, Ellis RA (eds): Advances in Biology of Skin, Vol 2. New York, Pergamon, 1961, pp 123–149
28. Harward TRS, Volny J, Golbranson FL, et al: Oxygen inhalation induced TcPO$_2$ changes as a predictor of amputation level. Int Soc Cardiovasc Surg (Proceedings of 32nd meeting, Atlanta) p 62, 1984

P. Holstein
and Niels A. Lassen

30

Methods for Prediction of Amputation Wound Healing Based on Regional Blood Flow or Blood Pressure Measurements

The importance of saving the knee in major amputations has stimulated the development of methods for determining the safe level of amputation. These techniques have also been applied to minor amputations on the foot, the failure of which causes loss of the limb. Ideally one single method should be used in mapping out circulation of the whole ischaemic limb. In our experience, however, no single method has yet been devised that is suitable both in major and in minor amputations. This paper presents the evidence for choosing among the presently available methods.

MAJOR LEG AMPUTATION

In selecting objectively the best major amputation level, viz. the below knee (BK), the through knee (TK), or the above knee (AK) level, we use Kety's local clearance method.[1] It is based on the washout of a depot of radioactive tracer recorded by a simple scintillation detector. This method determines regional blood flow. Moreover, by recording the external pressure required to stop the washout, the regional perfusion pressure is measured.[2]

The Tracers

The tracer should diffuse freely across the capillaries, so that its washout is a function of regional blood flow. Several radioactive tracers of this type can be used. Originally we used ^{133}Xenon dissolved in physiological saline. This tracer is, however, not practical because its high solubility in adipose tissue causes a slow wash-out. ^{131}Iodine labelled iodoantipyrine is almost equally soluble in all tissues and adipose tissue does not retard its washout rate. We have used it extensively but recently we have turned to the much cheaper ^{99m}Technetium (as the pertechnetate). This tracer diffuses well enough across the capillaries to be a flow limited tracer in the low range of flows of importance for amputation problems.[3]

DIAGNOSTIC TECHNIQUES AND ASSESSMENT
PROCEDURES IN VASCULAR SURGERY

© 1985 Grune & Stratton
ISBN 0-8089-1721-8 All rights reserved

The Injection

The radioactive tracer, contained in a volume of 0.1 ml saline, is injected intra-dermally using an 0.4 mm needle. The injectate contains 50 micrograms of histamine (as diphosphate) to ensure maximal local vasodilatation. This is important in order to ensure reproducible results of the maximal regional blood flow in the prevailing conditions. Histamine minimizes the effect of local trauma that also involves hista-mine liberation (but in much lesser amount). It also eliminates the effect of tem-perature on skin blood flow.

The exact amount of radioactivity injected is not important, as the washout rate is a relative measure, viz. the slope of the curve in a semilogarithmic plot. With ^{99m}Technetium we use 40–80 microCuries to ensure a good counting rate. As this dose is in the order of 1/1000 of doses given for other tracer methods the radiation hazard is correspondingly small: it is for practical purposes to be considered as completely negligible.

Regional Skin Blood Flow (SBF)

The washout rate is recorded by a scintillation detector coupled to a ratemeter with a logarithmic output, The recorded curve can be used to calculate the slope, i.e. the exponential coefficient k. Because the partition coefficient for ^{99m}Technetium is 1.0 (practically the same as for iodo-antipyrine), the skin blood flow is equal to k if expressed per gram of tissue. Or, using the conventional unit of 100 grams of tissue:

$$SBF = 100 \cdot k \text{ ml/100g/min} \qquad (1)$$

In practice k is obtained as the slope multiplied by 2.30, the natural logarithm to 10, as the ratemeter output is in decimal logarithm and not in natural logarithm.[4]

The semilogarithmic curve consists of three phases. For the first few minutes after the injection the washout is slow. The second, faster component is almost monoexponential and lasts until about 80 percent of the tracer has been washed out. In the third phase, the washout gradually decreases towards zero. The second com-ponent is used for slope reading (skin blood flow) and for recording of the external pressure required for making the curve horizontal (skin perfusion pressure). It is important to wait for the second phase on the curve, which in low blood flow/blood pressure circumstances may be delayed for 5–10 minutes. The slope of the curve used for blood flow determination can be determined by line drawing on the curve and usually no more than a 3–4 minutes part of the tracing should be employed since the rest of the second phase should be used for washout cessation pressure measurement.

Regional Skin Perfusion Pressure (SPP)

External counter pressure is applied by placing a conventional arm blood pressure cuff, so that it covers the depot.[2] In order to measure the local pressure over the injected skin area even more precisely, we usually employ in addition a 12×12 cm (inflatable part (11×11 cm) thin-walled plastic bag, that is interposed between the depot and the blood pressure cuff. The bag is filled with a small amount of air, so that it is slack and moulds to the labelled skin. The bag is connected to a mercury manometer by which the applied external counter pressure is recorded.

When a sufficiently long washout curve has been obtained for blood flow recording external pressure is applied and raised stepwise resulting in a stepwise decrease in washout rate. It is necessary to observe the curve for about 5 minutes at each step when approaching the horizontal level and using pressure increments of 5 mmHg, the SPP is taken to be the pressure midway between the highest pressure, where washout can still be discerned by eye and the washout cessation pressure.

Where to Measure Flow and Pressure

The sites of measurement, i.e. where the depot is injected, have been standardized: the anterolateral side of the calf about 10 cm below the knee joint, on the anterolateral part of the thigh 10 cm and 20 cm proximal to the knee joint. In most cases the situation is sufficiently elucidated by one measurement, i.e., at the standard site below the knee.

Measurement Conditions and Sources of Error

All measurements are made with the examinees in the supine position at room temperature about 25° C, so that the patients feel comfortable with light clothing. The arm blood pressure is measured repeatedly during the examination to secure that the systemic blood pressure remains constant. Pains may cause the blood pressure to rise considerably and may cause movements of the leg. An analgesic, for example Demerole, is given intravenously in repeated doses (25 mg) in practically all cases. A measurement that is painful for the patient is unacceptable and unreliable. The leg must be kept immobile at a constant distance from the detector and this demands proper fixation of the leg by sandbags. Edema of the skin is another source of error: external counterpressure squeezes the edema and the labelled fluid away giving a "false" clearance. This difficulty is overcome by inflating a cuff at the swelling to 40–80 mmHg for about 5 minutes. This must naturally be done before the skin is labelled.

Skin Blood Flow is not as Accurate as Skin Perfusion Pressure

In normal subjects the histamine augmented skin blood flow is about 12 ml/100g/min as measured with [99m]Technetium on the calf[3] and the skin perfusion pressure is a few mmHg above the systemic diastolic blood pressure.[2,5]

In 60 GK amputations the healing in relation to SBP and to SPP measured on the same tracing was significantly correlated to both parameters. The SPP, however, yielded the best prognostic index[6] with poor results, i.e. only 25 percent healed with SPP below 20 mmHg whereas 90 percent healed with SPP above 30 mmHg. The correlation between SBP and SPP is shown in figure 30-1. The scatter is great, but low SPP is associated with low SBP.

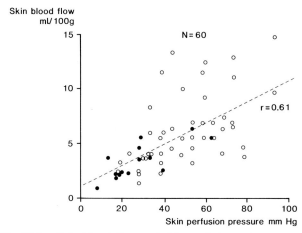

Fig. 30-1. Skin blood flow and skin perfusion pressure measured as the skin blood flow cessation counterpressure below the knee. 60 below knee amputations—open symbols successful amputation, closed symbols failure of wound healing.

BK Amputations: Clinical Level Selection
Compared to Skin Perfusion Pressure

In another series of 102 major leg amputations the level selection was based upon conventional clinical criteria. The results were afterwards compared with sealed SPP values as determined preoperatively[7] Table 30-1. Sixteen cases had been subjected to AK amputations and two cases to TK amputations. Of these, 15 had SPP values at BK level below 30 mmHg. The clinical findings leading to sacrificing the knee are listed in table 30-2.

In the remaining 84 cases primary BK amputation had been performed. Healing failed in 17 cases and was significantly correlated to SPP values (table 30-3). In only one patient with amputation failure and low perfusion pressure were signs of ichaemia present (an ischaemic ulcer on the calf). There was no difference in healing rate in relation to SPP between diabetic and nondiabetic cases.

This series demonstrates, that the surgeons to a large extent relied on clinical criteria, i.e. temperature demarcation lines, cyanoses, and ischaemic ulcers at the calf when sacrificing primarily the knee. And such clinical signs were also closely associ-

Table 30-1
Healingrates in Relation to Histamine Augmented
Skin Blood Flow (SBF) and Skin Perfusion
Pressure (SPP) in 60 BK Amputations

	SPP (mmHg)		
	<20 mmHg	20–29 mmHg	>30 mmHg
Healing rate	2/8 = 25%	8/12 = 67%	36/40 = 90%
	SBF		
	<2.5 ml	2.5 − 3.9 ml	>4 ml
Healing rate	5/11 = 46%	7/11 = 64%	34/38 = 90%

Table 30-2
Clinical Findings in Patients Selected for Primary AK (or TK) Amputation

No. of AK (or TK) amputations	Skin perfusion pressure at BK level (mmHg)	Skin at BK level Temperature demarcation	Cyanosis	Ulceration or necrosis	Other factors* contributing to AK level	Poor physical and mental condition
9	<20	3	4	6	3	5
6	20–30	1	1	2	2	2
3	>30	0	0	2	1	2

* Other factors: Severe oedema, 2 cases; steroid skin changes, 2 cases; paralysed leg (poliomyelitis), 1 case; uraemia, 1

Table 30-3
The Healing Rates in Relation to Skin Perfusion Pressure in 84 Cases Selected for Primary BK Amputation

SPP	<20 mmHg	21–30 mmHg	>30 mmHg
Without diabetes mellitus	0/6	4/9	34/35
With diabetes mellitus	1/3	2/4	26/27
Whole series	1/9	6/13	60/62
95% confidence limits	0–48%	29–75%	89–100%

ated with low SPP values. However, the series also demonstrated, that the absence of these clinical signs of ischaemia by no means is a guarantee against ischaemic failure of wound healing. For this reason objective measurements are necessary in selecting the correct level of amputation.

AK Amputations

Healing studies have also been made on AK amputations in relation to SPP as measured 10 cm above the knee.[8] Reamputation, i.e. resection of bone, was only occasionally necessary, even at low pressures. But healing was slow and wound

Table 30-4
The Healing Results in Relation to Skin Perfusion Pressure in 59 Cases of AK Amputation

SPP	<20 mmHg Primary healing	Healing within 2 months	Major wound complication	21–30 mmHg Primary healing	Healing within 2 months	Major wound complication	>30 mmHg Primary healing	Healing within 2 months	Major wound complication
Without diabetes mellitus	0	0	2	1	0	6	25	6	3
With diabetes mellitus	0	0	1	0	1	0	11	2	1
Whole series	0	0	3	1	1	6	36	8	4

complications were associated with a high mortality. In a series of 59 AK amputations there were severe wound complications (defined as total break down of the stump or healing delayed for more than three months) in as many as 9 out of 11 cases (table 30-4). The mortality in hospital was 24 percent, but cases with severe wound complications had a mortality of 50 percent. In the 6 cases who survived with major wound complications, healing was accomplished late, but within 5 months.

Thus a low SPP on the AK level implies that the surgeon has to decide whether an attractive long stump justifies the risk of delayed healing (and death), or whether a short and useless stump should be made in order to reduce these complications.

MINOR AMPUTATIONS ON THE FEET

Skin Perfusion Pressure?

Measurement with radioisotopes as injected intradermally on the dorsal side of the foot may be difficult in the ischaemic foot often with severe edema or infection. In a series of 134 minor amputations the SPP could only be measured in 43 cases.[9] These were 4 cases with SPP below 20 mmHg and these cases all failed to heal. However, in 39 cases with SPP above 20 mmHg only 19 healed and no level of SPP with a resonable garantee of success could be identified. In our experience, therefore, SPP is of limited value for selecting candidates for minor amputations on the feet.

Digital and Ankle Systolic Blood Pressure by Strain-Gauge

In the same series, systolic digital and ankle blood pressures were evaluated.[9] The results are shown in table 30-5 table 30-6. Digital pressures below 20 mmHg and pressures below 50 mmHg were associated with very poor healing. Digital pressures above 30 mmHg and ankle pressures above 100 mmHg were associated with healing in about 75 percent of the cases. We prefer the digital pressures because

Table 30-5

Healing Rates in Digital and Forefront Amputations
with and without Diabetes Mellitus (DM) in Relation
to the Systolic Ankle Pressure (SABP) as
Measured in 119 Cases

SABP	<50 mmHg	50–99 mmHg	≥100 mmHg
Without DM	0/2	8/17	7/10
With DM	0/3	18/32	40/55
Digital amputations	0/5	18/36	41/57
Transmetatarsal forefoot amputations	0/0	8/13	6/8
Total	0/5 (0%)	26/49	47/65 (72%)
Confidence limits (95%)	0–52%		60–83%

Table 30-6
Healing Rates in Digital and Forefoot Amputations
with and without Diabetes Mellitus (DM) in Relation
to the Systolic Digital Blood Pressure (SDBP)
as Measured in 110 Cases

SDBP	<20 mmHg	20–29 mmHg	≥30 mmHg
Without DM	1/7	6/7	8/12
With DM	3/16	7/15	43/53
Digital amputations	2/17	9/17	47/60
Forefoot amputations	2/6	4/5	4/5
Total	4/23 (17%)	13/22	51/65 (78%)
Confidence limits (95%)	5–39%		67–88%

the "grey zone" is narrow (20–29 mmHg), whereas in ankle pressures it is large (50–99 mmHg) comprising about 40 percent of the cases. Moreover, 9 percent of the diabetic cases had noncompressible arteries at the ankle due to medial sclerosis. The phenomenon causes ankle pressures to be nonreliable in diabetics. Fortunately this source of error does not invalidate digital pressures.

The high number of failures (about 25 percent) at reasonable arterial supply in diabetics ending up with major leg amputations, represents invasive infections often treated inadequately with antibiotics. This loss of limbs highlights the need for adequate profylacsis and therapy of ulcers in the diabetic neuropathic foot.

DISCUSSION

The materials presented show that the skin perfusion pressure is valuable in major amputation level determination, whereas systolic digital blood pressure is more practical in determining the prognosis on the feet.

Amputations in dysvascular patients should be made at the most distal level allowing healing to take place. Continued improvement in amputation surgery implies continued efforts to replace AK amputations with BK amputations whenever possible and to do TK amputations in many of the remaining cases. TK amputations are almost as favourable with regard to rehabilitation as the BK amputations[10] and it probably ought to be used on a wider scale.[11]

In diabetic patients the BK amputation can probably be replaced by Syme's amputation as popularized by Wagner and his group.[12] Reliable measurements, however, for this and similar proximal foot levels are in our opinion not at hand. It is hardly justified to try this level without objective measurements in as much as the clinical evaluation of the circulation in the diabetic foot can be most difficult.

We are continuously looking for methods that are simpler, faster, and more reliable than the isotope washout technique. Photoelectric recording of SPP is rapid, but it cannot be applied to all patients[13,14] and a careful selection of the skin area studied is necessary. Transcutaneous oxygen tension measurement correlates with SPP,[3] but in our experience this technique is less reliable than SPP measurements. Red cell velocity measurements in heated skin using the Laser Doppler technique should also be explored. In this context it should be noted, that one of the reasons for the reliability of the SPP method is probably that a pseudo-amputation[15] is made with the counter pressure cuff. Cessation of skin blood flow means that circulation distal to the cuff decreases although it does not stop completely. This pseudo-amputation should probably be included in measurements with other techniques.

REFERENCES

1. Kety SS: Amer Heart J 38:321, 1969
2. Holstein P, et al: Scand J Clin Lab Invest 37:649, 1977
3. Holstein P, et al: Clin Physiol 3:313, 1983
4. Lassen NA, et al: Lancet i:686, 1964
5. Holstein P, et al: Microvasc Res 17:71, 1979
6. Holstein P, et al: Acta Orthop Scand 50:49, 1979
7. Holstein P: Acta Orthop Scand 53:821, 1982
8. Holstein P, et al: Acta Orthop Scand 50:59, 1977
9. Holstein P: Acta Orthop Scand 55:227, 1984
10. Steen-Jensen J, et al: Acta Orthop Scand 54:101, 1983
11. Thyregod HC, et al: Prosth Orthot Int 7:61, 1983
12. Wagner FW: Foot Ankle 2:64, 1981
13. Stöckel M, et al: Acta Orthop Scand 52:405, 1981
14. Holstein P, et al: Scand J Clin Lab Invest 40:535, 1980
15. Lassen NA, Holstein P: Surg Clin Amer 54:39, 1974

PART VI

Upper Limb Ischaemia

Edward Housley

31

Immunology and Arterial Disease

When the body is exposed to an antigen an immune response occurs with production of humoral antibodies, or a cellular response with production of aggressive lymphocytes. Antigens may complex with circulating antibodies to form "circulating immune complexes." If not cleared by the reticulo endothelial system these complexes may deposit in blood vessel walls causing increased permeability, and activation of complement causing chemotactic attraction of leucocytes with inflammation and tissue damage. It seems likely that this is the mechanism responsible for most immunological disorders affecting arteries though cell mediated immune reactions, where sensitised lymphocytes release lymphokines causing similar reactions, may be responsible in some diseases. The immune response may be to an exogenous antigen, such as an organism or drug, or it may be an "autoimmune" response to part of itself, eg to DNA in systemic lupus erythematosus.

Some diseases affecting arteries seem to have an immunological aetiology and arterial diseases have not escaped the explosion of immunological research in the last few years.

My remit is to offer advice to the practising surgeon in his clinic or wards, not to write a treatise on the immunology of arterial disease. However I think a brief, but by no means comprehensive, survey of some recent work on the immunology of arterial disease would be of interest before discussing the practical aspects.

THROMBOANGIITIS OBLITERANS (BUERGER'S DISEASE)

This disease, occurring in young men, with inflammatory involvement of the arteries and veins would seem a likely candidate for an immunological aetiology.[1] In the last few years there has been some evidence to support this. Gulati et al[2] demonstrated arterial auto-antibodies in Indian patients with inflammatory arterial disease, resembling thromboangiitis obliterans as seen in the West, and also found

DIAGNOSTIC TECHNIQUES AND ASSESSMENT
PROCEDURES IN VASCULAR SURGERY

© 1985 Grune & Stratton
ISBN 0-8089-1721-8 All rights reserved

an increased prevalence of nonorgan specific antibodies. Adar et al[3] also found increased sensitivity of lymphocytes to collagen in patients with thromboangiitis obliterans again suggesting an immune aetiology. Attempts are also being made to demonstrate tobacco antibodies in these patients.

TAKAYASU'S ARTERITIS

In its more florid form, occurring in young women with systemic symptoms, abnormalities of plasma proteins, raised ESR, and inflammatory involvement of major arteries, an immune aetiology would again seem very likely. However, despite intensive research the evidence remains weak. Gyotoku et al[4] found circulating immune complexes in seven out of 29 cases. Numano et al[5] also found circulating immune complexes in 46% of their cases compared to 20% of controls. They did not regard this as good evidence of an immune aetiology in that over half their cases did not have increased circulating immune complexes and also the level of the complexes in the blood bore no relationship to the activity of the disease.

SYSTEMIC LUPUS ERYTHEMATOSUS (SLE)

This of course has long been known as an autoimmune disease. DNA–Anti-DNA antibody complexes circulate in the blood and deposit in small arteries, particularly in the kidneys, but also in the cutaneous and digital circulation. These complexes activate complement with inflammatory and particularly lymphocytic infiltration of the vessels causing increased permeability, further vessel damage, and thrombosis. Anti-nuclear antibody can be demonstrated by a relatively simple immunofluorescent technique, ie. the anti-nuclear factor test (ANF) and then, more specifically, the level of anti-DNA binding can be measured by radioimmunoassays. Measurement of serum complement levels is somewhat controversial but some believe that a fall in complement level indicates activity of the disease particularly renal vasculitis. Many other auto-antibodies can be demonstrated in SLE.

SCLERODERMA

This label covers a fairly wide range of disease from the very active autoimmune-like disease of sclerodermatomyositis with systemic symptoms, poly-myositis, plasma protein abnormalities, and raised ESR, through progressive systemic sclerosis, the classic multi-system sclerotic fibrosing disease affecting young women and often coming to fatal conclusion within a few years, to the apparently more benign CRST syndrome confined to the fingers and oesophagus that, although severely disabling, rarely seems to develop into anything more serious or cause death. Many workers have shown that a high percentage of patients with sclero-derma have positive ANF tests, particularly showing a "nucleolar pattern" on the test. The prevalence of a positive ANF depends on the selection of cases, ie. the more one has of the active progressive systemic sclerosis or sclerodermatomyositis variety, the higher the percentage of a positive ANF. In my experience in the CRST syndrome, which is the form of scleroderma most commonly presenting to vascular surgeons, a positive ANF is rare. More complex and sophisticated tests for anti-centromere antinuclear factor may be positive in up to 80% of patients.[6,7]

GIANT CELL ARTERITIS

The clinical picture of this condition with its association with polymyalgia rheumatica and response to steroid therapy is strongly suggestive of autoimmune disease. Papaioannou et al[8] have demonstrated circulating immune complexes in the acute phase.

CUTANEOUS VASCULITIS

This condition has many features of an immunological disease with its variable time course and intense inflammatory infiltration of cutaneous arterioles. Many studies have shown immune complexes deposited in the skin arterioles and capillaries. The complexes may consist of antibody with an extrinsic antigen such as drugs or organisms or auto-antigens such as DNA, when it is seen as part of SLE, and IgG when it occurs in rheumatoid arthritis. Circulating immune complexes have been demonstrated by Andrews et al.[9]

Where does this leave the practising vascular surgeon? Let us consider this under the heading of various disease patterns presenting in a vascular clinic.

Arteriosclerosis Obliterans

The patient presenting with intermittent claudication, rest pain or gangrene in whom it is clinically obvious that the aetiology is arteriosclerosis requires no immunological investigation.

Raynaud's Phenomenon

The majority of patients presenting with Raynaud's phenomenon show the classic primary form, ie. episodic digital vasospasm occurring in otherwise healthy young women and present for some years. In my opinion there is no convincing evidence of any underlying immunological disorder in these girls and they do not require any investigation. Allen[10] stated that if the Raynaud's has been present for two years without any ulcers or infarcts developing, it could be confidently labelled as primary Raynaud's phenomenon (or Raynaud's disease as he called it) and with this I would concur. Those who say otherwise forget that in a temperate climate approximately five percent of young women have primary Raynaud's phenomenon so that one would expect some patients developing secondary Raynaud's phenomenon in later life to give a history of Raynaud's going back to girlhood. They have developed secondary Raynaud's phenomenon in addition to their primary and it is not that the primary has become secondary. However, I have yet to meet even this as in my experience all patients with secondary Raynaud's have developed severe ischaemia, infarction of ulcers within one to two years of the first symptom of Raynaud's.

If a patient presents with secondary Raynaud's phenomenon should one undertake immunological investigation? I think there is no need to do any immunological investigation of patients whose Raynaud's is clearly due to scleroderma of the CRST or progressive systemic sclerosis variety. One may find a faintly positive ANF and minor abnormalities of ESR and plasma proteins in some patients, but these tests do not aid diagnosis or management. If the patient has systemic symptoms and other features suggesting polymyositis or sclerodermatomyositis or the Raynaud's phenomenon is not clearly due to scleroderma (or vibration white finger) it is worth doing a few simple screening tests for autoimmune disease, such as a full blood count with platelets, ESR and plasma protein electrophoresis, and more specific immunological tests, ie. ANF and RA latex tests. If abnormalities are found the patient should then be referred to a physician for further investigation and treatment. In my experience while working in a vascular clinic, such patients are rarely found. The impression that many patients with secondary Raynaud's have a definable immunological disorder comes from studies by rheumatologists and dermatologists who have studied patients in their own clinics where selection bias favours such patients.

Cutaneous Vasculitis

These patients usually present with multiple painful nodules, often ulcerating, mainly on the legs, feet, and hands. Systemic lupus erythematosus may be the cause so a full blood count, ESR, plasma protein, and antinuclear factor tests are indicated. If the ANF is positive anti-DNA binding levels should be measured, as, if SLE is diagnosed, medical treatment, usually with steroids, may be indicated. I do not think it worthwhile looking, at this stage, for circulating immune complexes or measuring complement levels as the interpretation of these tests is difficult and the tests themselves time consuming and expensive.

Arteritis of Major Vessels

These patients usually present with chronic occlusive disease of the major vessels, usually of the aortic arch, but sometimes the abdominal aorta or iliac vessels. If the patient is middle-aged or elderly and the symptom of claudication of the arms is accompanied by systemic symptoms and aching discomfort in the shoulder girdle muscles suggesting polymyalgia rheumatica, it is likely the pathology is giant cell arteritis. Investigations of value here are the ESR and temporal artery biopsy. These investigations should be undertaken urgently and steroids given to avert ophthalmic artery thrombosis. Looking for other immunological abnormalities is of no aid in diagnosis or management.

If the patient is a younger woman, particularly Asian, the diagnosis is likely to be a Takayasu type of arteritis. In younger patients systemic symptoms may be prominent, but immunological investigations, although interesting, do not really affect the diagnosis or management. The decision to use steroids depends on the activity of the disease as shown by clinical features, sedimentation rate, and plasma protein abnormalities rather than tests for circulating immune complexes. In more long-standing cases, particularly in middle age, secondary atherosclerotic changes have usually occurred and the disease seems to have become less active anyway and steroids are not indicated.

THROMBO-ANGIITIS OBLITERANS (BUERGER'S DISEASE)

Immunological investigation, again although interesting, has not reached the stage of being useful in diagnosis or management of thrombo-angiitis obliterans. The diagnosis remains clinical, ie. predominantly peripheral disease in a young male who smokes heavily supported, if possible, by typical angiographic findings and pathological examination of arteries in resected limbs or digits. Even if this disease has an immune basis, treatment with steroids or immunosuppressive drugs is not indicated as they are not effective and the disease responds well to giving up smoking.

In conclusion, although immunological research is shedding further light on the aetiology of some inflammatory arterial disease, in ordinary clinical vascular surgical practice immunological investigation remains confined to a search for SLE or rheumatoid disease in patients with secondary Raynaud's phenomenon or cutaneous vasculitis.

REFERENCES

1. Spittell JA: Thrombo-angiitis obliterans—an autoimmune disorder? Editorial. New Eng J Med 308:1157, 1983
2. Gulati SM, et al: Autoantibodies in thrombo-angiitis obliterans. Angiology 33:642, 1982
3. Adar R, et al: Cellular sensitivity to collagen in thromboangiitis obliterans. New Eng J Med 308:1113, 1983
4. Gyotoku Y, et al: Immune complexes in Takayasu's arteritis. Clin Exp Immunol 45:246, 1981
5. Numano F, et al: Circulating immune complexes in Takayasu's Disease. Lack of evidence of a causative role. Arch Intern Med 141:162, 1981
6. Tam EM, Rodnan GP, Garcia I, et al: Diversity of antinuclear antibodies in progressive systemic sclerosis: anticentromere antibody and its relationship to CREST syndrome. Arthritis Rheum 23:617, 1980
7. Catoggio LI, Bernstein EM, Black CM, et al: Serological markers in progressive systemic sclerosis. Ann Rheum Dis 42:23, 1982
8. Pappaioannou CC, Gupta RC, Hunder GG, et al: Arthritis Rheum 23:1021, 1980
9. Andrews BS, et al: Circulating and tissue immune complexes in cutaneous vasculitis. J Clin Lab Pharmacol 1:311, 1979
10. Allen EV, Brown GE: Raynaud's Disease: A critical review of minimal requisites for diagnosis. Amer J Med Sci 183:187, 1932

James S. T. Yao

32

Preoperative Assessment of Upper Extremity Ischemia

Unlike occlusive diseases affecting the lower extremities, where the etiology is either atherosclerotic or embolic, a wide variety of systemic and neurogenic diseases may cause ischemic symptoms of the hands. Evaluation of upper-extremity ischemia, therefore, requires a thorough history taking and a careful physical examination. Even so, the diagnosis may be difficult, and various tests may be needed to establish an accurate diagnosis.

At present, several noninvasive tests are helpful to detect arterial occlusion of the upper extremities, especially in the digital arteries. These are strain-gauge- and photo-plethysmography,[1-3] the transcutaneous Doppler ultrasound flow detection technique,[4-8] B-mode ultrasound scan of the peripheral arteries,[9] and the cold stimulation test.[10-13] The Doppler flow detection technique is of particular use in evaluation of the ulnar and digital arteries which, in general, are not accessible to physical examination. In combination with the cold stimulation test, these noninvasive tests are of value to separate Raynaud's disease from Raynaud's phenomenon. The discovery of arterial occlusion leads to arteriographic examination, which may offer definitive diagnosis in patients with hand ischemia.

The present chapter reviews the current concepts in preoperative assessment of upper-extremity ischemia.

DIAGNOSIS

History Taking

Multiple etiologic factors are responsible for hand ischemia. Therefore, a thorough history taking is absolutely necessary. Table 32-1 enumerates the various causes of hand ischemia.

The increasing use of cardiac catheterization and arterial lines for blood gas or pressure monitoring has produced a new spectrum of problems with thrombosis of

DIAGNOSTIC TECHNIQUES AND ASSESSMENT
PROCEDURES IN VASCULAR SURGERY

© 1985 Grune & Stratton
ISBN 0-8089-1721-8 All rights reserved

Table 32-1

Etiology of Upper Extremity
and Digital Ischemia

Atherosclerosis
    Arteriosclerosis obliterans
    Embolization
        Cardiac
        Atheromatous emboli

Arteritis
    Collagen disease
        Scleroderma
        Rheumatoid arteritis
        Systemic lupus erythematosus
        Polyarteritis
    Allergic necrotizing arteritis
    Takayasu's disease (autoimmune disorder)
    Buerger's syndrome
    Giant-cell arteritis

Blood dyscrasias
    Cold agglutinins
    Cryoglobulins
    Polycythemia

Drug-induced occlusion
    Ergot poisoning
    Drug abuse
    Chemotherapeutic agents

Occupational trauma
    Vibration syndrome
    Hypothenar hammer syndrome
    Bullman's hand
    Electrical burns

Thoracic outlet syndrome

Congenital arterial wall defects

Trauma
    Iatrogenic catheter injury
        Cardiac catheterization
        Arterial blood gas and pressure monitoring
        Arteriography
    Radiation injury
    Frost bite

Renal transplantation and related problems
    Azotemic arteriopathy
    Hemodialysis shunts

Aneurysms of the upper extremity

Modified from Yao JST, McDaniel MD, King TA: Arterial surgery of the upper extremity. Clin Surg Internat Vol. 8. Arterial Surgery. Bergan JJ Ed. Edinburgh, Churchill Livingstone, 1984, pp 201–224 With permission.

the hand arteries. The diagnosis is often apparent in these patients. The presence of atrial fibrillation is helpful in diagnosis of embolic occlusion. Although embolic occlusion is often accute, it may present with subacute or late manifestations of chronic ischemia. Of the diseases affecting the small arteries, autoimmune diseases, including scleroderma, lupus erythematosus, and mixed connective tissue diseases are the most common.

History taking must include occupational history because one of the frequently encountered causes of hand ischemia is occupational trauma. Occupational trauma includes the "vibratory white finger" in workers who use vibrating tools,[14] the hypothenar hammer syndrome,[15] and rarely, the bullman's hand.[16] Professional athletes, such as baseball players, may present with either digital artery occlusion or vascular complications due to thoracic outlet compression.[17]

A review of the patient's pharmacologic history is also helpful. The use of ergot derivatives for migraine has been known to cause upper-extremity ischemia.[18] Raynaud's symptoms may be due to the use of beta-blockers.[19] Chemotherapeutic agents, such as vinblastine, bleomycin, and cisplatin may also cause hand ischemia.[20] In addition, hand ischemia may develop as a result of high-dose dopamine infusion.[21]

A history of smoking must be sought in all patients who present with hand ischemia. The diagnosis of Buerger's disease may be made in a young adult if there is evidence of heavy smoking, collagen disease abnormalities are absent, and digital artery occlusion is demonstrated by arteriography.

A history of radiation therapy should alert the surgeon to consider radiation injury. Irradiation may cause damage to small vessels and large arteries. Within the first few years after radiation, patients often present with mural thrombus and embolization to the digital arteries. Late manifestations of radiation injury include fibrotic occlusion or accelerated atherosclerosis of the irradiated artery.

Clinical Examination

Clinical examination in patients who present with symptoms of hand ischemia must include evaluation of the thoracic outlet and the entire upper extremity. Palpation of the supraclavicular region may help to detect the presence of a subclavian artery aneurysm, or not infrequently, a cervical rib. Auscultation of the subclavian artery and listening for the presence of a bruit in neutral position and during various thoracic outlet maneuvers (exaggerated military, Adson, abduction, and external rotation) helps to establish the diagnosis of thoracic outlet syndrome. Arteries in the upper extremity are accessible to pulse palpation, and therefore, diagnosis of major arterial occlusion is seldom a problem. Examination of the hand must include the Allen test[22] to determine patency of the palmar arch. Palpation of the finger pulses is less reliable, but embolic phenomena involving the digital arteries are usually identified by the presence of petechial lesions or superficial gangrene of the finger-tip.

Apart from examination of the vascular system, a careful inspection of the joints of the hand and the skin may offer some diagnostic clues. Rheumatoid arteritis is not uncommon in patients with severe rheumatoid arthritis, in which a typical rheumatoid deformity may be apparent. Hyper- or abnormal mobility of a joint calls for the diagnosis of Ehlers-Danlos syndrome. The combination of weakness of the arterial wall and hyperextension of joints contributes to damage to the brachial artery.[23] Finally, abnormal elasticity of the skin, especially over the joint space, raises the possibility of pseudoxanthoma elasticum, which may accompany degeneration of the arterial wall and result in stenosis or occlusion.[24]

Laboratory Examination

In severe hand ischemia, especially when both hands are involved, a systemic cause of the arterial insufficiency should be sought. Ischemia due to collagen disease may be identified by appropriate serologic testing. Although patients with these conditions are seldom candidates for surgical intervention, it is important for interested surgeons to establish proper diagnoses.

In detection of scleroderma (systemic sclerosis) and its variant, the CRST syndrome, a battery of tests may be used. The features of the CRST syndrome include calcinosis, Raynaud's phenomenon, esophageal dysfunction, and telangiectasias. In this condition, a combination of physical examination, soft tissue roentgenograms, and esophageal motility studies may be revealing.

Systemic lupus erythematosus (SLE), another important cause of bilateral hand ischemia, is characterized by multisystem abnormalities caused by a variety of autoantibodies. The erythrocyte sedimentation rate is often elevated and remains so, even during disease remission. Rheumatoid factor may become positive in these patients.

In addition to collagen disease, arterities such as giant-cell arteritis or Takayasu's disease may cause upper-extremity ischemia. The diagnosis is aided by an elevation of sedimentation rate, the arteriographic findings, and to a greater extent, the absence of serologic abnormalities referable to collagen disease.

Not infrequently, blood dyscrasias may be the cause of upper-extremity ischemia. Blood dyscrasias include polycythemia vera, platelet dysfunction, hyperviscosity syndrome, intravascular coagulation, and abnormal serum proteins including cryoglobulin and cold agglutinins. A routine blood count, coagulation profile, cold agglutinins, and cryoglobulin tests will aid diagnosis. Bone marrow examination may be needed to establish the definitive diagnosis of polycythemia vera.

Noninvasive Testing

Noninvasive testing is used to detect arterial occlusion, especially of the digital arteries, and to determine the need for arteriography. Several noninvasive tests, including plethysmography and transcutaneous Doppler ultrasound flow detection, are now available for objective evaluation of hand ischemia. Of these techniques, Doppler flow detection is simplest.

Doppler Ultrasound

The Doppler examination of the upper extremity consists of both arterial waveform recording and analysis and pressure measurements. Bilateral examinations should be performed in view of the fact that many of the diseases affecting the hand are symmetric.[25] Often, the asymptomatic hand will have significant occlusion.

Since the axillary and brachial arteries are so superficially located, they lend themselves to Doppler examination throughout their entire course in the upper arm. Distal to the elbow, however, arterial signals are more difficult to obtain, and it is not until the wrist that both the radial and ulnar arteries become superficially situated once again.

In the hand, the palmar arches are best heard at the mid-thenar and hypothenar regions. The common digital vessels are heard at the base of the fingers, at their division into the proper digital arteries along the shaft of each finger. The waveforms are analyzed for their shape and contour, similar to examination of the lower extremity.

For segmental upper extremity pressures, a pneumatic cuff is placed at the upper arm, as it is routinely used for blood pressure recording. The arm pressure will represent the brachial pressure, which should be within 15 to 20 mmHg of the opposite extremity. A greater difference signifies either innominate, subclavian, axillary, or brachial artery stenosis. If brachial artery occlusion is suspected, a pressure cuff may be applied to the forearm and the pressure recorded in a similar manner, using the radial artery for signal detection. If there is a pressure drop of 15 mmHg or more, this signifies an obstruction distal to the brachial artery. A disparity of forearm pressures between the brachial and ulnar arteries suggests the presence of occlusion below the bifurcation of the brachial artery. For digital pressure measurement, a 2.5 cm cuff is placed at the base of the finger, and the return of Doppler signals following cuff deflation is monitored at the finger tip. The normal digital pressure index averages 0.97 ± 0.09 (range, 0.78–1.27).[1]

Patency of the palmar arch and digital artery examination. The palmar circulation is assessed by listening over the hypothenar and thenar eminences for the palmar arches. Patency of the palmar arch is assessed by the modified Allen test described by Kamienski and Barnes.[26] The Doppler probe is placed over the radial artery while compressing the ulnar artery. Should the waveform be obliterated, the arch is dependent on the ulnar artery for supply. If the pulse remains present, the arch is complete. The procedure is repeated by listening over the ulnar artery while compressing the radial artery. The Allen test can be repeated while listening at the base of each digit or along the proper digital vessels of each finger. In some cases, even though the arch appears patent, pulsatile flow will be lost to the digits.[27] Arterial obstruction distal to the palmar arch is best detected by digital pressure measurements. The presence of an arterial occlusion distal to the palmar arch is defined by a pressure gradient between the fingers of >15 mmHg, or a wrist-to-digit difference of 30 mmHg. These very distal occlusions are caused by emboli, Buerger's disease, or arteritis.

Tests for thoracic outlet compression. Since thoracic outlet compression is not primarily vascular in origin, the diagnosis cannot be made with Doppler ultrasound alone. A positive test will only suggest compression of the vascular structures within the thoracic outlet. The provocative maneuvers for thoracic outlet syndrome include the exaggerated military position, hyperabduction, the Adson maneuver, and adduction-external rotation. Arterial waveforms and pressures are first obtained in the resting position. The patient is then asked to assume an exaggerated military position with the shoulders back, closing the costoclavicular space. Radial or brachial arterial tracings are monitored during the maneuver. Next, the arm is placed in full hyperabduction, stretching the subclavian artery over the first rib. Finally, the Adson maneuver is performed by abduction and external rotation of the arm with the patient's head turned first toward the arm and then away. Here, the subclavian artery is stretched while the tone of the scalene muscles changes. It is often difficult to obtain a continuous tracing with the Doppler probe and, as a result photoplethysmography is more convenient. The photosensor is placed on the finger and changes in flow are observed during the various thoracic outlet maneuvers.

B-mode Scan

The high-resolution, real-time B-mode scan now available for carotid artery examination can be readily applied to assessment of the peripheral arteries of the

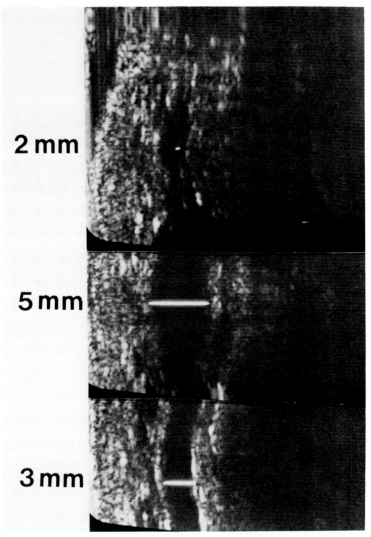

Fig. 32-1. B-mode scan of an aneurysm of the palm. The scan outlines the size of the aneurysm arising from the ulnar artery.

upper extremity. The technique is of particular use to examine catheter injury of the brachial artery. For patients with a pulsatile mass in the palm, the scan is helpful to detect aneurysm of the ulnar branch arteries (Fig. 32-1).

Cold Stimulation Test

Nielsen and Lassen[13] have advocated using local cooling and recording of digital artery pressures at various temperature ranges to detect critical closing of the artery. Others have suggested a variety of tests to record the response to cold as a means to confirm the presence of Raynaud's phenomenon. Of these tests, we have used the technique described by Porter.[11] The technique consists of recording the digital pulp temperature of each digit of both hands at room temperature with a cutaneous thermistor. The hand is then immersed in ice water for 20 seconds. Immediately thereafter, recording of digital temperature is done every five minutes until it returns to baseline, or until 30 minutes have elapsed. In 95% of normal digits, the temperature returns to baseline in 15 minutes. This test is useful to supplement digital pressure recording.

Radiologic Examination

Plain Roentgenogram

Plain roentgenogram of the hand is often helpful to establish a diagnosis, especially in the CRST syndrome. Diagnostic features of plain roentgenogram include rheumatoid deformity for rheumatoid arteritis and soft tissue calcification (calcinosis) for CRST syndrome. Calcified digital arteries seen on plain roentgenogram are characteristic for azotemic arteriopathy (Fig. 32-2). For thoracic outlet syndrome, plain X-ray of the thoracic outlet will detect rib abnormality, old fracture of the clavicle, and the presence of a cervical rib.

Arteriography

Transfemoral arteriography. Arteriography remains the most conclusive test for diagnosis of upper-extremity ischemia, and it must be done to determine operability if surgery is contemplated. The preferred method for arteriography of the upper extremity, including the hand, is transfemoral catheterization of the subclavian and brachial arteries, with selective contrast injection into these vessels. The innominate and subclavian arteries must be included in the examination. Bilateral examination is often needed to define the hand anatomy and its relationship to ischemia. The asymptomatic hand may provide important information on anatomical variations of the hand vasculature.

In addition to establishment of a diagnosis, arteriography defines variations of the normal anatomy of the brachial artery and its branches. Such variations are of surgical significance if an operative procedure is contemplated, since normal anatomical variations have been observed in the brachial artery and its branches, and in the palmar arch of the hand.

The origin of the radial and ulnar vessels has been noted to be variable by McCormack et al.[28] In 750 upper-extremity dissections, 139 specimens (18.5%) had variations in the brachial artery branching pattern. Most commonly, there was a high origin of the radial branch (14%), either from the axillary (2%) or midbrachial

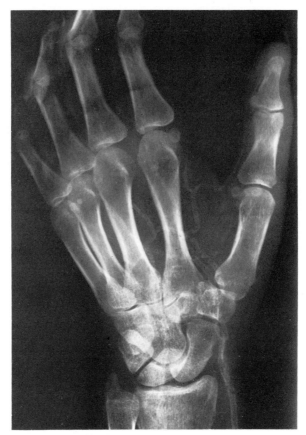

Fig. 32-2. Characteristic calcification of the radial and digital arteries in a diabetic patient with chronic renal failure (azotemic arteriopathy).

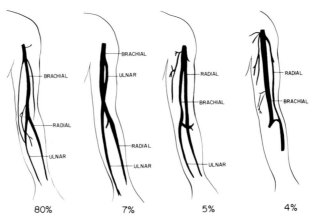

80%   7%   5%   4%

Fig. 32-3. Normal anatomical variation of the bifurcation of the brachial artery. From Yao JST, McDaniel MD, King TA: Arterial surgery of the upper extremity, in Bergan JJ (ed): Arterial Surgery. Clin Surg Internat Series, Vol. 8. Edinburgh, Churchill Livingstone, 1984, pp 201–224

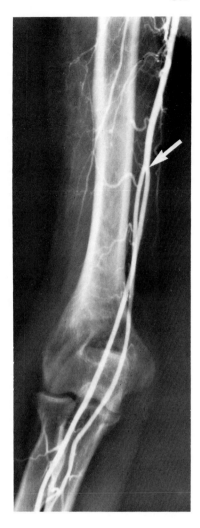

Fig. 32-4. High bifurcation (arrow) of the ulnar and radial artery.

(12%) artery (Figs. 32-3, 32-4). High origin of the ulnar artery was seen less frequently, being present in 2.6% of cases. Rare anomalies, such as an accessory brachial artery or partially duplicated radial artery, were also identified. Recognition of these anatomical variants is important if the origin of a bypass graft or a thrombectomy needs to be performed at the brachial artery.

The blood supply to the fingers depends on the integrity of the superficial and deep palmar arches. Of all arterial patterns of the upper extremity, the palmar arch is subject to most variation (Fig. 32-5). In a study by Coleman and Anson,[29] the superficial arch was found to be complete in 80% of cases. In this group, there were five subgroups identified. In Type A, the arch was formed by the ulnar artery and the superficial palmar branch of the radial artery (35.5%). In Type B, the arch was formed entirely by the ulnar artery (37%). In Type C, the arch was formed by an enlarged median artery (3%). In Type D, the arch was formed by the radial, median, and ulnar arteries (1.2%), and in Type E, the arch was formed by the ulnar artery joined by a vessel from the deep palmar arch at the base of the thenar eminence.

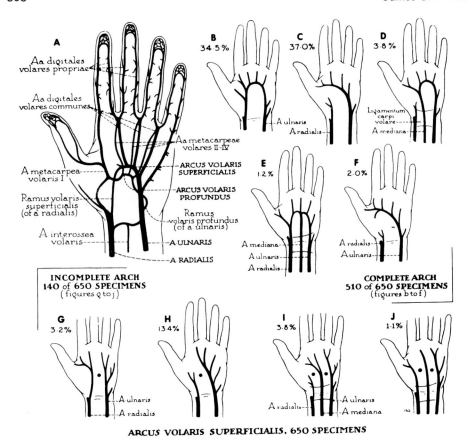

Fig. 32-5. Diagrammatic representation of the various patterns of normal palmar anatomy. From Coleman SS, Anson B: Arterial patterns in the hand based upon a study of 650 specimens. Surg Gynecol Obstet 113:409, 1961

Incomplete arches were present in the remaining 20% of individuals, and probably were one of the major underlying factors in the etiology of digital ischemia. An incomplete arch is defined as one in which the superficial arch does not anastomose with any radial branch, and the ulnar artery does not supply the thumb and radial aspects of the index finger. There are four subgroups of incomplete arches.[29] In Type A, the superficial palmar branches of both the radial and ulnar arteries supply the palm and fingers but do not anastomose (3.2%). In Type B, the ulnar artery forms the entire superficial palmar arch, but does not supply the thumb or index finger (13.4%). In Type C, the median artery reaches the hand to supply the digits, but does not anastomose with the radial or ulnar arteries, and the median artery supplies a branch to the thumb (3.8%). In Type D, the radial, median, and ulnar arteries all give origin to the superficial vessels, but do not anastomose (1.1%) (Fig. 32-6).

The deep volar arch is formed primarily by the terminal part of the radial artery and its anastomosis with the deep palmar arch of the ulnar artery. Normal variations include complete and incomplete arches. Of 500 arteriograms analyzed by

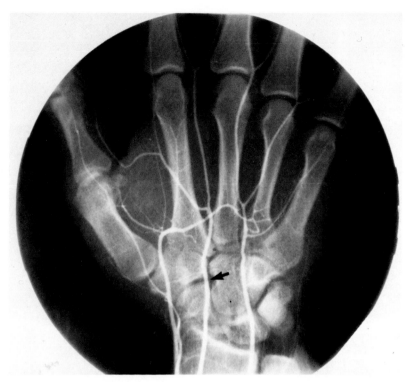

Fig. 32-6. Contribution of the median artery (arrow) to the palmar circulation, a normal variant.

Janevski,[30] the deep volar arch appeared in its entirety in 95.2% of the cases. This incidence is comparable to the anatomical analysis by Coleman and Anson,[29] who found a complete deep volar arch in 97.0% of the cases.

In our analysis of 44 patients with severe hand ischemia, we found that occlusion of the ulnar artery was most common in 25 of 51 hand arteriograms. Forty hands had digital artery occlusion; the radial artery was involved in only six instances. An incomplete palmar arch was very common. Of interest was the finding of symmetrical anatomical variation in the contralateral, asymptomatic hand. A mirror image was noted in 16 of 19 bilateral studies. We concluded, as have others, that digital ischemia often occurs in patients with abnormal palmar arch anatomy.

The location of the disease process defined by arteriography, together with certain characteristic arteriographic findings, helps to establish a definitive diagnosis. Atherosclerosis is common in the subclavian and innominate arteries, and ulcerating plaque in this region may cause embolization to the digits. With the exception of patients with chronic renal failure aand long-standing diabetes mellitus, however, it is rarely seen in the brachial or radial artery (Fig. 32-7).

In collagen disease, the digital arteries or palmar arch are commonly involved, with the third and fourth digits being affected in 80%–90% of patients.[31] Also, involvement of the ulnar artery occurs in 50% of patients, while the radial artery is often spared.

In rheumatoid arteritis, a hyperemic change (hypervascularity) is often seen

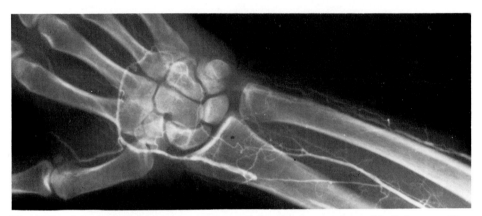

Fig. 32-7. Atherosclerotic occlusion of the radial artery in a patient with diabetes mellitus and chronic renal failure.

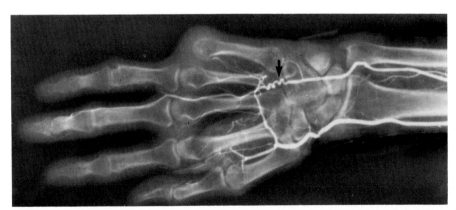

Fig. 32-8. Corkscrew artery (arrow) in a patient with rheumatoid arteritis and gangrene of the fifth finger. The fifth finger was amputated. Digital artery occlusion is seen in all remaining fingers.

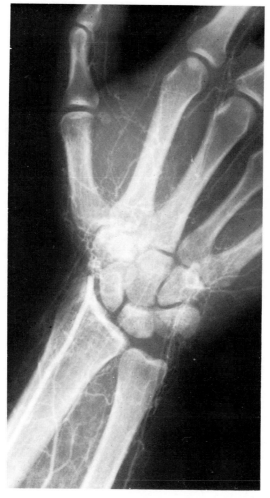

Fig. 32-9. Occlusion of the palmar arch and all digital arteries in young, male heavy smoker. The ulnar artery is also occluded.

around the joint space. Other characteristic arteriographic findings in rheumatoid arteritis include corkscrew formation (Fig. 32-8) and early venous filling.[32] It must also be noted that the subclavian and axillary arteries may demonstrate changes in rheumatoid arteritis.

Characteristic arteriographic findings in Buerger's disease (thromboangiitis obliterans) are occlusion of the small arteries of the digits with abundant collaterals (Fig. 32-9). In severe cases, both the radial and ulnar arteries are involved.

Giant-cell arteritis, though rare, has been reported to involve the subclavian and axillary arteries. The unique arteriographic findings are a long, segmental stenosis alternating with areas of normal or increased caliber; smooth, tapered occlusions; and absence of irregular plaques and ulcerations (Fig. 32-10). Takayasu's disease, another arteritis often associated with systemic symptoms, involves the

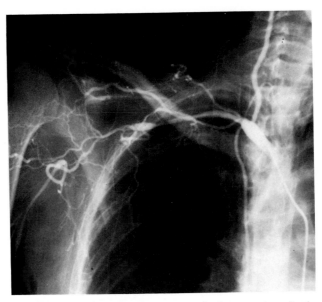

Fig. 32-10. Large, segmental, tapered stenosis of the subclavian-axillary artery in a patient with histologic confirmation of giant-cell arteritis.

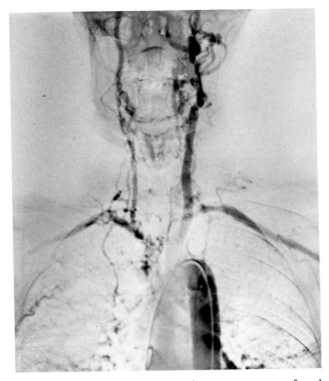

Fig. 32-11. A typical arteriogram in a young woman found to have Takayasu's arteritis. The innominate and left subclavian arteries are occluded.

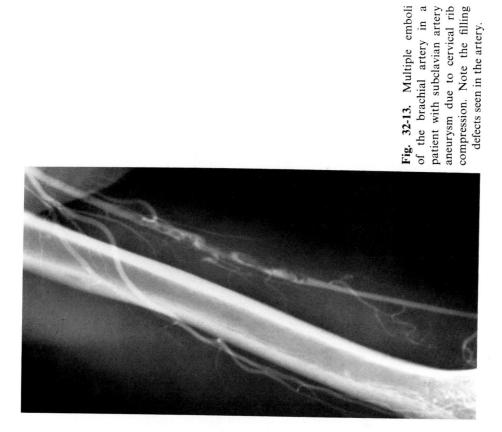

Fig. 32-13. Multiple emboli of the brachial artery in a patient with subclavian artery aneurysm due to cervical rib compression. Note the filling defects seen in the artery.

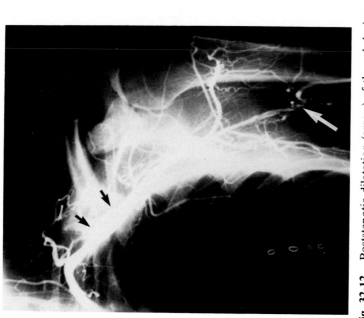

Fig. 32-12. Poststenotic dilatation (arrow) of the subclavian artery in a patient with hand ischemia due to thoracic outlet compression. The brachial artery is occluded due to embolization (white arrow).

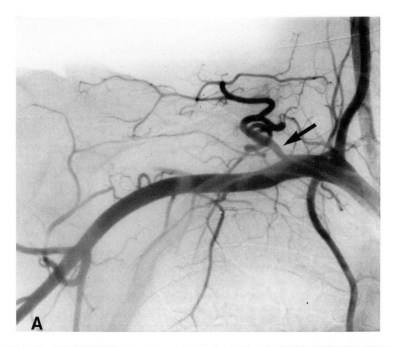

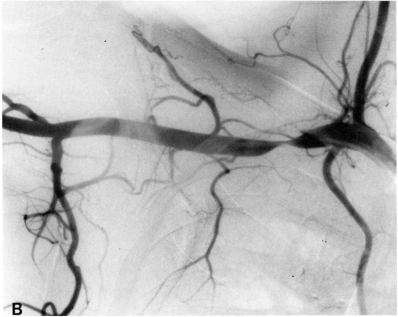

Fig. 32-14. Thoracic outlet compression of the subclavian artery in a professional baseball pitcher. (A) Neutral position. (B) Pitching position. Note the suprascapular artery, seen in neutral position (A), is also compressed in the pitching position.

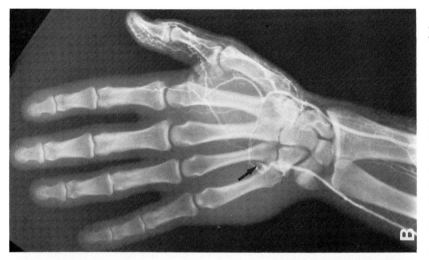

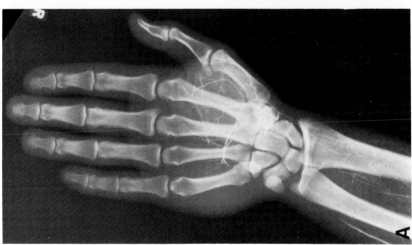

Fig. 32-15. Ulnar artery occlusion in a professional baseball player. (A) Intense spasm of the ulnar artery. (B) Relief of spasm by infusion of papaverine, a vasodilating agent. Note the occlusion of the ulnar artery (arrow).

major arteries arising from the thoracic aortic arch (Fig. 32-11). Quite often, both the subclavian and carotid arteries are involved in the disease process.

Arteriography plays an important role in the evaluation of vascular complications of the thoracic outlet syndrome. Arteriographic findings indicating the presence of damage to the subclavian artery are mural thrombosis, post-stenotic dilatation (Fig. 32-12), aneurysm formation, and embolization to the brachial, radial, or ulnar arteries (Fig. 32-13).

In severe ischemia, it is not unusual to find occlusion of both the radial and ulnar arteries, with the interosseous artery as the only remaining supply of blood flow to the hand. If bypass is contemplated, it is important to remember that there are anterior and posterior interosseous arteries in the forearm. A lateral projection must be made to determine the exact location of the remaining interosseous artery.

Positional arteriography.   Positional arteriography is done in patients suspected of having thoracic outlet compression. The arm is placed in any particular position which induces symptoms, and this position is used for the "stress" series. If the patient is unaware of a particular position that causes symptoms, the upper extremity is hyperabducted at the neck and the head rotated to face the contralateral side while the exposure is made. Attention must be paid to the exact site of compression, as well as the status of branches from the subclavian artery (Fig. 32-14).

Magnification hand arteriography.   Recently, Rösch et al[33] have advocated the use of cryodynamic hand arteriography to quantitate the degree of vasospasm of the hand vasculature. The arteriogram is performed with ice exposure and reserpine administration. The response to a vasodilating agent can also be noted (Fig. 32-15).

COMMENTS

The multiple and often disparate causes of upper-extremity ischemia require a thorough history taking and awareness of etiologic factors to derive a diagnostic and therapeutic plan. In the majority of cases, a complete history taking will provide a logical approach to the problem.

Once the diagnosis is made, the goal of preoperative assessment is to determine operability and the degree of ischemia. Systolic pressure recordings of the forearm and the fingers, readily available in most laboratories, are useful to establish the degree of ischemia. Further, the test provides objective documentation of improvement after surgical intervention. Of all preoperative tests, arteriography remains the definite examination. Characteristic arteriographic findings provide vital diagnostic information, and the site of the disease process determines operability and the surgical approach.

With the exception of occlusion of the digital arteries or palmar arch, lesions involving larger arteries are amenable to surgery. The type of surgical procedure depends on the extent of the disease process. Thromboendarterectomy with vein patch is useful when a short segment of artery is involved. For more extensive disease processes, the use of autogenous vein for bypass appears to be the best choice. Again, the origin and the distal anastomosis of the bypass graft depend on the arteriographic findings. If the subclavian artery is involved in the disease process, the common carotid artery may serve as the inflow. The distal anastomosis will depend on refilling of the radial, or ulnar, or interosseous artery. When the interosseous artery is the only remaining patent artery, a lateral projection must be made. The lateral projection will determine the exact location of the interosseous artery.

For vascular complications of the thoracic outlet syndrome, arterial damage such as irregular arterial wall, poststenotic dilatation, or aneurysm seen on arteriography dictates the need for an interposed vein graft with exclusion or resection of the diseased segment. If there is evidence of distal artery involvement due to embolization, the need for a concomitant bypass graft depends on the status of the distal arteries and the degree of ischemia. Thrombectomy may be attempted at the time of proximal bypass graft, if embolization is of relatively recent onset. In the event that no demonstrable arterial damage except compression to the subclavian artery is seen, the site of compression depicted by arteriography will also help to determine the surgical approach. The exact site of compression can be located by noting the distance from the internal mammary artery, the thyrocervical trunk, and the vertebral artery. In addition to compression to the subclavian artery, attention must be paid to the suprascapular artery, which may be compressed in the stress position. Compression of the suprascapular artery may contribute to symptoms related to the shoulder muscles. For surgical intervention, the supraclavicular approach allows a close inspection of the subclavian artery and its branches. Using this approach, scalenectomy is performed to ensure that the suprascapular artery is freed from compression.

In summary, surgical correction offers the best way to relieve ischemic symptoms of the upper extremity. To achieve maximal therapeutic effect, a careful preoperative assessment, especially the judicious use of arteriography, is needed.

Acknowledgment

This work was supported in part by the Conrad Jobst Foundation, the Seabury Foundation, and the Northwestern Vascular Foundation.

REFERENCES

1. Sumner DS: Noninvasive assessment of upper extremity ischemia, in Bergan JJ, Yao JST (eds): Evaluation and Treatment of Upper and Lower Extremity Circulatory Disorders. Orlando, Fla, Grune & Stratton, 1984, pp 75–95
2. Pearce WH, Ricco J-B, Yao JST: Upper extremity vascular diagnosis, in Zwiebel WJ (ed): Introduction to Vascular Ultrasonography. Orlando, Fla, Grune & Stratton, 1982, pp 215–227
3. Nielsen PE, Bell G, Lassen NA: The measurement of digital systolic blood pressure by strain gauge technique. Scand J Clin Lab Invest 29:343, 1972
4. Yao JST, Gourmos C, Irvine WT: A method for assessing ischemia of the hand and fingers. Surgery 135:373, 1972
5. McNamara MF, Takaki HS, Yao JST, et al: A systematic approach to severe hand ischemia. Surgery 83:1, 1978
6. Balas P, Tripolitis AJ, Kaklamanis P, et al: Raynaud's phenomenon. Primary and secondary causes. Arch Surg 114:1174, 1979
7. Gundersen J: Segmental measurement of systolic blood pressure in the extremities including the thumb and the great toe. Acta Chir Scand Suppl 426, 1972

8. Downs AR, Gaskell P, Morrow I: Assessment of arterial obstruction in vessels supplying the fingers by measurement of local blood pressures and the skin temperature response test, correlation with angiographic evidence. Surgery 77:530, 1975

9. Neiman H, Yao JST, Silver J: Gray scale ultrasound diagnosis of peripheral arterial aneurysms. Radiology 130:413, 1979

10. Hirai M: Cold sensitivity of the hand in arterial occlusive disease. Surgery 85:140, 1979

11. Porter JM: Raynaud's syndrome and associated vasospastic conditions of the extremities, in Rutherford RB (ed): Vascular Surgery. Philadelphia, Saunders, 1977, pp 597–604

12. Hoare M, Miles C, Girvan R, et al: The effect of local cooling on digital systolic pressure in patients with Raynaud's syndrome. Br J Surg 69(Suppl):527, 1982

13. Nielsen SL, Lassen NA: Measurement of digital blood pressure after local cooling. J Appl Physiol 43:907, 1977

14. Ashe WF, Cook WT, Old JW: Raynaud's phenomenon of occupational origin. Arch Environ Health 5:63, 1975

15. Conn J, Bergan JJ, Bell JL: Hypothenar hammer syndrome: Posttraumatic digital ischemia. Surgery 68:1122, 1970

16. Brady MP, O'Sullivan DJ: Bullman's hand: An unusual occupational lesion. J Cardiovasc Surg 16:157, 1975

17. Blackburn D, Peterson LK, Flinn WR, et al: Noninvasive assessment of occupational "white finger." Proc 3rd Int Symposium on Hand-Arm Vibration, Ottawa, May 18–20, 1981

18. Henry LG, Blackwood JS, Conley JC, et al: Ergotism. Arch Surg 110:929, 1975

19. Eliasson K, Danielson M, Hylander B, et al: Raynaud's phenomenon caused by beta-receptor blocking drugs. Improvement after treatment with a combined alpha-and beta-blocker. Acta Med Scand 215:333, 1984

20. Vogelzang NJ, Bosl GJ, Johnson K et al: Raynaud's phenomenon: A common toxicity after combination chemotherapy for testicular cancer. Ann Intern Med 95:288, 1981

21. Alexander CS, Sako Y, Mikulic E: Pedal gangrene associated with the use of dopamine. New Engl J Med 293:591, 1975

22. Allen EV: Thromboangiitis obliterans: Methods of diagnosis of chronic occlusive arterial lesions distal to the wrist with illustrative cases. Am J Med Sci 178:237, 1929

23. Bowers WH, Spencer JB, McDevitt NB: Brachial artery rupture in Ehler-Danlos syndrome: An unusual cause of high median nerve palsy. J Bone Joint Surg 58A:1025, 1976

24. Wahlqvist ML, Fox RM, Beach AM, et al: Peripheral vascular disease as a mode of presentation of pseudoxanthoma elasticum. Aust NZ J Med 7:523, 1977

25. Yao JST: In discussion of Erlandson, EE, et al: Discriminant arteriographic criteria in the management of forearm and hand ischemia. Surgery 90:1034, 1981

26. Kamienski RW, Barnes RW: Critique of the Allen test for continuity of the palmar arch assessed by Doppler ultrasound. Surg Gynecol Obstet 142:861, 1976

27. Little JM, Zylstra DL, West J, et al: Circulatory patterns in the normal hand. Br J Surg 60:652, 1973

28. McCormack LJ, Cauldwell EW, Anson BJ: Brachial and antebrachial arterial patterns: A study of 750 extremities. Surg Gynecol Obstet 96:43, 1953

29. Coleman SS, Anson BJ: Arterial patterns in the hand based upon a study of 650 specimens. Surg Gynecol Obstet 113:409, 1961

30. Janevski B: Angiography of the Upper Extremity. The Hague, Martinus Nijhoff, 1982

31. Bookstein JJ: Arteriography, in Pozanski AK (ed): The Hand in Radiologic Diagnosis. Philadelphia, Saunders, 1974, pp 65–77

32. Wegelius U: Angiography of the hand. Clinical and postmortem investigations. Acta Radiol, Suppl 315, 1972

33. Rösch J, Porter JM, Gralino B: Cryodynamic hand angiography in the diagnosis and management of Raynaud's syndrome. Circulation 55:807, 1977

Gordon Heard

33

The Clinical Demonstration of Sympathetic Activity in the Limbs

The place of sympathectomy in the treatment of hyperhidrosis is undisputed. Its role in Raynaud's disease diminishes with increasing recognition of the importance of underlying primary and systemic diseases. In the ischaemia of occlusive vascular disease the value of sympathectomy either alone or in conjunction with arterial reconstruction is now seriously questioned by many vascular surgeons. While sympathetic release has been found to dilate the arterio-vascular anastomoses, it has not been proved to increase skin capillary flow. On the other hand the advent of chemical sympathectomy by the injection of Phenol has led to a resurgence of its popularity with those who continue to regard sympathetic denervation as helpful.

Supposed evidence of the benefits of sympathectomy is unsatisfactory, being largely anecdotal and poorly controlled, both as regards the clinical response and the effectiveness of the attempted autonomic blockade, the latter particularly in the case of chemical sympathectomy, which has been shown to have a significant failure rate. In the evaluation of sympathetic blockade, objective study of both the disease state and the therapeutic manoeuvre is mandatory. It is with the latter in mind that these methods of clinical demonstration of sympathetic activity in the limbs are presented.

METHODS

As is well known, the activity of the sympathetic nervous system in the limbs is twofold, namely vasomotor and sudomotor. Each of these provides a means of study.

The Vascular Response

Vasomotor activity is vasoconstrictor. It is shown to be present when an increasing cutaneous circulation is brought about by release of vasoconstrictor tone. The latter may be induced reflexly by body heating, by sympathetic drugs or locally by surgical or chemical "sympathectomy."

DIAGNOSTIC TECHNIQUES AND ASSESSMENT
PROCEDURES IN VASCULAR SURGERY © 1985 Grune & Stratton
ISBN 0-8089-1721-8 All rights reserved

379

Although more sophisticated techniques such as venous occlusion plethysmography, isotope clearance or Doppler ultrasound might be used, the resulting increase in cutaneous blood flow is more simply observed by measurement of changes in skin temperature either by thermography or the use of thermistors.

A clear-cut local increase in skin temperature under properly controlled conditions is usually meaningful. There are, however, a number of fallacies.

1. In severe peripheral vascular disease the circulation may be insufficient to provide any increase in flow.
2. When generalized vasodilatation is produced (e.g. by drugs or by body warming) blood might be diverted elsewhere rather than to the area beyond an arterial occlusion where, on the contrary, the circulation could be reduced despite relaxation of vasomotor tone (the borrowing and lending phenomenon.)
3. Sedation alone might bring about sympathetic release and warming of the extremities. This could wrongly be thought to indicate successful sympathetic blockade. Clearly it is important to contrast the observations with others simultaneously recorded in a control limb and in a controlled environment.

The Sudomotor Response

Sweating in an extremity is evidence of local sympathetic innervation.

Demonstration of Local Sweating

The traditional technique is to use a powder that will change colour when it becomes moist, as does a mixture of starch and iodine. When sweating is provoked, usually by body heating, any area of sympathetic denervation will be mapped out. (Fig. 33-1)

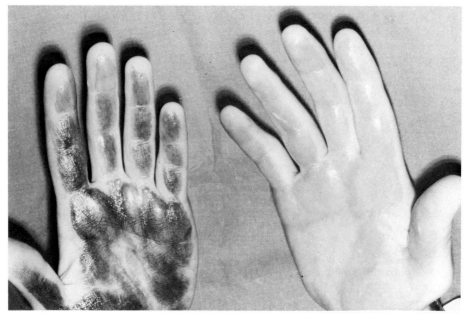

Fig. 33-1.   Absence of sweating demonstrated by use of starch and iodine powder.

A more convenient though less graphic method of demonstrating the moistness or dryness of the skin is to use a simple meter to measure the resistance of the skin to the passage of an electric current.

A multimeter can be used or a meter readily constructed (Fig. 33-2). The instrument shown in Figure 33-2 consists of a battery with milliameter in circuit. The

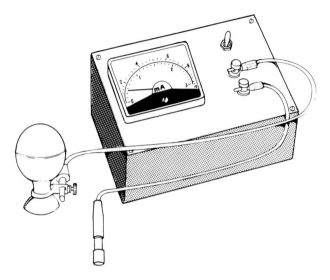

Fig. 33-2. A simple meter suitable for demonstrating gross skin resistance.

suction electrode is the fixed one and the other is used as a testing probe. The latter is a dry disc of conductive metal, which is used to test skin surface conductivity on the extremity under study. The fixed electrode is placed with jelly to ensure the good electrical contact. Skin when dry will offer considerable resistance but when moist will allow free passage of a current. This is gross skin conductivity and not to be confused with resistance changes related to P.G.R. (vide infra).

Under reasonably warm conditions there is often enough spontaneous sweating to demonstrate the contrast between a normal and sympathectomized area. Otherwise, if the patient is cold and calm it may be necessary to apply body heating to induce normal sweating in the innervated area.

The Psychogalvanic Response

In the extremities, electrical currents can be demonstrated. The possible sources of these currents are the sweat glands and the cutaneous vasculature. The evidence favours a main origin in the depolarization accompanying the presecretory activity of the cells of the sweat glands.

The term psycho-galvanic response (P.G.R.) has been applied to changes in these currents and also to changes in resistance with similar time relations. These changes occur in response to a variety of stimuli such as conversation, pin prick, a bright light in the eyes, taking a deep breath, and coughing.

The effect of the stimulus depends upon the mental reaction that it induces. For this reason P.G.R. has been much explored in psychiatric fields and has been used in lie detection and in monitoring the emotions.

The reflex can be abolished by interruption of the sympathetic pathways and is therefore a useful means of demonstrating sympathetic activity or denervation.

The response is, however, depressed by sedation and abolished by sleep and anaesthesia.

The P.G.R. is very easily elicited using an electrocardiograph machine[1]. The recording is made using Standard Lead 1, which makes use in electrocardiography of the right leg (R.L.), left arm (L.A.) and right arm (R.A.) leads. The grounding lead (R.L.) is attached to the forearm or calf while the left (L.A.) and right arm (R.A.) leads are placed on the ventral and dorsal surfaces of the hand or foot, using E.C.G. electrodes and electrode jelly. (Fig. 33-3).

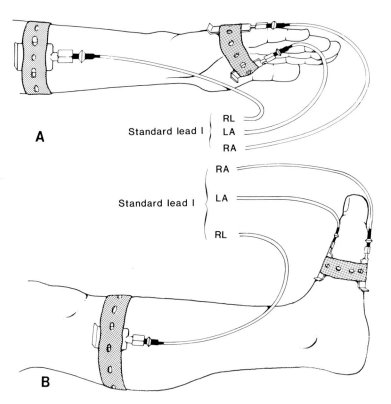

Fig. 33-3. Disposition of electrodes by which P.G.R. can be elicited using an electrocardiograph machine in the hand (A) and in the foot (B).

The E.C.G. recording shows the variation in electrical potential that follows stimulation, either at a normal paper speed of 25 mm/sec. (Fig. 33-4) or preferably, if within the machine's capability, at a reduced speed of 2.5 mm/sec. (Fig. 33-5). At the slower speed the changes are better appreciated.

We have found in studies comparing P.G.R. with the more commonly used methods of observing sympathetic activity, that its sensitivity is similar to that afforded by measurement of gross skin conductivity, but it does not require heating

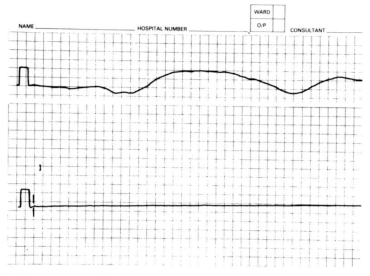

NAME _____ HOSPITAL NUMBER _____ WARD / O/P   CONSULTANT _____

Fig. 33-4. The upper trace illustrates P.G.R. at normal E.C.G. (Paper speed 25 mm/sec.).

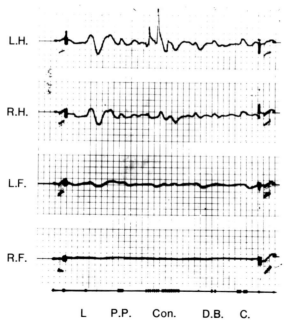

L.H.

R.H.

L.F.

R.F.

L   P.P.   Con.   D.B.   C.

Fig. 33-5. Changes in potential occurring in the extremities in response to light (L), pin prick (P.P.), conversation (Con.), deep breathing (D.B.), and coughing (C). The right leg (R.F.) had been sympathectomized (Paper speed 2.5 mm/sec.).

383

of the patient. On the other hand, it is not suitable for "mapping out" areas of sympathetic denervation. Neither gross skin conductivity nor P.G.R. are as sensitive in indicating sympathetic denervation as the vascular response when the vasculature is normal. P.G.R. is particularly useful in affording rapid evidence of the effectiveness of a sympathetic block in an ischaemic limb.

APPLICATION

These tests can be considered in relation to four questions that might arise in clinical practice.

Has the Patient Undergone Sympathectomy in the Past?

When both limbs are present and a normal limb is available for comparison, skin temperature tests may be meaningful. The other limb, however, might be cooler on account of poor contralateral blood flow because of more extensive vascular disease. Severe vascular occlusion in the sympathectomized limb may lead to a cold ischaemic extremity with no evidence of a vascular response despite sympathetic denervation.

The vascular response when evident is maximal in the early days following denervation and diminishes after an interval when temperature elevation above that of the "normal" limb may not be striking.

If sympathectomy has been bilateral, skin temperature comparisons will be unhelpful.

If sweating is present the limb is not the site of sympathetic denervation. However, if there is not sweating this is only significant if sweating is present in the contralateral limb or if sweating still fails to occur after thorough body heating has resulted in marked sweating elsewhere.

Provided the patient is not sedated, asleep or anaesthetized the P.G.R. will be present if the sympathetic pathways are intact.

Has Sympathetic Blockade Been Successful?

Immediate assessment. In measurement of skin temperature changes it is desirable that the patient should be in equilibrium with stable environmental conditions. It is also necessary, whenever possible, to compare temperature changes with those in the contralateral limb. A vascular response may, as has been indicated, be absent in severe peripheral vascular disease, even though the blockade has been successful.

When sympathetic blockade has been recent, time will be required for moisture produced *before* denervation to evaporate and for the area to become dry. For this reason simple gross electrical resistance measurements may be misleading.

If the patient is sedated or anaesthetized for the procedure, the P.G.R. will be abolished irrespective of the success or failure of the block.

Later assessment. If the contralateral limb is actively sweating, demonstration of dryness by gross resistance measurement on the relevant side will be conclusive.

The P.G.R. remains independant of a vascular response and independant of active sweating and is therefore the most certain of the methods available.

Has Sympathetic Blockade Persisted?

In assessing the value of methods of sympathetic blockade, permanence of effect is an important aspect. The ability to reliably determine sympathetic activity is clearly desirable.

Is There Autononic Neuropathy?

In certain diseases, notably diabetes, neuropathy may result in sympathetic denervation of a limb. The demonstration of sympathetic activity in such patients is most readily accomplished by the P.G.R.

CONCLUSION

Over the years sympathectomy has been widely used in the management of vascular disorders and the advent of chemical sympathectomy by the injection of phenol has led to a resurgence of popularity.

There is considerable disagreement as to the place of these procedures in different conditions. Further, chemical sympathectomy is by no means a certain undertaking and might often be technically unsuccessful.

Proper evaluation demands controlled clinical studies and it is important that these should include demonstration of the success or persistence of sympathetic denervation.

REFERENCE

1. Lewis LW: Evaluation of sympathetic activity following chemical or surgical sympathectomy. Curr Res Anesth. 34:334, 1955

PART VII

Arterio-Venous Malformations

Giorgio Biasi, Paolo Pignoli,
Sergio Miani, and Ugo Ruberti

34

Detection and Classification of Arterio-Venous Malformations

The management of vascular malformations is based on a comprehensive understanding of the hemodynamics and natural history of these conditions, which represent a broad range of anatomical and functional disorders.

Vascular malformations have been classified by Malan and Puglionisi[1-3] as predominantly venous, arterial, arteriovenous, and mixed (Table 34-1). The venous variety, which is the more frequent, is characterized by the presence of venous stasis and its sequelae. The pure arterial angiodysplasias are rare and are represented by dysplastic arterial trunks. Arteriovenous angiodysplasias more frequently present an arteriovenous shunt that is an abnormal communication between an artery and a vein, and allows blood to be totally or partially diverted away from the peripheral capillary bed. Depending on the magnitude of the shunted blood flow, an arteriovenous fistula (AVF) may be hypoactive or hyperactive. The communicating channel, through which the shunting results, may be microscopic (microfistolous connection) or macroscopic (macrofistolous connection). The communication may be unique or multiple. The activity of an AVF may change with time as a result of spontaneous evolution or treatment. Because of complex hemodynamic angiogenetic factors, hypoactive AVF may become hyperactive after the existing equilibrium has been changed by surgical therapy. Congenital AVF may be circumscribed or diffuse, involving large portions of a limb, head, and viscera.[4-6]

Congenital AVF are present at birth, however they may become apparent later in the second or third decade often related by the patient to some minor physical trauma or developing during puberty or pregnancy as part of the more general trophic changes. Congenital AVF are frequently associated with bony and soft tissue hypertrophy, which seems to be a secondary feature resulting from the altered hemodynamics induced by the AVF (increased oxygen tension, increased venous pressure, increased arterial inflow). The creation of an AVF in a growing child results in bony and soft tissue hypertrophy. These vascular malformations do not show a sex prevalence.

DIAGNOSTIC TECHNIQUES AND ASSESSMENT
PROCEDURES IN VASCULAR SURGERY

© 1985 Grune & Stratton
ISBN 0-8089-1721-8 All rights reserved

TABLE 34-1
Classification of congenital
angiodysplasias

Venous dysplasias
  phlebectasic dysplasias
    regional phlebectasias
    phlebectasias with hypoplasia of the deep veins
    genuine diffuse phlebectasias
  phlebangiomas
    superficial
    deep
  phlemangiomatosis
    superficial
    deep
    possible associations of the three preceding forms

Arterial dysplasias
  troncular arterial dysplasias

Arterial and associated venous dysplasias
  genuine phlebarteriectasia
  angiodysplasia with arterio-venous shunts:
    troncular arteriovenous fistulas
    arteriovenous angiomas

Mixed angiodysplasias
  troncular haemolymphatic dysplasias
  haemolymphangiomas
  complex forms

   * Malan E, Puglionisi A: Congenital angiodysplasias of the extremities. J Cardiovasc Surg 5:87, 1964. With permission.

Congenital AVF must be differentiated from acquired AVF, which may be traumatic or iatrogenic. The traumatic AVF are the effect most often of a penetrating injury (frequent in the military and traffic context) or blunt trauma. The border between a congenital AVF and an acquired one resulting from a minor blunt trauma may not be clear.

The pathophysiology of each AVF determines the clinical symptoms as well as the natural course of the condition. The evaluation of an AVF is based on the clinical examination, noninvasive tests, and contrast angiography. These investigative methods are complementary and add informatiion to each other.

This chapter is a review of the clinical findings that should alert the physician about the presence of an AVF and of the current noninvasive methods to confirm the diagnosis, functionally evaluate its state, and monitor its evolution.

Because both the local and systemic manifestations of an AVF result from the induced hemodynamic alterations, the pathophysiology of this condition will be synthetically described in order to define the parameters that functionally characterize the lesion.

HEMODYNAMICS OF AVF

The proximity of an AVF with respect to the heart and the resistence of the connecting channel(s) are the critical anatomic factors influencing the magnitude of the shunt and the effect of this on central and peripheral hemodynamics. The resistence of the connecting channel(s) is dependent on the overall cross section area and the number and tortuosity of the involved vascular formations. An AVF is a system composed by units that play a different role and present peculiar anatomic and functional characteristics. The main components of this system (Fig. 34-1) are:

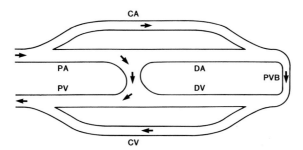

Fig. 34-1. Schematic representation of a congenital AVF (PA = proximal artery, DA = distal artery, CA = collateral arteries, PVB = peripheral vascular bed, DV = distal vein, PV = proximal vein, CV = collateral veins).

(1) the proximal artery, (2) the distal artery, (3) the collateral arteries, (4) the communicating channel, (5) the distal vein, (6) the proximal vein, (7) the collateral veins, and (8) the peripheral vascular bed.

The presence of an AVF is associated with the following hemodynamic phenomena[7-9]:

1. An increase in the proximal artery blood flow volume, blood flow velocity, and arterial pulse. These changes are the result of the increase in blood flow that occurs (for the Ohm's law) because of the decrease in resistance, with a constant the pressure gradient, which is maintained due to the compensatory activity of the heart.
2. A decrease in the distal artery blood flow volume, blood flow velocity, and arterial pulse. These phenomena are the consequence of the diversion of blood through the AVF from the peripheral vascular bed. If the shunt is large, a condition of peripheral ischemia may be present and the peripheral arterioles vasodilate to increase blood flow volume and oxygen delivery to these tissues. The peripheral ischemia stimulates the development of collateral arteries that add flow to the distal artery. If the resistance through the AVF is lower than through the peripheral vascular bed, blood may flow cephalad away from the periphery in the distal artery, which therefore may show a centripetal rather than a centrifugal blood flow. This flow again is wasted with respect to the peripheral tissue metabolic demands.
3. The development of collateral arteries with an increase in their blood flow volume and velocity. The development of these arteries is more pronounced

than that expected with an obstructive lesion inducing the same degree of ischemia. Many theories have been proposed to[10,11] explain the development of
collateral circulation.

4. An increase in the proximal vein blood flow volume, blood flow velocity with
   arterialization of the flow pattern. This occurs to accomodate the flow coming
   from the shunt and it is accomplished by an enlargment of the vein size
   resulting from the large compliance of the vein wall. This dilatation allows the
   pressure in this vein to be relatively unchanged unless a proximal outflow obstruction develops.

5. The development of collateral veins. This occurs because at the level of the
   fistula the vein pressure is high (reflecting the arterial pressure transmitted by
   the shunt) and a relative obstacle to the venous return from the peripheral bed
   develops. The high venous pressure is transmitted toward the peripheral part
   of the distal vein because the valves, with the passing of time, becomes incompetent.

6. An increase in peripheral venous pressure, resulting from the factors discussed
   at point 5. The magnitude of this venous hypertension is dependent on the
   balance between collateral veins development, shunted blood flow volume, and
   obstruction to proximal vein outflow.

7. An increase in the oxygen tension of the venous blood draining from the AVF.
   This occurs because saturated arterial blood by-passes the peripheral capillary
   bed and is directly mixed with the venous blood coming from the periphery.
   The magnitude of the shunt determines the level of oxygen tension in the
   venous blood collected in the proximal vein.

8. The development of disturbed flow at the level of the communication and in
   the proximal artery. The high velocity of the blood flow elevates the system
   "Reynold's number"[12] and turbulence may occur. This fluidodynamic phenomenon is clinically manifested by a thrill and by a bruit. The turbulence may
   play a role in the pathogenesis of the anatomic alterations (tortuosity, wall
   thickening, atheroma formation) frequently found in the AVF.

9. A decrease in total peripheral resistance related to the presence of the communication that presents a very low resistance as compared to that offered by the
   peripheral vascular bed.

10. An increase in cardiac output. Owing to the decrease in total peripheral resist-
    ance a normal mean blood pressure is maintained by an increase in the heart
    rate and stroke volume. The hyperkinetic state resulting from the presence of
    an AVF may lead to heart failure.

11. An increase in the circulating blood volume. This occurs because the enlarg-
    ment of the veins and of the arteries increases the blood "container" of the
    body; a salt retaining mechanism is activated to enlarge the plasma volume
    until a new equilibrium is developed between the container (the vascular bed)
    and the contained (the blood).

These hemodynamic phenomena are associated with anatomical changes of
cardiovascular structures. The proximal artery and vein enlarge, become tortuous,
and wall thickening occurs. The heart enlarges until failure supervenes.

The magnitude of the described hemodynamic changes depends on the activity
of the AVF. As the resistence of the peripheral circulation is changed owing to

spontaneous or induced modifications of the AVF connecting channels, a new equilibrium is reached in the same way it has been found in acute experimental preparations of AVF.[13-15]

The closure of the AVF by manual compression when feasible or by surgery determines locally a decrease in proximal artery and vein blood flow volume, an increase in the distal artery blood flow and pressure, and a decrease in distal vein pressure with an overall amelioration of the peripheral vascular bed perfusion. Systematically the closure of the AVF induces a decrease in heart rate (Nicoladoni-Branham sign), stroke volume and cardiac output.[16]

DIAGNOSTIC PROBLEMS

The vascular surgeon, faced with the potential presence of a congenital AVF, should answer the following questions:

1. Is it really present?
2. Is it diffuse or localized?
3. Is it associated with other vascular lesions or malformations?
4. Is there peripheral ischemia?
5. Is there venous hypertension?
6. What is the activity of the shunt?
7. What is the size (macroscopic to microscopic) of the connecting channel(s)?
8. What is the short term and long term local and systemic prognosis?
9. Which are the involved arteries and veins?
10. What is the best treatment?

The answers to these questions are based on clinical and instrumental data that have to be collected by appropriate investigations.

The clinical findings associated with the presence of a congenital AVF are: an increase in length and girth of an extremity, the presence of a continuous bruit and thrill, varicose veins (which cannot be explained on the basis of the usual incompetent vein valves), pulsatile veins, cutaneous hemangioma, the Branham sign, a higher cutaneous temperature (unless there is peripheral ischemia and coolness), secondary venous ulcers and dermatitis, pallor of the ischemic peripheral vascular bed, and signs of heart failure. Patients with congenital AVF may complain of pulsation, throbbing, heaviness, and increased warmth of the affected part. Hemodynamically hypoactive AVF may be silent and can be detected only by instrumental methods.

PRINCIPLES OF NONINVASIVE VASCULAR TESTING

The procedures aimed at the noninvasive evaluation of a congenital AVF are based on the use of the continuous wave Doppler, the strain gauge plethysmograph, and the small part real time scanner. Cuffs of different sizes and a manometer are required for pressure measurements.

The Continuous wave (CW) Doppler allows the evaluation of the blood flow velocity pattern in the vessel(s) insonified by the exploring beam.[17] The presence or absence of blood flow may be appreciated. The characteristics of the audible signal reflect the blood flow velocity pattern. The behaviour of the velocity as function of time may be defined as well as the distribution of the velocities of the flowing red blood cells at a given time. A laminar flow is associated with a low number of velocities (i.e. red blood cells travel at the same speed). A disturbed flow is characterized by the presence of red blood cells flowing at different speeds and this phenomenon generate a characteristic Doppler signal.[18] Direction sensitive Doppler allows us to define the mean direction of the insonified flowing blood with respect to the ultrasound probe. More sophisticated Doppler systems allow the graphical presentation of the audible signal for visual analysis and detection of the presence of simultaneous flows with opposite directions.[19,20]

The CW Doppler may be used to monitor blood flow while performing systolic pressure measurements. The Doppler device detects blood flow resumption when the pressure in the occluding cuff equals the systolic pressure.

More complex Doppler Systems (Pulsed Doppler, Duplex Systems, Multigate Pulsed Doppler)[21] may be useful, however, they probably do not add very significant information to what we can obtain with the cheaper and easy-to-use CW Doppler.

The strain gauge plethysmograph allows the detection and measurement of the circumference changes due to the pulsatile activity of the heart (pulse plethysmography) or to the temporary occlusion of the venous outflow induced by a cuff (vein occlusion plethysmography).[22] The plethysmograph may be calibrated and the absolute changes in limb or digit cross section may be measured.[23] The magnitude of the arterial pulse is related to blood flow volume, especially in the digits. However, only vein occlusion plethysmography allows the noninvasive measurement of blood flow volume in a digit or limb. The strain gauge plethysmograph may be used to monitor blood flow during pressure measurements.[22]

The small part real time scanner generates an image that is a cross section of the insonified region.[24] The ultrasonic pulse propagates through the tissue and is backscattered from acoustic interfaces (i.e. gradients in acoustic impedence), which are represented by the capsulae of the organs and other relatively macroscopic structures. A small part high resolution scanner must be used in order to visualize small structures like arteries and veins. Low frequency abdominal scanner may be used to evaluate deep visceral vessels. The lumen as well as the vessel wall may be visualized in superficial vessels.

THE DOPPLER AND PLETHYSMOGRAPHIC EVALUATION OF AN AVF

The presence of an AVF, suspected on the basis of the clinical findings, may be documented evaluating with noninvasive methods the hemodynamic parameters that are known to be altered and comparing the results of our exploration with those expected theoretically. The potential variability of the hemodynamic changes due to the wide range of anatomic and functional forms of AVF should also be taken into account.

The presence of an increased mean blood velocity in the proximal artery, as compared with the controlateral side, is a typical finding of the Doppler evaluation of an AVF. In peripheral arteries normally the diastolic flow is very low due to the high peripheral resistance. The decrease in the peripheral resistance induced by the AVF generates a high diastolic flow, similar to that found in the internal carotid artery, which shows an high diastolic velocity in the Doppler signal (Fig. 34-2). The relatively high mean velocity is associated with a high Reynold number and the presence of a disturbed flow. This is represented in the spectrum of the Doppler signal by a broadening of the frequency content. The laminar flow present in a normal artery shows red blood cells travelling with a very similar velocity at a given time (Fig. 34-2). These findings obviously depend on the magnitude of the shunt.

An increase in the mean blood flow, however, may be found in other conditions (inflammation, hyperkinetic states), which can be ruled out on the basis of the clinical findings.

The occlusion of the communicating channel(s) of the AVF or of the proximal vein decreases the blood flow volume and velocity in the proximal artery that may be monitored with the Doppler probe. A decrease in velocity with the compression of some suspected area is an hallmark of the presence of an AVF.

The arterial pulse, which can be measured by the strain gauge plethysmograph, is generally increased proximally to an AVF. A decrease in this parameter is expected after AVF occlusion. The measurement of the segmental systolic pressure shows higher values in the limb with an AVF than in the controlateral limb. This may be due to the enlargement of the artery, which reduces the pressure gradient from the heart, and to a cuff artifact induced by the increased circumference of the hypertophied limb.[26]

The quantification of the blood flow volume in the proximal artery could be useful to estimate the magnitude of the shunt. However, the noninvasive evaluation by vein occlusion plethysmography of the proximal artery blood flow is very difficult because the occlusion of the venous outflow, in the presence of an AVF, requires the inflation to a suprasystolic pressure, owing to the increased proximal vein pressure. Under these circumstances the arterial inflow in the proximal artery is impeded and the measurement is therefore impossible.[28]

The blood flow velocity may be reduced at the level of the peripheral artery. The comparison with the controlateral side may allow the Doppler evaluation of the changed velocity. However, the problems related with the correct estimate of the Doppler beam incident angle make the evaluation of the decrease in velocity rather inaccurate.

The level of peripheral hypoperfusion may be appreciated more correctly measuring the systolic pressure in the distal artery or in a more peripheral location like a digit. The Doppler or a plethysmograph may be used. The plethysmographic method may allow the measurement of lower systolic pressure when used in the DC operating mode.[27] A peripheral hypotension as well as a reduced arterial pulse (Fig. 34-3) are important markers of ischemia and may indicate the need of a reconstructive vascular procedure with ligation of the AVF. A systolic pressure lower than 40 mmHg indicates a borderline tissue viability.[25] A low peripheral systolic pressure may be due to other conditions than an AVF. The more frequent cause of peripheral hypotension is obstructive arterial disease. In this case, however, the compression of a suspicious lesion or of a large varicose vein does not increase the peripheral pressure. In some cases it is not possible to selectively compress the connecting channel

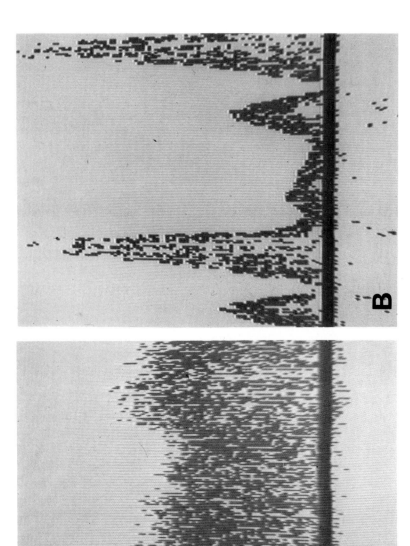

Fig. 34-2. The Doppler spectrum of the signal from a normal peripheral artery (B) and from the proximal artery of an AVF circuit (A).

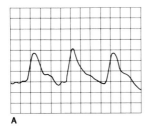
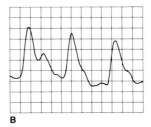

A   B

Fig. 34-3.   The arterial pulse evaluated with the strain-gauge
plethysmograph from a digit located distally to an AVF (A)
and from a digit of the controlateral normal limb (B).

of an AVF and some interference may be exerted on the blood flow of the proximal
and collateral arteries. Under these circumstances the peripheral pressure may
actually decrease with manual compression. The finding of a normal peripheral
pressure and arterial pulse does not rule out the presence of an AVF but only
indicates that blood is not diverted away from the periphery because the AVF is
hypoactive.

   If peripheral resistance is high as compared with that induced by the communicating channel of the AVF circuit, blood may flow in a retrograde cephalad direction in the distal artery from the collateral arteries. This flow inversion may be
detected with a direction sensitive CW Doppler if the distal artery may be insonified
by proper positioning of the exploring probe. AVF occlusion results in a change in
flow direction.

   In an AVF the proximal vein blood velocity shows a pulsatile (Fig. 34-4)
pattern that is normally absent in a normal superficial vein. It is synchronous with
the heart beat rather than with the ventilation.[30] The manual compression of the
fistula normalizes the proximal vein blood flow velocity pattern. The presence of a
pulsatile flow in a superficial vein should alert about the presence of an AVF. The
communicating channel(s) may be located following the course of the vein with the
Doppler probe until a distinct high frequency arterial velocity signal is found. The
manual compression of this area should induce the disappearance of the pulsatile
flow in the vein distally to the communication. The presence of several communications, however, results in a more difficult, if not impossible, localization of the
arterialization points.

   In the distal vein the blood pressure may be normal in chronic AVF. Indeed the
large compliance of the vein wall may allow enlargement of the vessel to accomodate the increased blood flow without a significant increase in the vein blood pressure. However, any increase in the vein blood pressure interferes with capillary
exchanges and[29] edema may result when the capabilities of the lymphatic drainage
system are overcome. Venous pressure may be measured by a cuff and a CW
Doppler; when the cuff pressure is a bit lower than the venous pressure a characteristic wind-like sound is heard.

   The intraoperative use of a sterile probe of the CW Doppler may allow monitoring the effect of vessel clamping on peripheral hemodynamics. The systolic pressure and the arterial pulse may be evaluated at the level of the distal artery and
peripheral vascular bed. In obscure cases the surgeon may try the hemodynamic

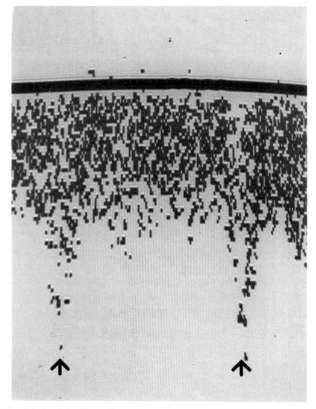

Fig. 34-4. The Doppler spectrum of the signal from a proximal vein of an AVF circuit.

effects on the peripheral vascular bed of the planned surgical procedure before ligating and cutting the vessels. Under these circumstances the risk of peripheral ischemia may be reduced.

After surgery the noninvasive tests are useful to evaluate with the clinical findings the result of the procedure. They play a role in the follow up of the patient. This may be particularly important in the patient with congenital AVF, which may show an unpredictable evolutive potential.

RADIONUCLIDE EVALUATION OF AVF

The quantitative estimation of the shunt flow with respect to the proximal artery flow may be performed using radionuclide labelled microspheres.[31] This method allows the confirmation of the existence of an AVF in those cases that present multiple microscopic communications. In these patients it is impossible to identify the individual components of a typical AVF circuit and the compression of the fistula, to induce the characteristic hemodynamic changes, is impossible. Under these circumstances, the Doppler evaluation of the AVF may be impossible or of very difficult interpretation.

The method is based on the direct passage into the venous system through the shunt of 15–30 micron microspheres injected in the artery proximal to the AVF. The percentage of microspheres that flow through the shunt is dependent on the magnitude of the shunt. In practice, the radioactivity over a lung region resulting from the shunted microspheres is compared with the radioactivity over the same area induced by a known amount of microspheres injected in a peripheral vein and completely trapped in the lung. To perform the measurement a scintillation camera and a 3M brand albumin microspheres kit are required. Three counting are performed in the same lung area. The first after the injection of the suspending solution in a peripheral vein (to determine the contribution of unbound radioactive tecnetium). The second after the injection of labelled microspheres in the artery presumed to nourish the AVF and the third after intravenous injection of labelled microspheres in a peripheral vein. Counting of radioactivity present in the syringes after injection allows estimation of the true injectate. Different formulas assist in the calculation from the measured parameters of the percentage of proximal artery blood flow that is shunted.

MEASUREMENT OF THE OXYGEN TENSION IN THE VENOUS BLOOD

A simple method to confirm the presence of an AVF relies on the comparison of the oxygen tension of blood drained from a vein that receives blood directly from an artery through an AVF with that from a vein of the controlateral supposed normal limb. Because of the shunt, saturated arterial blood mixes with that coming from the peripheral vascular bed and therefore the oxygen tension is higher than normal.[32]

B MODE AND DUPLEX SYSTEM EVALUATION OF AVF

B mode real time imaging may be used to detect the presence of venous dilatation, which may suggest the presence of an AVF.[33] The same technique may allow the evaluation of arterial dysplasias. The presence or absence of valves may be shown in dysplastic collector veins.

The role of B mode imaging in the study of congenital AVF is less impressive than its use in the evaluation of AVF surgically performed for hemodialysis. The formation of parietal thrombus may be documented before complete occlusion occurs and early antithrombotic medical or surgical treatment may be suggested[34] (Fig. 34-5).

Duplex System allows the Pulsed Doppler evaluation of a small volume of flowing blood. The position of the sampled volume may be known from the B mode image. The Doppler evaluation of the component vessels of an AVF circuit may be simplified by the anatomic knowledge of the region under study. Doppler imaging was found to be useful to image a femoro-femoral AVF to the point that arteriography was not performed before surgical intervention.[35]

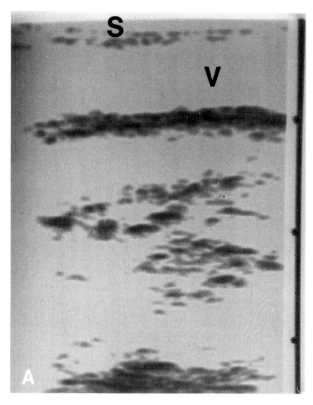

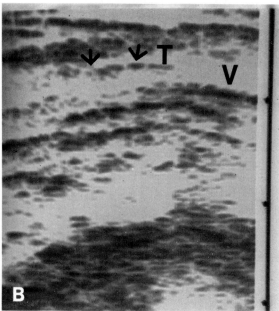

Fig. 34-5. B mode real time image of a varicose vein located distally to an AVF communication. (A) without thrombus, (B) with a parietal thrombus (arrows).

CONCLUSION

The typical classification of congenital arteriovenous malformations is still that proposed in 1964 by Malan and Puglionisi.[36,37] Such classification is made on a morphological basis. Other authors have classified the lesions taking into account the hemodynamic disturbances caused by the arterio-venous shunt.[38] The present availability of noninvasive techniques may be useful to better characterize the hemodynamics of those lesions that are difficult to treat. Indeed, the frequent diffuse involvement makes a radical excision impossible or a hazard for the remaining tissues. A nonradical excision is frequently followed by the development of previously dormant microscopic communications. Therefore, a conservative approach should be followed with careful follow-up of the patient to detect clinical and instrumental signs suggestive of progression, unless a very localized lesion is amenable of radical excision.

REFERENCES

1. Malan, E, Puglionisi A: Congenital angiodysplasias of the extremities. Generalities and classification. Venous dysplasia. J Cardiovasc Surg 5:87, 1964
2. Malan E, Puglionisi A: Congenital angiodysplasias of the extremities. arterial, arterial and venous, and hemolymphatic dysplasias. J Cardiovasc Surg 6:255, 1965
3. Malan E: Vascular malformations (Angiodysplasias). Carlo Erba Foundation. Milan, 1974
4. De Takats G: Vascular anomalies of the extremities. Surg Gynecol Obstet 55:227, 1932
5. Callander CL: Study of arteriovenous fistula with an analysis of 447 cases. Ann Surg 71:428, 1920
6. Coleman CC: Diagnosis and treatment of congenital arteriovenous fistulas of the head and neck. Am J Surg 126:557, 1973
7. Strandness DE, Sumner DS: Arteriovenous fistula, in Hemodynamics for Surgeons, New York: Grune & Stratton, 1975, p. 621–663
8. Sumner DS: Hemodynamics and pathophysiology of arteriovenous fistulas, in Rutherford RB (Ed.): Vascular Surgery, Philadelphia, WB Saunders Company, 1977, pp. 737–767
9. Barnes RW: Non invasive assessment of arteriovenous fistula. Angiology 29:621, 1978
10. D'Silva J, Fouche RF: The effect of changes in flow on the caliber of the large arteries. J Physiol 150:23P, 1960
11. John HT, Warren R: The stimulus to collateral circulation. Surgery 49:14, 1961
12. Attinger EO, Sugawara H, Navarro A, et al: Pulsatile flow patterns in distensible tubes. Circ Res 18:447, 1966
13. Sabiston Dc, Theilen EO, Gregg DE: Physiologic studies in experimental high out-put cardiac failure produced by aortic-caval fistula. Surg Forum 6:233, 1955
14. Ingebrigtsen R, Krog J, Leraand S: Circulation distal to experimental arteriovenous fistulas of the extremities: a polarographic study. Acta Chir Scand 125:308, 1963
15. Nakano J, De Schryver C: Effects of arteriovenous fistula on systemic and pulmonary circulations. Am J Physiol 207:1319, 1964
16. Longo T, Pignoli P: The behaviour of the Nicoladoni Branham sign at rest and under effort. Angiology 32:797, 1981
17. Strandness DE, Schultz RD, Sumner DS, et al: Ultrasonic flow detection, a useful technique in the evaluation of peripheral vascular disease. Am J Surg 113:311, 1967

18. Satomura S: Study of flow patterns in peripheral arteries by ultrasonics. J Acoust Soc Japan 15:151, 1959
19. Johnston KW, Maruzzo BC, Cobbold RS: Errors and artifacts of Doppler flowmeters and their solution. Arch Surg 112:1335, 1977
20. McLeod FD: Directional flowmeter. Proc Ann Conf Eng Med Biol 9:27, 1967
21. Phillips DJ, et al: Detection of peripheral vascular disease using the Duplex Scanner III. Ultrasound Med Biol 6:205, 1980
22. Sumner DS: Digital Plethysmography, in Rutherford RB (Ed.): Vascular Surgery, Philadelphia, WB Saunders Company, 1977, p. 73
23. Whitney RJ: Measurement of volume changes in human limbs. J Physiol (London) 121:1, 1953
24. Janowitz WR: Small parts Scanning. Radiology/Nuclear Medicine Magazine, August 1981
25. Sumner DS: Diagnostic evaluation of arteriovenous fistulas, Rutherford RB (Ed): Vascular Surgery, Philadelphia, WB Saunders Company, 1977, p. 767
26. Kirkendall WM, Burton AC, Epstein FH, et al: Recommendations for human blood pressure determination by sphygmomanometers. Circulation 36:980, 1967
27. Mason DT, Braunwald E: A simplified plethysmographic system for the measurement of systemic arterial pressure and peripheral blood flow. Am Heart J 64:796, 1962
28. Hurwich BJ: Plethysmographic forearm blood flow studies in maintenance patients with radial arteriovenous fistulae. Nephron 6:673, 1969
29. Starling EH: On the absorption of fluids from the connective tissue spaces. J Physiol 19:312, 1896
30. Lewis J, Hobbs J, Yao J: Normal and abnormal femoral vein velocities, in Roberts C (Ed.): Blood Flow Measurements, London, Sector Publishing Ltd., 1972, pp 48–52
31. Rhodes BA, Rutherford RB, Lopez-Majano V, et al: Arteriovenous shunt measurements in extremities. J Nucl Med 13:357, 1972
32. Veal JR, McCord WM: Congenital abnormal arteriovenous anastomoses of the extremities with special reference to diagnosis by arteriography and by the oxygen saturation test. Arch Surg 33:848, 1936
33. Williams DB, Foulk WS, Johnson CM: Splenic arteriovenous fistula. Mayo Clin Proc 55:383, 1980
34. Scheible W, Skram L, Leopold GR: High resolution real time sonography of hemodialysis vascular access complications. Am J Radiol 134:1173, 1980
35. Blumoff RL, Kupper C: Ultrasonic arteriography of femoral arteriovenous fistulae. Bruit 5:39, 1981
36. Lindenauer SM: Congenital arteriovenous Fistula, in Rutherford RB (Ed.): Vascular Surgery, Philadelphia, WB Saunders Company, 1984, p. 904
37. Malan E, Tardito E, Sala A: Arteriovenous fistulae, in Haimovici H (Ed.): Vascular Surgery, New York, 2nd Edition, McGraw Hill, 1984, p. 533
38. Machleder H: Vascular Malformations, in Moore SW (Ed.): Vascular Surgery, Orlando, Fla, Grune & Stratton, 2nd Edition, 1984

David J. Allison
and Anne P. Hemingway

35

Arterio-Venous Malformations: Arteriography and Embolization

A large number of different surgical and histologic classifications exist for arterio-venous malformations, and these include a bewildering variety of descriptive terms for the various lesions that are grouped under this heading. Angiographically, however, a somewhat simplistic approach to classification permits the great majority of these malformations to be allotted to one of three principal groups and these are considered in turn below. These groups are based on the angiographic appearances of the lesions and do not necessarily correspond to any histologic features. While a number of malignant neoplasms of vascular tissue exist and many malignant neoplasms arising primarily from nonvascular tissue exhibit abnormal vascularity, the three categories considered below are concerned only with those lesions consisting of benign collections of abnormal blood channels.

GROUP 1. PREDOMINANTLY ARTERIAL OR ARTERIOVENOUS LESIONS

These malformations are always very conspicuous angiographically and consist of tortuous enlarged feeding arteries and prominent draining veins. Abnormal communications usually exist between the arteries and veins (macrofistulae) and the degree of arteriovenous shunting occurring in the lesion will depend on the number and size of these communications. Rapid shunting is shown arteriographically by fast flow through the arteries, very early or immediate venous filling, and rapid clearing of the contrast medium injection bolus. Vascular detail within the lesion itself is often very poorly demonstrated because of the dilution of the contrast medium and its rapid evacuation into the venous system (Fig. 35-1). Clinically these lesions are manifest as pulsatile swellings or space-occupying lesions and there is commonly a bruit on auscultation. The lesions may cause local pressure effects, local gigantism, trophic changes in soft tissues, distal ischaemia, haemorrhage, pain, and disfigurement. Lesions in or near the ear may cause tinnitus. The decrease in periph-

DIAGNOSTIC TECHNIQUES AND ASSESSMENT
PROCEDURES IN VASCULAR SURGERY

© 1985 Grune & Stratton
ISBN 0-8089-1721-8 All rights reserved

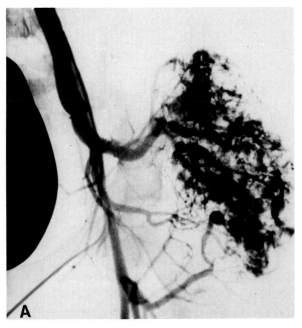

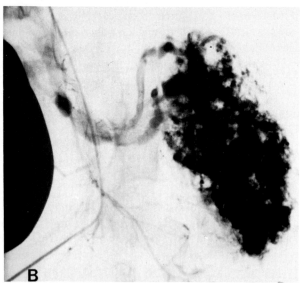

Fig. 35-1. AVM of the buttock in a 17-year-old girl. The feeding arteries break down into a meshwork of abnormal vascular spaces (A), which are drained by prominent veins (B). The lesion was successfully eradicated by a series of three embolization procedures. From Crainger RG and Allison D: Diagnostic Radiology: a textbook of organ imaging (in press): with permission of Churchill Livingstone, London

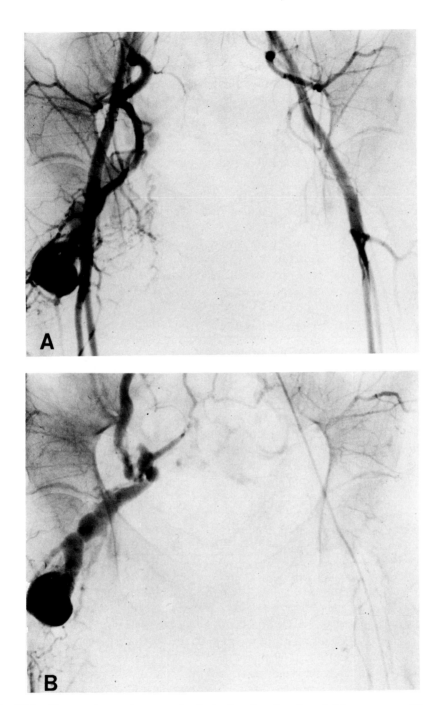

Fig. 35-2. Traumatic arteriovenous fistula in the gluteal region. A false aneurysm fills early in the injection sequence (A) and drains immediately into a massive vein (B). From Crainger RG and Allison D: Diagnostic Radiology: a textbook of organ imaging (in press): with permission of Churchill Livingstone, London

eral resistance caused by such malformations leads to an increase in cardiac output that may become massive and ultimately cause cardiac failure.

Degenerative changes in the arteries supplying the lesion may lead to aneurysm formation.[1] Some Group 1 lesions exhibit less marked shunting on arteriography and are much easier to demonstrate in detail because the arteriovenous communications are small enough to allow staining of the abnormal vascular bed of the malformation by the contrast medium (Fig. 35-1). The flow is still large through such lesions, however, and prominent arteries and draining veins are apparent. Acquired arteriovenous shunts such as the A-V fistulae caused by trauma, surgery, or biopsy procedures are usually very localized lesions with a relatively wide communication between artery and vein; on arteriography the vein fills almost immediately following the arterial injection of contrast medium in such lesions (Fig. 35-2).

Successful arteriography in fast-flow lesions requires rapid early filming to demonstrate the site(s) of shunting, and in most cases a pressure injection of contrast medium from a pump is necessary to achieve adequate vascular opacification. It is very easy to mistake large 'arterialized' veins for feeding arteries, and the films should be carefully scrutinized to establish the exact sequence and direction of vascular filling. Digital subtraction angiography if available is particularly useful when investigating fast-flow arteriovenous malformations (AVMs), and rapid sequence 105-mm filming or cine radiography may also be helpful.

GROUP II. PREDOMINANTLY CAPILLARY OR SMALL-VESSEL MALFORMATIONS

Malformations affecting predominantly the capillaries or other very small vessels are difficult to demonstrate radiologically, and few such lesions require investigation as this rarely influences treatment; arteriography does not, for instance, contribute to the clinical management of a capillary naevus ("port wine stain"). There are a few exceptions to this general rule, however, one of the most notable being angiodysplasia.[2] Angiodysplasia is a disorder of the microvasculature of the gastrointestinal tract, occurring predominantly in late middle age and old age. The lesions consist of ectasia of small vessels (arterioles, venules, capillaries) in the mucosa and submucosa of the bowel (normally the caecum and ascending colon). These lesions act as miniature shunts and can be demonstrated by selective visceral angiography (Fig. 35-3).

The lesions of Osler-Weber-Rendu disease (hereditary haemorrhagic telangiectasis) can be shown by arteriography and this is sometimes useful in localizing specific lesions causing problems such as epistaxis or gastrointestinal haemorrhage when embolization is being considered as a possible mode of treatment. Successful angiography for small-vessel malformations depends primarily on achieving sufficiently selective catheterization of the vascular bed under examination. This is because lesions are small and may easily be obscured by overlying vessels in other vascular beds if these have also been opacified. Care must be taken not to induce spasm in the artery selected for catheterization; small-vessel lesions may fail to opacify in the presence of a reduced perfusion pressure and be missed entirely. Filming sequences for small vessel lesions do not need to be particularly rapid, but should continue for up to 20 seconds following the injection of contrast medium;

some of these abnormalities become more conspicuous in the later stages of an injection sequence as contrast medium accumulates in the abnormal vessels and spaces of the lesion. Subtraction angiography, magnification arteriography, and pharmacoangiography may be useful in some circumstances in the investigation of small-vessel abnormalities.

GROUP III. PREDOMINANTLY VENOUS ABNORMALITIES

Venous (cavernous) malformations consist of collections of dilated veins and abnormal vascular spaces or channels on the venous side of the capillary bed. Clinically they are non-pulsatile, can be compressed easily, and exhibit gravity-dependent filling. When superficial they often give a blue discolouration to the overlying (or affected) skin, and this, together with the mass effect can be extremely disfiguring, especially if the face is affected.

Arteriography of venous malformations is usually fairly disappointing: the lesions frequently appear entirely normal in the early stages of the filming sequence as the arteries supplying such lesions are not necessarily increased in either number or size (sometimes, of course, they are). There is no significant increase in flow demonstrable arteriographically and the only abnormal finding may be staining of unusual vessels or venous spaces in the late stages of the study. If it is anatomically possible, retrograde venography may be a feasible technique for showing the abnormality if a clinical indication exists for doing so.

The angiomas that occur in association with dyschondroplasia (Maffucci's syndrome) and other rare disorders are usually predominantly venous in nature. They may contain phleboliths which show on plain films, but angiography is usually unrewarding and rarely indicated.

ARTERIOGRAPHY

There are a number of points that should be considered in relation to the arteriography of AVMs. The first question is whether or not the investigation is indicated at all. If there is no real prospect of any definitive treatment for the lesion concerned, or arteriography seems unlikely to contribute any clinically significant information (eg, in the case of a predominantly venous or lymphatic abnormality), then an arteriogram may not be necessary. In some such cases it may be that no investigation is indicated; in others a different investigation such as venography, lymphography, ultrasonography, enhanced CT scanning, or MR scanning may be more appropriate.

If arteriography is the procedure of choice the principles of the investigation are: to localize the lesion (if it is deep-seated); to define its extent and its degree of involvement with neighbouring structures; to define its feeding vessels; to show all the collateral routes of supply (actual and, as far as possible, potential); to show the size, site, and number of any significant arteriovenous communications; and to define the draining veins from the lesion. It is of course not always possible to achieve all these aims, but a substantial proportion of them can be fulfilled in most patients. It is important to begin the investigation with an arteriogram that is not

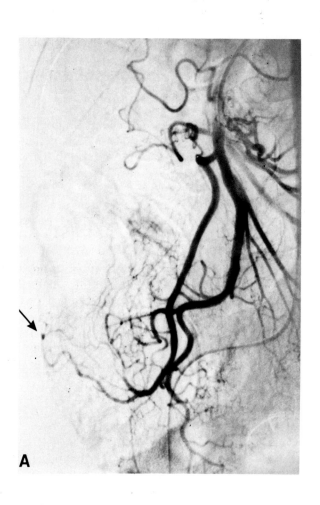

A

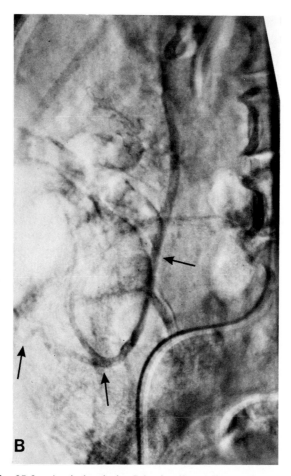

B

Fig. 35-3. Angiodysplasia. Selective ileo-colic arteriogram in
a 50-year-old man with chronic obscure gastrointestinal bleeding. A dilated tortuous artery fills an abnormal vascular 'lake'
(arrow) in the arterial phase of the study (A). A prominent
early-filling vein (arrows) is seen draining the lesion in a later
film (B). From Crainger RG and Allison D: Diagnostic
Radiology: a textbook of organ imaging (in press): with permission of Churchill Livingstone, London

too selective in nature, as important collateral feeding vessels may be missed in this way. An AVM in the upper thigh for instance, supplied predominantly by vessels from the deep femoral artery, may also receive blood from the gluteal or pelvic arteries and these branches of supply will only be seen if the internal iliac artery is opacified. Once all the vessels of supply have been identified, selective studies of individual arteries may be necessary to obtain more detailed information about the lesion with the higher local concentrations of contrast medium that can be achieved in this way, and in the absence of any overlying obscuring opacification of neighbouring vascular territories. With Group I lesions large volumes of contrast medium injected at a fast rate and a very rapid filming sequence may be necessary to delineate the lesion adequately. It is not possible to obtain an adequate study of a Group I lesion of any size without an automatic injection pump; a hand injection will simply not achieve adequate opacification of a fast-flow lesion unless DSA is available. In the case of very fast shunts, 105-mm pictures (6 frames per second) or even cine radiography may be necessary to display the anatomy of the abnormality; other techniques for achieving this include the use of balloon catheters on either the arterial or venous side of the lesion to slow the flow during the period of contrast opacification, or the use of a limb tourniquet if the AVM is in one of the extremities. Low osmolality contrast media should be used in preference to conventional media and great care should be taken during diagnostic arteriography not to damage any of the vessels feeding an AVM, as this may compromise any subsequent attempt to embolize the lesion. As in all types of vascular study, multiple views taken in different projections may be extremely valuable. In the case of Group II and III lesions, the filming sequence should be sufficiently long to demonstrate any late staining of abnormal vessels via 'slow flow' malformations.

With the information derived from the arteriogram the radiologist and vascular surgeon should be able to decide on the potential benefits and risks of treating the lesion and the relative merits of embolization alone, surgery alone, embolization followed by surgery, or, in occasional cases, surgery followed by embolization.

EMBOLIZATION

Group I Lesions

As a general rule Group I lesions (fast-flow arteriovenous communications) are best treated by embolization, though in some cases it is advisable to follow the embolization by a surgical biopsy or complete excision while the vascularity of the lesion is reduced.[3] This is particularly important when the histologic nature of the lesion is in doubt. An important exception to the general rule of embolization being the preferred 'first-line' treatment in Group I lesions is when the A-V communication is wide and short. This occurs particularly in acquired A-V shunts (eg, traumatic femoral artery-vein fistula). In such cases the risk of venous (pulmonary) embolization during embolization is so great that a direct surgical approach is usually simple and safer.

The principles of embolization in the treatment of an AVM are straightforward (much more straightforward than putting them into practice!). They are that all the vessels feeding the lesion should be blocked as close to the lesion as possible, that the 'nidus' of the lesion should if possible be embolized (to minimize the likelihood or recurrence), that no emboli should pass through the lesion into the venous circulation during the procedure, that the principal access vessels to the feeding vessels should be left patent at the end of the procedure (to allow for a return trip if necessary), and that the arteries feeding neighbouring or downstream structures should be neither damaged nor embolized during the procedure. If the AVM is itself in a structure of vital functional importance (eg, a kidney), then a further consideration is of course that the function of that organ or structure should be preserved insofar as this is possible commensurate with the complete eradication of the AVM. In some cases a clinical decision may have to be made as to whether the total elimination of an AVM or the preservation of some function in a particular organ is the more important consideration.

Numerous different types of material are available for embolization:[4] these include sterile absorbable gelatin sponge, steel coils, lyophilized human dura mater, polyvinyl alcohol sponge, ethyl alcohol, hypertonic dextrose solution, detachable balloons, and polymerizing liquids such as acrylates or polyurethanes.

A detailed discussion of the different indications and criteria for using these materials is beyond the scope of this article: in general, however, the smaller particulate emboli (eg, fragmented sterile absorbable gelatin sponge) are useful for getting into the nidus (core) of a lesion or the small vessels near it. The larger emboli (eg, steel coils, detachable balloons) are used for blocking large vessels in situations where there are no small distal vessels to trap smaller particulate emboli (eg, caroticocavernous fistula), or where the nidus of a lesion has previously been blocked with small emboli but a major feeding vessel is still patent. Liquid emboli are used when the lesion to be embolized is either itself composed of very fine vessels or is fed by very small arteries along which only liquid emboli will pass. Liquid emboli can be mixed with particulate emboli to increase the thrombogenic potency of the injected solution and they can also be used alone in situations where only very small calibre catheters can be introduced into a vascular bed for technical reasons. Liquid emboli are very much more likely than particulate emboli to pass into neighbouring vascular beds through fine collateral vessels and should never be used in situations where this could be hazardous.

In fast-flow lesions it can be extremely difficult to obtain vascular obstruction by embolization without allowing some emboli to pass through into the venous circulation. Occasionally it can help to reduce the flow with arterial or venous balloons, or by the use of a tourniquet, but extreme care should always be exercised to avoid pulmonary embolism when dealing with such lesions. As mentioned above, in some Group I lesions (particularly the very localized acquired A-V fistulae), surgery may well be the treatment of first choice. In other lesions, particularly those with multiple feeding arteries or in difficult anatomical situations, surgery may be dangerous or impossible, and embolization has to be attempted despite the potential risk of venous embolization. It is often stated that major feeding vessels to AVMs should never be embolized to allow future access if recurrence occurs. This is not strictly true: it is sometimes impossible permanently to occlude the flow to a lesion without embolizing a major feeder but this should only be done after the core and distal bed within the AVM have been embolized with smaller particles. Embolization of the feeding artery may then be a crucial step in preventing its subsequent recanalization. It is of course important never to embolize the principal artery

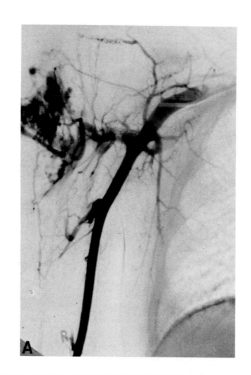

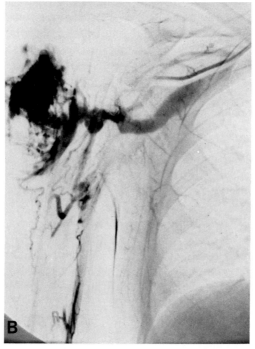

412

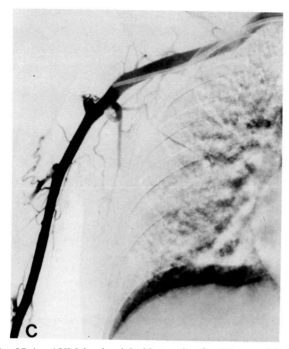

Fig. 35-4. AVM in the deltoid muscle of a 16-year-old girl. The abnormal vessels fill from branches of the axillary artery (A). A densely staining nidus is seen in a later film, together with prominent draining veins (B). After successful embolization the lesion is no longer opacified at arteriography (C). From Crainger RG and Allison D: Diagnostic Radiology: a textbook of organ imaging (in press): with permission of Churchill Livingstone, London

giving access to an entire region containing an AVM as this will make it impossible to return to embolize on a subsequent occasion; it would be unwise for instance completely to occlude the external carotid artery or the hypogastric artery in the respective cases of a facial AVM or a buttock AVM.

It should be emphasized that embolization of an AVM is often better performed in several stages rather than at one prolonged attempt.[5] The multistage technique reduces the risk of massive tissue necrosis, and the likelihood of contrast medium overdosage. It also means that the operator returns fresh to what may be an extremely difficult technical task, and is likely to achieve a better final result. The ideal AVMs for embolization are the slower-flow lesions that form a subdivision of Group I (Fig. 35-4). These lesions still carry preferential flow relative to the normal surrounding structures, but the vessels break down into a fairly fine abnormal meshwork of arterioles that stains densely at arteriography and traps injected emboli. Once this meshwork is thrombosed the lesion is unlikely to recur.

A special problem exists with regard to pulmonary AVMs[6] since any emboli passing through such a lesion will end up in the systemic circulation: a far more dangerous situation than that is in systemic AVMs where the lungs exist as a safety net to trap any emboli inadvertently passing through during the procedure. For this

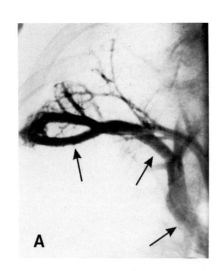

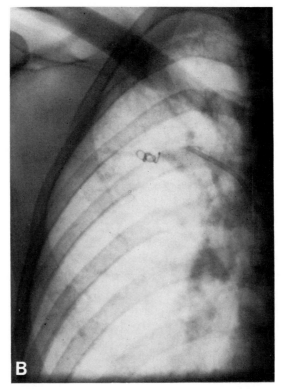

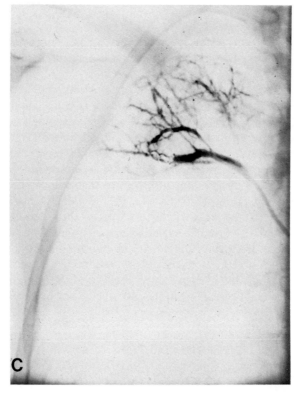

Fig. 35-5. Pulmonary AVM. A selective arteriogram shows a feeding artery and an enlarged draining vein (arrows) that fills almost instantly (A). A steel coil has been selectively inserted close to the site of the fistula (B). A postembolization study (C) shows abolition of the shunt with preservation of perfusion in the surrounding normal lung. From Crainger RG and Allison D: Diagnostic Radiology: a textbook of organ imaging (in press): with permission of Churchill Livingstone, London

reason particulate emboli and liquid emboli cannot be used in pulmonary AVMs; the only safe embolic agents are detachable balloons or steel coils. The balloon or coil must be large enough to block the malformation on the arterial side, but not so large as to block an unduly great proportion of the regional pulmonary bed (Fig. 35-5).

GROUP II LESIONS

Arterial embolization is not an effective form of treatment at present for capillary lesions such as port wine stains. For certain localized small-vessel malformations such as the lesions of hereditary telangiectasis, arterial embolization is effective when a specific lesion is causing a clinical problem (eg, a lesion in the nose causing epistaxis). Embolization is not used for angiodysplasia because of the risk of bowel infarction.

GROUP III LESIONS

Arterial embolization is not generally effective in venous malformations; the presence of a normal or near-normal capillary bed prevents the emboli reaching the abnormal vascular spaces, which therefore remain patent. Reducing the arterial supply to such a lesion may indeed make it worse because it may appear more cyanosed following embolization and become more of a disfigurement, especially if it is a facial lesion. There are three ways in which embolization may be used to cure these lesions in the future: Firstly, work on new liquid emboli agents with controlled setting characteristics may produce a fluid which sets preferentially in the immediate post-capillary region of the circulation; secondly, a considerable volume of experimental work is being directed towards the percutaneous obliteration of venous lesions using imaging guidance to place a fine needle in the abnormal vascular spaces; and thirdly, it may be possible to embolize these lesions using a venous catheter approach. With currently available embolic agents, however, this is very hazardous because of the risk of pulmonary embolization. At the present time the best treatment for Group III lesions appears to be complete surgical excision; unfortunately, this is not possible in many cases, because of the size and position of the lesion, or the risk or serious scarring in the case of facial or other exposed lesions.

COMPLICATIONS OF EMBOLIZATION

The complications of embolization are listed in Table 35-1. Of these the two complications most likely to occur during the embolization of AVMs are the inadvertent embolization of vessels other than those supplying the lesion, and the passage of emboli through the malformation into the venous circulation. Even if one of these complications does occur, it is unlikely in most cases to result in any serious clinical sequelae, provided it is immediately recognized and no further accidents are allowed to occur. The morbidity of carefully conducted procedures is in fact very low. The above statement does not of course apply to embolization of lesions in or near the CNS, where the inadvertent embolization of any normal tissue may have disastrous consequences. Embolization in the carotid[7,8] and spinal territories should only be attempted by experienced neuroradiologists.

PREEMBOLIZATION SURGERY

Prior to embolization surgeons had no alternative but to attempt to control AVMs using surgical techniques (in those cases where some treatment was mandatory). The techniques included surgical excision, the direct injection of sclerosants (without imaging control), or the ligation of major feeding and/or draining vessels. The latter technique was unfortunately associated with a very high incidence of recurrence or failure owing to the rapid enlargement of collateral feeding vessels to the lesion and should no longer be employed if embolization is technically feasible. Surgical ligation of a feeding vessel makes its subsequent embolization

Table 35-1
Complications of Embolization

General
    Usual hazards of super-selective angiography
    Contrast medium reactions

Specific
    Immediate
      Pain
      Nausea
      Inadvertent embolization of normal structures
      Pulmonary embolization through A-V shunts
      Adherence of catheter tip to vessel wall (bucrylate)
      Reaction to embolic material
    Delayed
      Pain
      Fever   } 'post embolization syndrome'
      Leucocytosis
      Infection
        Local
        Systemic
      Tissue necrosis (unintentional)
      Extension of thrombosis beyond embolized area
      Release of humoral substances from infarcted endocrine tissue
      Renal failure

extremely difficult, as the collateral feeding vessels may be impossible to catheterize, or may be too small or tortuous to carry emboli to the actual lesion without first themselves becoming occluded (Fig. 35-6). In such cases it may be necessary to perform a second operation to bypass the ligature or otherwise restore access to the major feeding vessel so that a subsequent embolization becomes feasible. It is just as important that an inexperienced radiologist should not insert a coil or balloon into a major feeding artery without first eradicating flow in the more distal vessels of supply; the effect is otherwise the same as a surgical ligature: ineffective and a hindrance to proper treatment.

The correct approach to the management of an arteriovenous fistula is for the patient to be assessed jointly by a vascular surgeon and a radiologist with experience in embolization. They can decide whether any investigation is indicated and if it is, select the most appropriate method (arteriography, venography, CT, etc). If on clinical assessment embolization seems likely to be the preferred form of treatment for a particular lesion a decision can be taken for the radiologist to proceed directly to embolization without further consultation if the diagnostic arteriogram confirms the clinical impression. If doubt exists clinically as to the correct mode of treatment (ie, surgery, embolization, both, or none), further joint consultation can take place after the results of diagnostic investigations are available, when a final decision can be made. It cannot be emphasized too strongly that the key to safe and effective treatment of these lesions is the closest possible cooperation between surgeon and radiologist.

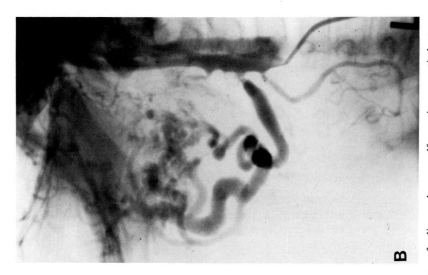

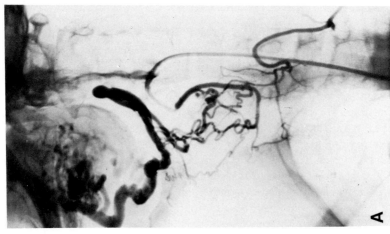

Fig. 35-6. Lingual AVM. The lingual artery feeding a large malformation was tied at a previous surgical operation. A selective angiogram (A) shows that lingual flow continues via collaterals from the superior thyroid artery; these vessels are too small to be used for embolization of the malformation. At a repeat surgical operation the lingual artery has been grafted back on to the external carotid artery (B).

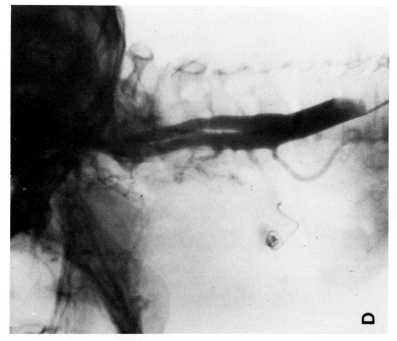

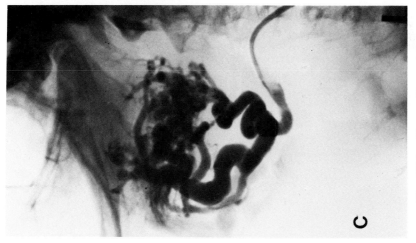

Fig. 35-6. The malformation can now be approached via the graft (C) and successfully embolized (D). From Crainger RG and Allison D: Diagnostic Radiology: a textbook of organ imaging (in press): with permission of Churchill Livingstone, London.

REFERENCES

1. Phillips JF, Yao JST: Congenital vascular malformations, in Neiman HL, Yao JST (eds): Angiography of Vascular Disease. New York, Churchill Livingstone, 1985, p 393
2. Boley SJ, Sammartano R, Adams A: On the nature and etiology of vascular ectasia of the colon: degenerative lesions of ageing. Gastroenterology 72:640, 1977
3. Allison DJ: Therapeutic embolization. Br J Hosp Med 20:707, 1978
4. Allison DJ: Interventional radiology. Rec Adv Radiol Med Imaging 7:139, 1983
5. Athanasoulis CA: Transcatheter arterial occlusion for arteriovenous fistulas and malformations of the trunk, pelvis and extremity, in Athanasoulis CA, Pfister RC, Greene RE, et al (eds): Interventional Radiology. Philadelphia, WB. Saunders 1982, p 203
6. White RI, Mitchell SE, Barth KH, et al: Angioarchitecture of pulmonary arteriovenous malformations. AJR 140:681, 1983
7. Kendall B, Moseley I: Therapeutic embolization of the external carotid tree. Neurol Neurosurg Psychiatr 40:937, 1977
8. Berenstein A, Kricheff II: Neuroradiologic interventional procedures. Sem Roentgenol 16:79, 1981

PART VIII

Venous

Simon G. Darke
and M. R. Andress

36

The Value of Venography in the Management of Chronic Venous Disorders of the Lower Limb

Patients with chronic venous disorders can, for convenience, be divided into those with primary varicose veins and those with complex problems. The latter group comprises the skin changes of venous insufficiency culminating in ulceration; and the syndrome of pain and swelling of the leg. These may occur separately, or co-exist.

It is neither practicable nor necessary to submit patients with primary varicose veins to venography. For the remainder, this investigation remains an important means of assessment. Although the information is to a great extent qualitative, venography is of value because it is the principle investigation by which the wide variety of possible abnormalities can be identified, distinguished, and assessed. These include post-phlebitic valvular damage and luminal stenosis or occlusion; ankle perforating vein dysfunction; superficial and deep femoral vein incompetence; and to some extent, long and short saphenous incompetence.

This paper reports the role that venography has played in a consecutive series of patients with complex venous disorders, in the identification of these lesions and correlating them with the clinical state. It provides the means to recognise certain groups of patients and to develop a strategy for management.

CLINICAL MATERIAL

Over a 30-month period, a consecutive series of patients with chronic venous disorders has been studied. These patients were referred to one surgeon with an interest in arterial and venous disorders. A total of 594 patients have been assessed. Table 36-1 shows the categories into which these patients have been divided. Those with primary and uncomplicated varicose veins are not considered further.

All those with "ulcer" had current ulceration or lesions that had only healed within the previous three months. Those designated as having the "pain and swelling" syndrome had both measurable calf oedema (and in some, the thigh as well)

DIAGNOSTIC TECHNIQUES AND ASSESSMENT
PROCEDURES IN VASCULAR SURGERY

© 1985 Grune & Stratton
ISBN 0-8089-1721-8 All rights reserved

Table 36-1
30-Month Study—Consecutive Series

Total No. of patients	594
Patients with primary varicose veins	466
No saphenous incompetence 46	
Saphenous incompetence 420	
Patients with complex disorders	128 (145 limbs)
48 limbs ulcer	(26 women, mean age—56)
52 limbs ulcer pain and swelling	(22 women, mean age—54)
45 limbs pain and swelling alone	(22 women, mean age—40)

and described pain in excess of the ache that may be associated with primary and uncomplicated varicose veins.

All these patients have been studied by clinical assessment, Doppler ultrasound, to demonstrate saphenous and popliteal vein incompetence,[1] and by ascending and descending venography. Three groups of patients were identified on clinical grounds and are studied and compared:

1. There were 42 patients with 48 limbs with ulcer alone. In 14 limbs there was a past history of deep vein thrombosis, and in 16 limbs a family history of similar disorders.
2. There were 46 patients with 52 limbs with ulcer and pain and swelling as well. In 20 limbs there was a family history of similar disorders and in 15 a past history of deep venous thrombosis.
3. There were 39 patients with 45 limbs with isolated pain and swelling syndrome. They tended to be a little younger than the other groups. In 17 limbs there was a family history of a similar disorder. There was a past history of deep venous thrombosis in 11 legs.

METHODS

Technique of Venography

The use of tilting X-ray tables and T.V. screening has made venography simpler, quicker, and more accurate. It can be performed on an Out-patient basis without prior preparation. The techniques employed are based on those described by Lea Thomas.[2]

Ascending Venography

A 21 or 23 gauge Butterfly needle is used, depending on the size of the vein. With the table tilted feet down and a tourniquet just above the ankle, this is inserted pointing distally into a dorsal foot vein. In case of difficulty it is often helpful to immerse the foot in warm water for a few minutes beforehand. If the foot is swollen, pressure with the thumb or fingers will often displace the oedema fluid, allowing a vein to be located. The needle is held in place with adhesive paper tape. Occasionally only the long saphenous vein just anterior to the medial malleolus can be found. Providing the needle is introduced with the point facing down towards the foot, this can be used successfully.

After checking needle position by instilling saline, and with the ankle tourniquet still in place, 50 mls of contrast medium are then injected under screen control with the table tilted approximately 50 degrees, feet down. The assistant injects and checks for extravasation while the Radiologist watches the venous filling on the T.V. screen.

The combination of the distally directed needle, the tourniquet above the ankle

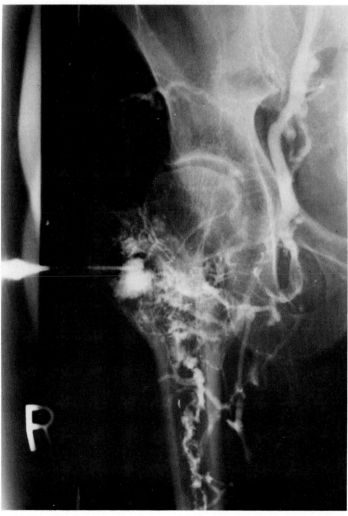

Fig. 36-1. A per-trochanteric inter-osseous venogram for femoral vein occlusion, showing external iliac vein reconstitution.

adjusted to occlude the superficial venous return, and the table tilt, ensure filling of the deep venous system. Mixing of the contrast medium and blood helps to avoid artefacts due to layering. Exposures are made using 43×35 cm films, split lengthwise into 2 or 3, when optimum filling is seen. Only AP projections are required, although it is sometimes useful to turn the leg to an oblique position to show overlapping veins more clearly. If the contrast medium is passing upwards in the superficial veins rather than in the deep venous system the ankle tourniquet is tightened and the table tilted more upright. A further tourniquet applied above the knee may help to encourage filling of the veins in the lower leg by restricting the upward flow of the medium. Once the veins of the lower leg have been demonstrated the table is lowered in stages to slightly head down to show the veins of the upper leg and pelvis as medium passes upwards.

Incompetent perforating veins can be identified on the screen during filling and early films taken to show the site and direction before the picture is obscured by contrast entering superficial vessels. Contrast which has entered superficial veins via incompetent perforators low down may obscure possible incompetent perforators higher up in the leg. If so, the contrast can be flushed out with saline and another tourniquet applied above the level already demonstrated to be incompetent. Further injections check for incompetence further up.

Generally, 50 mls of medium is sufficient to examine the leg by ascending venography. Once the films have been exposed, the contrast medium is flushed from the veins with saline and by exercising the calf muscles.

If it is impossible to locate a vein in the foot or ankle, intra-osseous venography via the medial malleolus can be employed, but this has not been necessary in our series. Where the common femoral vein is occluded a similar technique may be required to demonstrate reconstitution of pelvic veins. See Figure 36-1.

Descending Venography

The common femoral vein in the groin is punctured directly using a disposable Potts-Cournard needle. The femoral artery is palpated and local anaesthetic injected just medial to it, with the patient supine. The needle is then introduced and a slight resistance felt as it enters the vein. The stilette is removed and a connecting tube and syringe filled with saline are attached. Gentle suction is applied as the needle is slowly withdrawn until venous blood flows freely into the tubing. It is rarely necessary to advance the needle using the blunt stilette. If any abnormality has been seen in the pelvic veins on the ascending venogram, further pictures can be taken with the patient supine at this stage. The needle is secured with adhesive tape.

Initially in this series the table was brought almost upright at this stage but this may cause displacement of the needle in obese patients. Provided venous pressure is raised effectively by a valsalva manoeuvre, it has not proved necessary to tilt the table more than 30 degrees feet down. Some patients find it difficult to carry out a valsalva manoeuvre, thus the patient is asked to blow into a 10 cc syringe barrel attached to a sphygomanometer (Fig. 36-2). Sustaining a fixed 40 mmHg pressure standardises the procedure,[3–5] while 50 ml of contrast medium are injected.

The needle position is checked. Pictures are taken on 43×35 cm films, split lengthwise into 2 to show any retrograde flow and its extent. The needle is flushed with saline to clear contrast.

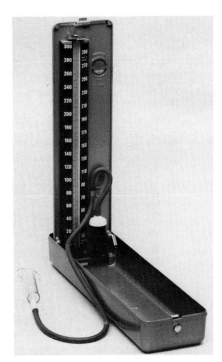

Fig. 36-2.   Sphygomanometer with a 10cc syringe
barrel attached.

Contrast Medium

Initially in this series, Meglumine Iothalomate (Conray 280) was employed for both ascending and descending venography, but a change was later made to the lower osmolality Sodium/Meglumine Ioxaglate (Hexabrix 320). A further change is now being made to use a non-ionic contrast medium such as Iopamidol (Niopam) or Iohexol (Omnipaque). It has been shown that there are less side effects in venography with these media including a significant reduction in thrombosis diagnosed by radio-active fibrinogen.[6,7]

INTERPRETATION

All venograms illustrated depict the right side, to facilitate orientation.

Ascending Venography

In the normal system the deep veins fill with smooth outlines and valves, visible as thin bicuspid structures. In post-thrombotic states the veins are occluded or may have recanalised with an irregular lumen and damaged or destroyed valves. Collateral veins may be shown bypassing blocks, in place of, or in addition to, recanalised veins. (See Figs 36-3, 36-4 and 36-5, showing post-phlebitic changes in calf, thigh, and pelvis.)

In incompetent perforating veins contrast passes in reverse from deep to superficial veins and these may be dilated and tortuous and lacking normal valves. There

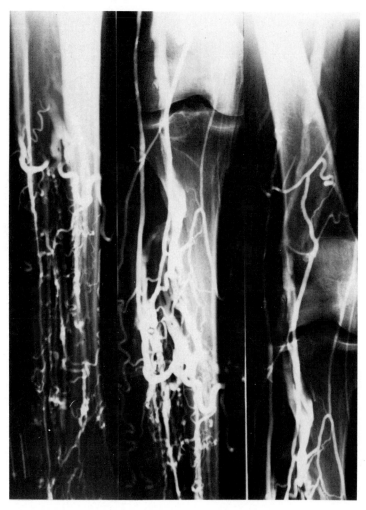

Fig. 36-3. Post-phlebitic damage in the calf veins, with incomplete recanalisation and tortuously dilated collateral circulation.

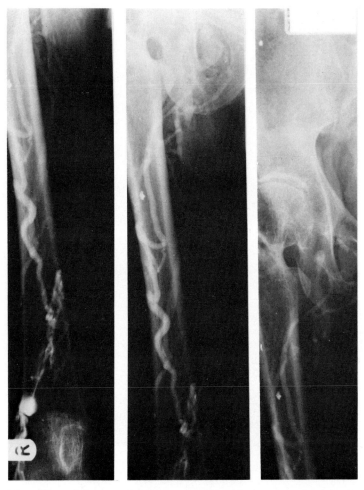

Fig. 36-4. Non-filling of the superficial femoral vein, with dye ascending via abnormal collateral circulation.

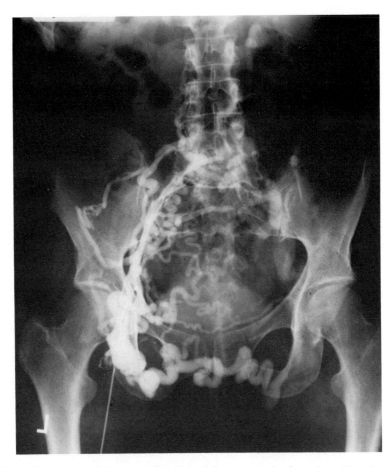

Fig. 36-5. Collateral circulation crossing the pelvis as a result of previous iliac thrombosis, demonstrated by a direct femoral stab.

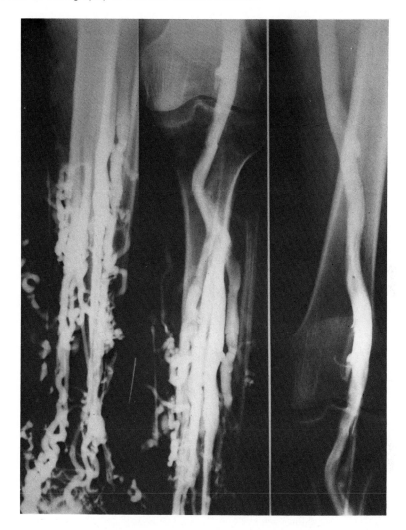

Fig. 36-6. Calf/ankle perforator incompetence.

may be a dilatation at the other end of such a vein where it joins a varicose super-ficial tributary. The perforating veins arise mainly from the posterior tibial veins medially and from the peroneal veins laterally. (See Fig. 36-6). Landmarks on the films can be employed to allow positions to be related to the leg.

Descending Venography

This is used to assess valvular competence in the superficial and deep femoral vein and saphenous veins. A little contrast can flow down past normal valves due to the specific gravity of the contrast medium, the tilted position, and the force of

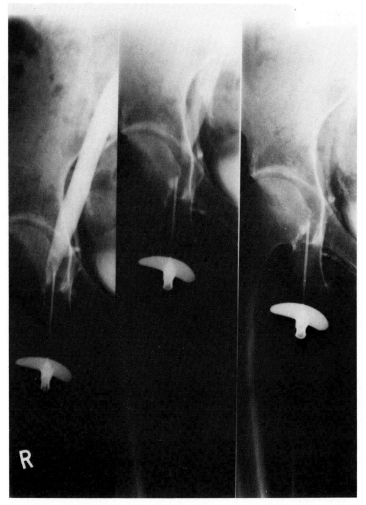

Fig. 36-7. Normal descending venogram, with rapid ascent of dye and clearance on injection.

injections. This leakage is often held up completely at a valve lower in the vein. Thus an attempt to quantify the degree of reflux has been made, as follows[8,9]:

> *Grade 0*—no reflux beyond upper femoral vein; see Figure 36-7.
> *Grade 1*—reflux, but not beyond proximal thigh.
> *Grade 2*—reflux to level of knee.
> *Grade 3*—reflux to below knee.
> *Grade 4*—reflux to the calf; see Figure 36-8.

In marked incompetence the contrast may pass to the calf and out through incompetent perforating veins into superficial veins of the saphenous systems. (See Fig. 36-11.)

Taheri et al[10,11] have pointed out that there is a group of patients who have a competent common femoral and upper superficial femoral valves but incompetent

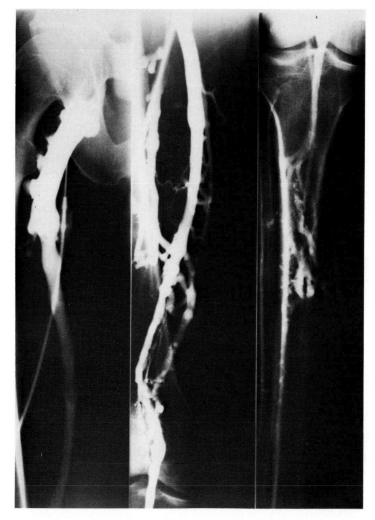

Fig. 36-8. Grade IV reflux, principally in the superficial femoral vein to mid-calf level.

popliteal valves below this. To demonstrate this it is necessary therefore to inject dye by retrograde catheterisation through the trans-brachial route. We have no experience of this procedure but this group of patients would seem to correlate with those in our series with Doppler evidence of popliteal reflux but "normal" conventional descending venograms, (vide infra).

RESULTS AND CONCLUSIONS

The results will be considered in two ways—an independent analysis of each abnormality, and secondly the various combinations of these abnormalities as they occur in the clinical situation.

Previous Deep Vein Thrombosis

Venographic evidence of previous deep vein thrombosis, although not quantifiable, can be separated anatomically into changes in the calf, thigh, and iliac systems. (See Figs. 36-2, 36-3, 36-4.) Of the 145 limbs studied this was present in 31. It was confined to the calf in 10, present in calf and thigh in 9, calf thigh and iliac system in 3, thigh alone in 5, iliac system alone in 3, and thigh and iliac systems in 1. There was no difference in the incidence and distribution between the three groups of patients, and details of this are given in Table 36-2. Included among these cases with

Table 36-2
Incidence and Distribution on Venographic Evidence
of Previous D.V.T.

	All limbs	Ulcer alone	Ulcer, pain and swelling	Pain and swelling alone
Total limbs studied	145	48	52	45
Calf alone	10	4	3	3
Calf and thigh	9	3	3	3
Calf/thigh/iliac	3	2	0	1
Thigh alone	5	2	3	0
Iliac alone	3	0	2	1
Thigh and iliac	1	0	1	0

a damaged deep venous system are 2 due to trauma. Figure 36-3 shows a patient who suffered a gunshot wound in the thigh some years previously.

Correlation of History of Previous D.V.T. with Venographic Evidence

In 11% of limbs studied there was a history of previous deep vein thrombosis, which was confirmed on the venogram. In a further 11% there was no history of previous deep vein thrombosis but positive findings on the venogram. In 17% of the limbs studied there was a history of previous D.V.T. but the venogram was normal. This implies that a history of a D.V.T. as evidence is unreliable, although those with a history but no venographic evidence may have undergone recanalization and restoration of function.[12] Furthermore it is possible that venography underestimates post-phlebitic damage. The presence of venographic changes, when present, are clear, and false positives unlikely but the extent of false negatives is difficult to estimate. This may be a limitation of the sensitivity of venography.

Association Between Venographic Post-Phlebitic Change and Femoral Incompetence

It has been reported that incompetence of the femoral valves occurs both as a consequence of previous thrombosis, and spontaneously due to inherent weakness of the vein or valve wall.[13] There were a total of 65 limbs in which Grade II or more severe reflux was demonstrable. Only 15 of these exhibited co-existant post-phlebitic damage on venography. Of those with Grade III or more severe reflux there were 32 limbs, in 7 of which previous deep vein thrombosis was identified. These data suggest, in common with previous authors,[14] a congenital or acquired weakness in the vein or the vein valve as the more common process.

Association Between Post-Phlebitic Change and Superficial Varicosities and Sapheno-Femoral Incompetence

This is relevant because of the inappropriate use of compression stockings or misplaced surgery in obliterating collateral varicosities that have developed secondary to deep vein thrombosis. Of the 31 limbs in which deep vein thrombosis was identified 15 had varicosities; 11 with sapheno-femoral incompetence, of which 2 were recurrent. There was no specific association between varicosities and occlusion of the deep thigh veins as opposed to damage at other sites. Venographically demonstrable post-phlebitic damage is not therefore inevitably associated with "secondary" varicose veins.

Incompetence of the Superficial and Deep Femoral Veins

Table 36-3 shows the incidence of Grade II or greater reflux in the superficial femoral vein alone; the superficial and deep femoral vein; and in the deep femoral vein alone, in the three groups of patients studied. A total of 65 limbs out of the 145 studied exhibited incompetence. In 54 this was confined to the superficial femoral vein. In 8 was this in both superficial and deep femoral veins. (See Fig. 36-9.) If indicated, therefore, the former group of patients would be suitable for transposition of the superficial to the deep femoral vein. Finally there were 3 patients in which the

Table 36-3
Femoral Incompetence

	Ulcer	Ulcer, pain and swelling	Pain and swelling
Total No. Limbs	48	52	45
S.F.V. alone	16	22	16
S.F.V. + D.F.V.	0	5	3
D.F.V. alone	0	0	3

S.F.V.—Superficial femoral vein
D.F.V.—Deep femoral vein

only identified abnormality was incompetence of the deep femoral vein itself. These patients complained of pain and swelling in the thigh. Examination revealed oedema, warmth, and dilated varicosities confined to the thigh. The authors have been unable to find a description of this recorded in the literature.

The distribution of femoral incompetence as a whole between the three groups of patients showed no differences but when assessed in the context of an association with the other abnormalities there are findings of relevance that are discussed below.

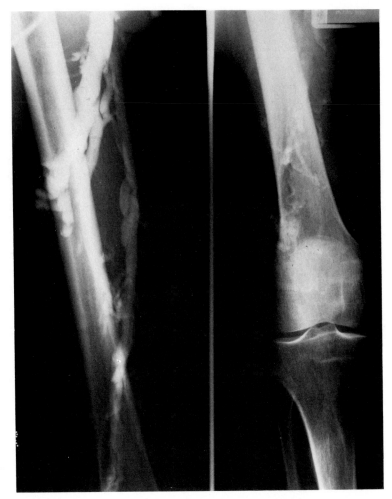

Fig. 36-9. Reflux down the superficial femoral vein, but more prominently in the deep femoral vein, the terminal tributaries of which are dilated and varicose.

Correlation of Venographic Evidence of Superficial Femoral Incompetance with Doppler Evidence of Popliteal Reflux

Of the 65 patients with femoral incompetence of Grade II or greater severity, 49 had associated reflux in the popliteal vein on Doppler. There were a further 19 patients with Doppler evidence of reflux, but without venographic evidence of valvular dysfunction higher up. Details of the distribution of patients with superficial, deep, and popliteal incompetence in the 3 groups of patients is shown in Table 36-4.

This degree of correlation between these two means of investigation is of relevance. It implies that what is demonstrated on X-ray is of haemodynamic significance. Furthermore, the Doppler popliteal reflux test is simple, non-invasive, quick, and easy to perform. It can be used to screen patients. (There were no patients

Table 36-4

Correlation Between "Venographic Incompetence" of the Superficial Femoral Vein (S.F.V.) Deep Femoral Vein (D.F.V.), and "Ultra-Sound Incompetence" of the Popliteal Vein (P.V.)

	Ulcer alone		Ulcer, pain and swelling		Pain and swelling		Total	
	Number	Percent	Number	Percent	Number	Percent	Number	Percent
	48	100	52	100	45	100	145	100
S.F.V. + P.V.	9	17	20	39	10	23	39	27
P.V. alone	6	11	6	11	7	16	19	13
S.F.V. alone	7	15	2	4	6	11	15	10
S.F.V. + P.V. + D.F.V.	0	0	5	10	3	7	8	5
D.F.V. + P.V.	0	0	0	0	2	4	2	1
D.F.V.	0	0	0	0	1	2	1	0.5
S.F.V. + D.F.V.	0	0	0	0	0	0	0	0

within the group designated as having primary and uncomplicated varicose veins in whom popliteal incompetence was demonstrated.)

Age and Sex Distribution and Family History of Venous Problems in Patients with Grade III + Incompetence Unassociated with Venographic Evidence of Previous D.V.T

If an inherent or congenital defect of the vein or valve wall exists in this group of patients, it is possible that some confirmation might emerge in a study of associated age, sex distribution, and family history of comparable disorders. This however, was not the case.

There were a total of 25 patients for analysis in this category, of which 14 were female, and a family history of a similar condition was present in 10 of these. The mean age was 53. This and the sex distribution and family history were not dissimilar to the group as a whole.

Descending Venography and Saphenous Incompetence

Recent authors,[15,16] have emphasised the limitations of traditional clinical methods in diagnosing sapheno-femoral incompetence. When compared with incompetence assessed at the time of surgical division, Doppler assessment correlated more closely, although there were a number of "false positives" on the latter technique. It can be argued, however, that reflux of blood on declamping at the time of transection of the long saphenous vein may be insensitive. This test is employed in the supine anaesthetised patient. With the patient conscious, erect, and exercising, the degree of competence might be different. Thus it may be inappropriate to allocate "false positives" to the Doppler test.

How should incompetence of the sapheno-femoral junction be judged? It seems likely that the more tests that are applied then the more "incompetence" will be demonstrated. Descending venography provides a further test. Although it is impractical to employ this technique in all patients with suspected incompetence, it is of interest to assess the correlation with "Doppler incompetence" in the patients studied here. Table 36-5 summarises the outcome of this analysis. In 55 patients

Table 36-5
Diagnosis of Sapheno-Femoral
Incompetence

	Number	Percent
Total No. of limbs	145	100
Doppler evidence alone	27	18.5
Doppler and Venographic evidence	55	38.0
Venographic evidence	12	8.0
All	94	64.5
Recurrent*	12*	8.0

* 10 associated with Grade II plus S.F.V. incompetence.

there was correlation between the two techniques; in 27 there was Doppler evidence alone; and in a further 12 limbs there was evidence only on venography. This casts doubts on the sensitivity of both the Doppler and venography to identify incompetent valves.

Recurrent Saphenous Incompetence

Descending venography can provide information on the morphology of recurrent sapheno-femoral incompetence. There were 12 limbs in which this was demonstrated. In 10 of these this was associated with Grade II or greater reflux in the superficial femoral vein. Figure 36-10 illustrates the typical appearance when this situation exists, with dilated and tortuous varicosities emanating from the common

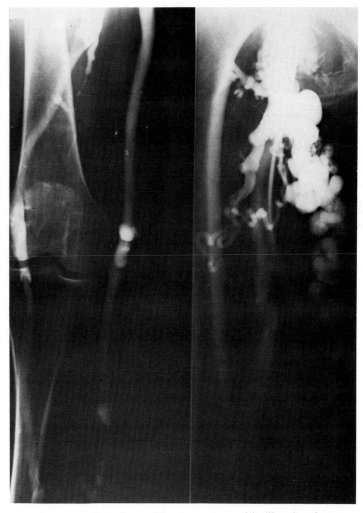

Fig. 36-10. Recurrent sapheno-femoral incompetence, with dilated and tortuous varicosities emanating from the groin. This is associated with Grade III superficial femoral vein reflux.

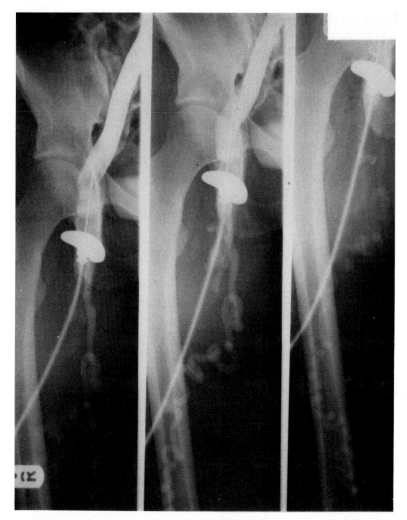

Fig. 36-11.   Recurrent sapheno-femoral reflux down a solitary tributary.

femoral. This might represent a reconstitution of veins and the co-existence of deep incompetence seems relevant. This is in contrast to the situation shown in Figure 36-11, where a solitary vessel of normal appearance has reestablished communications between the femoral and the subcutaneous veins. In these it seems likely that a tributary was missed at the time of the original operation. These data suggest two different processes in the recurrence of sapheno-femoral incompetence.

Figure 36-12 shows recurrent short saphenous incompetence in association with superficial and popliteal vein incompetence. The contrast medium refluxes down the deep veins and through tortuous dilated veins in the popliteal fossa, similar to the situation seen in the groin.

Figure 36-13 illustrates further information that may emerge. Dye does not descend down the long saphenous vein, which is competent, but through an incompetent superficial femoral and out through the thigh perforator. Simple saphenous ligation at groin level, therefore, would be ineffective.

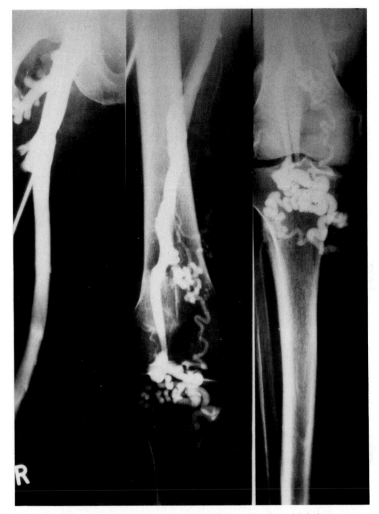

Fig. 36-12. Grade III reflux down the superficial femoral vein which in turn communicates with dilated and tortuous varicosities in the popliteal fossa, contributing to recurrent short sapheno-popliteal incompetence.

Ankle Perforator or Communicating Vein Incompetence

Incompetent perforating ankle veins were demonstrated in all but 2 of the limbs with ulcer alone, and all but 4 with ulcer and pain and swelling. It is difficult both to quantify this finding and to assess its relevance. In 33 of the 45 limbs, with the isolated pain and swelling syndrome, perforator incompetence was identified.

Clinical Relevance of Venographic Findings

These abnormalities which have been described may occur in isolation in the individual limb. In general, however, combinations of abnormalities occurred and these are now described in detail in the patients with ulcer and those with the pain and swelling syndrome alone.

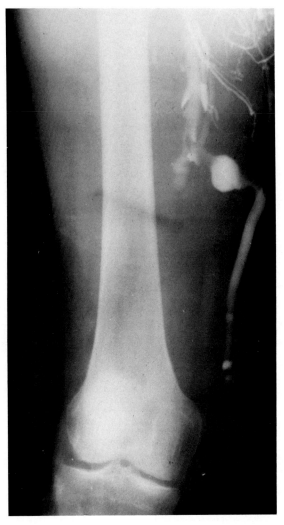

Fig. 36-13.   A descending venogram with dye refluxing down the superficial femoral vein and through a dilated and incompetent mid-thigh perforator, and filling the long saphenous vein.

Limbs with Venous Ulceration, with/without Pain and Swelling Syndrome

There were a total of 100 limbs studied in this group. The combinations of abnormalities are shown in Table 36-6. In 29 limbs there was a combination of saphenous (only 2 short saphenous) and perforator incompetence. There were 23 patients with post-phlebitic damage; 11 with associated superficial femoral incompetence in addition to a variety of saphenous and popliteal incompetence. There were 6 limbs with perforator incompetence alone. The remainder exhibited a combination of deep incompetence, perforator incompetence, and, in some, saphenous incompetence.

Table 36-6

Incidence, Venographic and
Doppler Incompetence
Ulcerated Limbs with or
without Pain and Swelling

Total Number limbs studied	100
Perf. alone	6
Perf. saph.	29
Perf. saph. S.F.V. P.V.	16
Perf. saph. S.F.V.	7
Perf. saph. P.V.	8
Perf. S.F.V. P.V.	11
Phlebitic ± other	23

NB: Perf. = Perforator; Saph. = Sapheno-
femoral (2 short saphenous); S.F.V. =
Superficial femoral vein; P.V. = Popliteal
vein (Doppler)

Limbs with Isolated Pain and Swelling Syndrome

There were 45 limbs studied. The combinations are listed in Table 36-7. For the
purposes of simplicity of analysis, the presence of ankle perforating incompetence
has been ignored as it is thought that this is unlikely to be of relevance in this
syndrome.

Table 36-7

Venographic Abnormalities—Limbs with Pain and Swelling
Syndrome (Perforator incompetence excluded)

	Number	Percent
Total number limbs	45	100
Isolated femoral incompetence	14	31
Isolated saphenous incompetence	10*	22
Post-phlebitic changes ± other	8	18
Multiple incompetence	7	15
Isolated popliteal incompetence	3	6.5
Saphenous and popliteal incompetence	3	6.5

* 3—short saphenous vein incompetence

There were 14 patients in which the only abnormality was incompetence of the
deep femoral system, and thus it seems this abnormality was a causative factor.
There were 9 limbs in which symptoms could only be ascribed to saphenous incompetence, (short saphenous in one). There were 8 patients in whom there was post-
phlebitic damage. In 2 this was an isolated finding; in 2 it was associated with both
long saphenous and femoral incompetence; in 1 there was recurrence of saphenous
incompetence; in 2 there was co-existant popliteal incompetence; in 1 isolated
femoral incompetence, and in 1 femoral and popliteal incompetence. There was 6

patients with incompetence in the popliteal vein, and in 3 limbs this was associated with saphenous incompetence. In the other 3 this was an isolated finding. There were a further 7 patients with a wide variety of abnormalities.

DECISION TO OPERATE AND CHOICE OF PROCEDURE

The surgical options are limited and sometimes contraindicated or of doubtful value. Venography may need to be supplemented by haemodynamic studies before treatment strategy can be defined. A detailed consideration of both these and the surgical procedures is outside the remit of this Chapter. In general terms, however, the operative measures are considered in sequence as they seem to apply to the groups of patients that have been recognised by venography.

Saphenous Ligation

In the authors' view this simple procedure remains the main therapeutic tool, appropriate to over 30% of cases. Its use in venous ulceration has been presented in more detail.[17] In 29% of the limbs with ulcer, saphenous and perforator incompetence were the only abnormalities. Preoperative dorsal foot vein pressure measurements before and after application of a tourniquet, which occludes the long saphenous vein, indicate that groin ligation and limited stripping re-establish relatively normal pressures and incompetence is of secondary importance. This group of patients are the easiest to treat, with the best chance of a successful outcome.

Twenty-three percent with ulcer combine saphenous and perforator incompetence with femoral reflux, without evidence of previous D.V.T. These limbs are currently under further scrutiny. However, if pressure studies suggest improved function with saphenous ligation, then it is reasonable to undertake this first. There are, however, a proportion of patients within this group that are not apparently improved by this approach. If conservative measures have failed, further procedures may be indicated, (vide infra).

For limbs with pain and swelling syndrome, the same policy is adopted. Those with symptoms associated solely with saphenous incompetence can be expected to improve. However, those with associated femoral incompetence are more difficult to manage, and the approach is similar to those with ulcer.

Ankle Perforator Ligation

Recent authors,[18] have argued the value of this procedure in venous ulceration. In this series, only 6% of limbs with ulceration had angle perforator incompetence as the only identifiable abnormality. In these perforator ligation is the logical approach.

One of the problems in assessing this abnormality is that it is demonstrable in most patients with ulcer, usually in association with other abnormalities. When co-existent with saphenous incompetence we treat the former condition first. When present with femoral incompetence, then perforator ligation is a reasonable option if healing cannot be achieved by saphenous ligation or by other more conservative measures. It should be undertaken before surgery of the femoral veins is considered, (vide infra). Perforator ligation is less likely to be effective in the presence of post-phlebitic damage.[19-21]

Surgery for Incompetence of the Superficial and Deep Femoral Vein

A surgical approach to this venographically demonstrable reflux was described as long ago as 1948 by Bauer,[22] who resected a segment of popliteal vein. The long-term results of this were disappointing.[23] Linton and Hardy[24] ligated the superficial femoral vein at a point below the union with the deep femoral. This approach would only seem of merit where valves in the associated deep femoral vein are competent—flow would thus be re-routed via a competent system. Psathakis[25] reported that a substitute valve might be devised using a tendon sling. More recently, interest has re-emerged with the suggestion that the valve itself might be repaired if not damaged by previous thrombosis.[26,27] Jones et al[28] have reported modifications of this technique. Alternatively, the incompetent superficial femoral vein can be transposed to the deep femoral vein[26] or onto the long saphenous vein.[29] Finally, a competent valve from the axillary or brachial vein can be interposed either at knee or groin level, provided the arm valves are not also incompetent.[10]

It is beyond the scope of this communication to assess the relative merits for these procedures; but in technical terms incompetence of this nature can be corrected in the short term, in some instances.[8,10,11,27,29,30] Follow-up on some of these patients has proved disappointing.[31]

In the authors' view surgery of this nature should be the last area to which attention is directed. Only when severe intractible ulceration persists after appropriate saphenous and perforator ligation and the usual conservative measures, and in the presence of at least Grade II reflux, should it be considered. There should be preoperative haemodynamic studies to confirm dysfunction. In the authors' experience this sort of case is unusual. We have operated on patients with femoral incompetence, both with the "primary" form and secondary to previous thrombosis, but under the latter the operation may be difficult to perform.

With respect to the pain and swelling syndrome the presence of femoral and popliteal reflux as an isolated abnormality is identifiable. Most of these patients can be treated with reassurance and compression stockings. Only rarely is surgery of this magnitude indicated for this syndrome. It should be preceded by haemodynamic studies to confirm the relevance of the venographic appearances.

The syndrome of thigh symptoms with isolated deep femoral incompetence described above has been treated by the authors by ligation of this vein at its junction with the superficial femoral vein. This has achieved a satisfactory outcome in the short term.

Reconstruction for the Occlusive Sequelae of Previous Thrombosis

In our experience this is infrequently feasible or indicated. When the pain and selling syndrome is associated with iliac occlusion or stenosis, the cross-over saphenous graft has been found to be of value.[32.33] This should be preceded by appropriate venous, capacitance, and outflow studies to demonstrate obstruction.[34] Other procedures have been described to alleviate post-phlebitic damage in the thigh.[35-37] In our series, cases for this sort of reconstruction were not apparent, principally because of poor proximal or distal vessel unsuitable for anastomosis.

ACKNOWLEDGEMENTS

We should like to thank Mr. B. Jennings for the photographic work and Mrs. L. A. Clynes for secretarial assistance.

REFERENCES

1. Nicolaides AN, Miles C, Zimmerman H: The non-invasive assessment of venous insufficiency, in Greenhalgh RM (ed): Hormones and Vascular Disease. Bath, Pitman Press, 1981, pp 219–237
2. Lea Thomas M: Phlebography of the lower limb. Edinburgh, Churchill Livingstone, 1982
3. Ferris EB, Kistner RL: Femoral vein reconstruction in the managements of chronic venous insufficiency. Arch Surgery 117:1571–1579, 1982
4. Lundstrom B, Ostermann G: Assessment of deep venous insufficiency by descending phlebography. Acta Radiologica 24:375–379, 1983
5. Lea Thomas M, Keeling FP, Ackroyd JS: Descending phlebography: A comparison of three methods and an assessment of the normal range of deep vein reflux (in Press) 1984
6. Lea Thomas M, Walters HL: Metrizamide in Venography. Br Med J Part II:1036, 1978
7. Walters HL, Clemerson J, Browse NL, Lea Thomas M: 125.I fibrinogen uptake following phlebography of the leg. Comparison of ionic and nonionic contrast media. Radiology 135 3:619–621, 1980
8. Kistner RL: Transvenous repair of the incompetent femoral vein valve in venous problems in Bergan JJ, Yao JST (eds): Chicago Year Book Medical, 1978, pp 492–509
9. Herman RJ, Neiman HL, Yao JST, et al: Descending venography: A method of evaluating lower extremity venous valvular function. Radiology 137 (i): 63–69, 1980
10. Taheri SA, Lazar L, Elias SM: Surgical treatment of post-phlebitic syndrome. Br J Surg 69 (Suppl.): 59–62, 1982
11. Taheri SA, Lazar L, Elias SM: Status of vein valve transplant after 12 months. Arch Surg 117:1313–1317, 1982
12. Lindhagen A, Bergquist D, Hallbook T: Deep venous insufficiency after post-operative thrombosis diagnosed with 125.I labelled fibrinogen uptake test. Br J Surg 71:515–519, 1984
13. Kistner RL: Primary venous valve incompetence of the leg. Amer J Surg 140:218–224, 1980
14. Raju S: Venous insufficiency of the lower limb and stasis ulceration. Ann Surg 197:688, 1983
15. McIrvine AJ, Corbett CRR, Aston ND, et al: The demonstration of sapheno-femoral incompetence; Doppler ultrasound compared with standard clinical tests. Br J Surg 71:506–508, 1984
16. Chan A, Chisholm I, Royle JP: The use of directional Doppler ultrasound in the assessment of sapheno-femoral incompetence. Aust NZ J Surg 53:399–402, 1983
17. Sethia KK, Darke SG: Long saphenous incompetence as a cause of venous ulceration. Br J Surg 71:754–755, 1984

18. Negus D, Friedgood A: The effective management of venous ulceration. Br J Surg 70:623–627, 1983
19. Recek E: A critical appraisal of the role of ankle perforators for the genesis of venous ulcers in the lower leg. J Cardiovasc 12:45, 1971
20. Burnand KG, Lea Thomas M, O'Donnell E, et al: Relation between post-phlebitic changes in the deep veins and results of surgical treatment of venous ulcers. Lancet 1:936–938, 1976
21. Burnand KG, O'Donnell TF, Lea Thomas M, Browse NL: The relative importance of incompetent communicating veins in the production of varicose veins. Surgery 82:9, 1977
22. Bauer G: The aetiology of leg ulcers and their treatment by resection of the popliteal vein. J Internat Chirugie 8:937–961, 1948
23. Lindhagen A, Hallbook T: Venous function in the leg 20 years after ligation and partial resection of the popliteal vein. Acta Chir Scand 148:131–134, 1982
24. Linton RR, Hardy IB: Post-thrombotic syndrome of the lower extremity—treatment by interruption of the superficial femoral vein and ligation and stripping of the long and short saphenous veins. Surgery 24:452, 1948
25. Psathakis N: Has the "substitute valve" of the popliteal vein solved the problem of venous insufficiency of the lower extremity? J Cardiovasc Surg 9:64, 1968
26. Kistner RL: Transvenous repair of the incompetent femoral vein valve in venous problems in Bergan JJ, Yao JST (eds): Chicago Year Book Medical, 1978, 492–509
27. Kistner RL, Sparkuhl MD: Surgery in acute and chronic venous disease. Surgery 85:31–43, 1979
28. Jones JW, Elliott F, Kerstein MD: Triangular venous valvuloplasty. Arch Surg 177:1250–1251, 1982
29. Queral LA, Whitehouse WM, Flinn WR, et al: Surgical correction of chronic deep venous insufficiency by valvular transposition. Surgery 87:688–695, 1980
30. Huse JB, Nabseth DC, Bush HL, et al: Direct venous surgery for venous valvular insufficiency of the lower extremity. Arch Surg 118:719–723, 1983
31. Johnson ND, Queral LA, Flinn WR, et al: Late objective assessment of venous valve surgery. Arch Surg 116:1461–1466, 1981
32. Palmar EC, Esperon R: Vein transplants and grafts in the surgical treatment of the post-phlebitic syndrome. J Cardiovasc Surg 1:94–107, 1960
33. Dale WA: Cross-over vein graft for relief of ilio-femoral venous block. Surgery 57:608, 1965
34. Killewich LA, Martin R, Cramer M, et al: Pathophysiology of venous claudication. J Vasc Surg 1:502–511, 1984
35. Warner R, Thayer TR: Transplantation of the saphenous vein for post-phlebitic stasis. Surgery 35:867–876, 1954
36. Husni EA: In situ sapheno-popliteal bypass graft for incompetence of the femoral and popliteal veins. Surg Gynaecol Obstet 130:279–284, 1970
37. Husni EA: Venous reconstruction in post-phlebitic disease. Circulation 43–44 (Suppl. 1):147–150, 1971

Andreas P. Barabas
and R. Macfarlane

37

The Use of Peroperative Venography in the Management of Difficult Primary and Recurrent Varicose Veins

It is common for varicose veins to recur after treatment. In one study of 222 limbs treated by surgery, 45% of the patients required additional treatment within one year.[1] Poor operative technique and incorrect preoperative diagnosis are often blamed, but recurrence rates are high in specialists as well. In a random trial of 500 patients comparing "enthusiastic injection-compression treatment" with expert surgery, Hobbs[2] found a failure rate at six years of 14% for surgery and 76% for compression sclerotherapy. Many of the remainder, while showing some improvement, required further treatment. High failure rates probably reflect the general ignorance of the aetiology of superficial varicose veins of the legs.

In recent years venography has played an increasing role in the management of varicose veins. Standard preoperative venography using a single injection into the dorsum of the foot is useful for the assessment of deep veins,[3] but swamping of the superficial veins with contrast makes accurate localisation of the perforating veins difficult. However, when clinical examination indicates likely sites for connections between superficial and deep veins, more selective studies are possible; gastrocnemius veins,[4] mid-thigh perforators,[5] and vulval varicosities[6] have all been successfully demonstrated by venography.

Venography may also be performed at operation, and Hobbs[7] has described a technique for accurate localisation of the saphenopopliteal junction. Intraosseous venography has also been used to identify incompetent calf perforators.[8] In both these techniques venography is performed as a separate procedure before towelling the legs for surgery. Skin-markers must be used to relate the venogram to the leg at operation.

Our technique differs from those previously described in being truly peroperative. We use roentgenogram equipment already available in the operating theatre for cholangiography and orthopaedic surgery. For several years it has been an integral part of all difficult varicose vein surgery, just as operative cholangiography is part of surgery for gallstones. It has been found to be both simple and safe.

DIAGNOSTIC TECHNIQUES AND ASSESSMENT
PROCEDURES IN VASCULAR SURGERY

© 1985 Grune & Stratton
ISBN 0-8089-1721-8 All rights reserved

PATIENTS

Peroperative venography is only suitable for patients with superficial varicose veins: either difficult primary or recurrent. Those with varicose veins secondary to deep-vein thrombosis are excluded on clinical grounds, or in doubtful cases, with the aid of deep-vein venography. We have used peroperative venography in approximately 100 legs, including in almost all varicose veins recurring after surgery, in all explorations of the popliteal fossa, and in patients with equivocal tourniquet tests.

Patients admitted for surgery are first assessed clinically. If after tourniquet tests and Doppler studies there is no doubt about the source of incompetence, venography during operation is not required. Venography is only used to answer diagnostic questions unsolved by clinical examination. These questions will give a guide to the sites of injection of contrast material during the operation. For instance, where varicose veins can be controlled in the thigh, attention is focused on groin and mid-thigh regions rather than the popliteal fossa.

Preparation for venography includes consent for radiology and the exclusion of iodine sensitivity. The varicose veins are marked with indelible ink.

EQUIPMENT

The radiologic equipment used is a Philips C arm image intensifier, although any other suitable equipment already available in the operating theatre will serve equally well for venography (Fig. 37-1). In the majority of cases, we only screen during venography, but in cases of special interest, or if a permanent record needs to be kept, the equipment easily adapts to take films as well. Theatre personnel take the usual precautions against exposure to radiation.

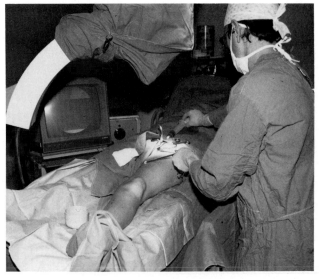

Fig. 37-1. Radiologic equipment.

TECHNIQUE OF PEROPERATIVE VENOGRAPHY

Apart from being placed on a radiolucent operating table, preparations are exactly the same as for varicose vein surgery without radiology. Under general anaesthetic and after standard skin preparation and draping, an 18-gauge metal cannula with a bulbous tip is inserted and tied into one of the marked varicosities. Contrast suitable for venography (initially we used 65% Urografin, but more recently Isopaque Amin 200) is then injected via a disposable syringe and connecting tubing (Fig. 37-2), and its progress monitored via the image intensifier. Points of interest may be marked on the skin using long artery forceps with a dental swab dipped in Bonney's Blue.

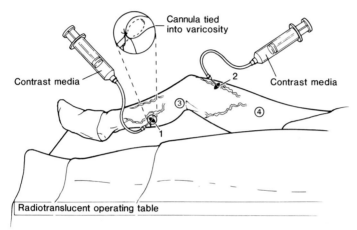

Fig. 37-2. 1 and 2 show sites of injection of contrast media. The site marked 3 is used for better visualisation of the saphenopopliteal junction, and site 4 for injection at the "T" junction.

Sites of Injection

In all patients with below-knee varicosities, at least one site is selected for injection at the watershed area between short and long saphenous veins (Fig. 37-2) at about mid-calf level. Contrast media is injected upwards to see whether it will preferentially fill the short or long saphenous system. If short saphenous incompetence is strongly suspected either on clinical grounds or after the first injection into a calf varicose vein, a further injection is usually made closer to the popliteal fossa. The exact site of the saphenopopliteal junction is thus identified and marked on the skin for later exploration. Injection from the "watershed mid-leg" site can be made easily downwards as well, and will show ankle perforators. However, as we use this technique mainly in primary varicose veins with normal deep veins, we rarely require to demonstrate these.

In all patients with varicosities above knee, at least one injection of contrast is made into a prominent thigh varicosity, in the direction of the groin. Commonly, contrast enters the deep vein via the nearest mid-thigh perforator. Either occlusion of the mid-thigh perforator by pressure, or exploration of this site and a second injection ("The T junction injection") is then required to see if there is a connection with the femoral vein in the groin.

If a major superficial vein is followed for considerable distances, repositioning of the cannula is often useful, as this reduces the number of minor tributaries that become swamped with contrast.

In most cases, one or two sites of injection suffice to answer all diagnostic questions and to aid surgery. In a few cases, further injections of contrast have to be made, the sites of which differ according too diagnostic or operative needs. Some examples of these often interesting and challenging cases will be described later.

Selective injections go a long way to reduce the problem of interpretation of venography, but two further simple procedures are worth describing; firstly, compression of the skin with artery forceps ("The 3-D effect"), and secondly, calf squeezing.

Compression with Artery Forceps

Even with selective injection of contrast, difficulties may arise correlating the X-ray picture and the anatomical position in the leg, because of the two dimensional nature of radiology. Veins identified on the venogram but which have not been already marked on the skin may be accurately located from a two-dimensional image by compression of the overlying skin with the artery forceps (Fig. 37-3).

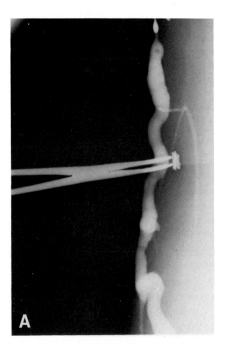 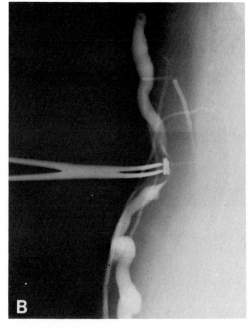

Fig. 37-3. (A) Artery forceps lie in the plane of the vein on roentgenogram, but have not localized it on the skin. (B) Vein correctly located in three dimensions. With permission of the Department of Medical Illustration, Ipswich Hospital, Ispwich, England.

Squeezing the Calf

Especially with recurrent varicose veins, a network of varicosities may overlie the deep vein. In the anaesthetized patient, the flow of contrast in the deep veins is often sluggish, and pin-point localization between the varicosities and the deep vein is therefore difficult. We have found that squeezing the calf will immediately clear all contrast from the deep vein and allow exact visualization of the junction (Fig. 37-4).

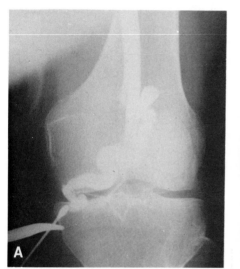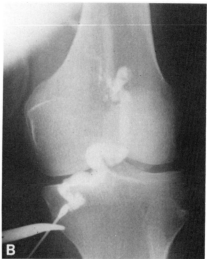

Fig. 37-4. Recurrent short saphenous incompetence: (A) Contrast filling the deep vein, (B) Saphenopopliteal junction pinpointed after squeezing the calf to flush out the deep vein. With permission of the Department of Medical Illustration, Ipswich Hospital, Ipswich, England.

Following venography, connections between superficial varicose veins and deep veins are ligated, and the superficial varicose veins avulsed. One hundred mL of contrast should be available for radiology, and bilateral screening time should not exceed five minutes.

RESULTS

In this chapter we do not propose to give a detailed analysis of all results, but to show examples of how this investigation helped in the management of specific groups of patients.

Saphenopopliteal Junction

This is a difficult area, even at first operation, because of the wide variation in location of the junction. Hobbs[7] has described a method for accurate localization of the saphenopopliteal junction and this has been widely accepted by others.[9] Peroperative venography too is ideal to locate it precisely (Fig. 37-4).

Groin Recurrence

In line with other studies on recurrent varicose veins,[10,11] a varicose tributary connecting with the groin is the most common finding in our experience. We have been surprised to find how often this occurred, when recurrence appeared to arise in mid-thigh level, and even after most rigorous clinical testing no clear evidence of a connection to the saphenofemoral junction could be found. This is probably because of the subfascial course of the veins in the upper thigh. However, even in those cases where there is a strong clinical suspicion of recurrence in the region of the groin, venography is still of considerable value. The surgeon is able to explore the severely scarred fossa ovalis with much greater confidence once the site of connection is both proved and localized.

Mid-thigh Perforators

Particular caution is needed when investigating the "T junction" area. The patient in Figure 37-5a developed recurrent varicose veins following surgery to strip the long saphenous vein. An ascending peroperative venogram shows to mid-thigh perforators (black arrows) as the apparent source of recurrence. (The deep vein here

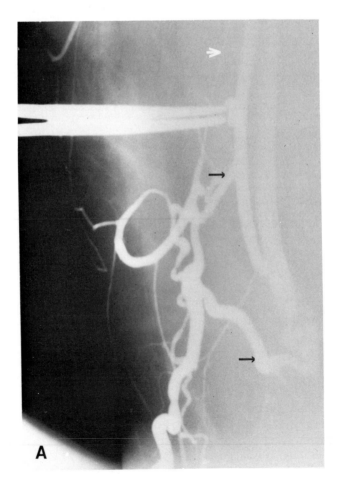

A

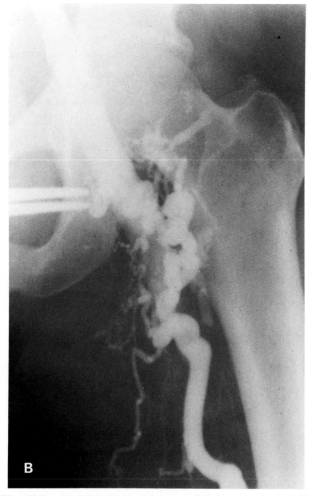

Fig. 37-5. (A) Mid-thigh perforators (Black arrows), and (B) groin recurrence. See text for details. With permission of the Department of Medical Illustration, Ipswich Hospital, Ipswich, England.

is double; a not uncommon finding.[3]) When these perforators had been ligated a further venogram was performed. Figure 37-5b now clearly shows the main source of recurrence in the groin. This vein is barely seen on the first film (white arrow) because of the rapid flow to the deep vein through the perforators. It is for this reason that a repeat study is necessary after mid-thigh perforators are ligated. Alternatively they can be temporarily occluded by compression.

Vulval Varicosities

These may appear either after previous groin exploration or as a primary condition in association with the pelvic congestion syndrome.

The patient in Figure 37-6a had previously had bilateral flush saphenofemoral ligations and the long saphenous vein stripped. She presented with extensive vulval

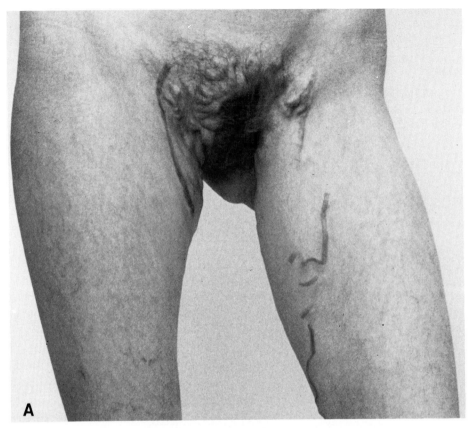

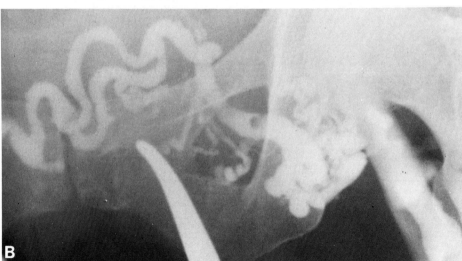

Fig. 37-6. (A) Extensive vulval varicose veins extending onto the anterior abdominal wall. (B) Peroperative venogram demonstrating the connection with the femoral vein in the groin. With permission of the Department of Medical Illustration, Ipswich Hospital, Ipswich, England.

varicosities extending on to the anterior abdominal wall. A peroperative venogram both confirmed patent femoral and iliac veins, and that the recurrence was entirely in the groins (Fig. 37-6b). After flush ligations, reinjection showed no connection with the pelvic veins.

In contrast, injection of vulval varicosities in a similar patient who had previously had two groin explorations, confirms communications with the pelvic veins (Fig. 37-7). In addition to dealing with the connection to the femoral vein, attention in such patients is also needed to the internal pudendal, obturator, and round ligament veins.[6]

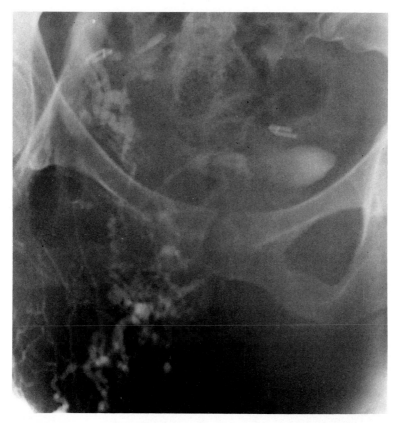

Fig. 37-7. Peroperative venogram of a patient with vulval varicosities demonstrating connections with the pelvic veins. With permission of the Department of Medical Illustration, Ipswich Hospital, Ipswich, England.

Selective Preservation of the Long Saphenous Vein

Controversy exists about whether the long saphenous vein should ever be removed in cases of varicose veins, as it may be required later for bypass grafting. Further weight for preservation of the long saphenous vein is added by the evidence that there is an association in middle-aged men with atherosclerotic disease.[12] However, a controlled trial of preserving or removing the long saphenous vein in

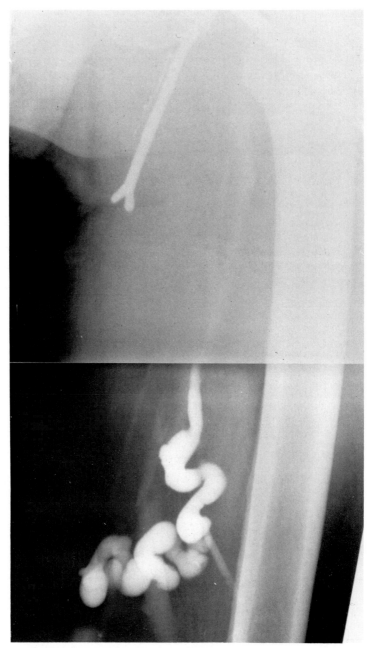

Fig. 37-8. (Top) competent long saphenous vein, and (bottom) varicose veins arising from a mid-thigh perforator. With permission of the Department of Medical Illustration, Ipswich Hospital, Ipswich, England.

cases of severe varicosities has clearly shown that there is a higher recurrence if the vein is not removed.[13] Venography may provide a solution to this problem, and we are currently engaged in a study using operative venography in selecting patients in whom the long saphenous vein can be spared. The descending peroperative venogram (Fig. 37-8) confirms a competent long saphenous vein, and an ascending injection from the knee locates the perforator, at mid-thigh level, responsible for the varicose veins.

DISCUSSION

Peroperative venography is a simple technique to master, and can be used on all but the smallest varicosities. Superficial thrombophlebitis and deep venous thrombosis are well recognized complications of venography,[14] but we have experienced neither of these. This is probably because most of the contrast stays in the superficial system, and these veins are subsequently avulsed.

Venography does not add significantly to the length of operation once the technique is familiar. The veins that are cannulated already require avulsion, and by using the image intensifier there is no delay while waiting for films to be developed. Accurate localization of connections with the deep veins allows the incision to be placed precisely at the correct point, and a confident diagnosis, combined with accurate localization, is of great benefit when reexploring groin or popliteal fossa.

We believe that venography during surgery is both more logical and more effective than other techniques previously described. The procedure is painless, does not require double preparation of the legs, and is performed by the surgeon who has specific diagnostic questions to be answered. There is no need to use skin markers, rulers, or lateral views to relate the leg to the two-dimensional X-ray film. In addition, the effectiveness of operation can be confirmed by repeating the injection after the connections with the deep veins have been tied. As Figure 37-5 has shown, single-injection venography does not always give the full picture.

Of nonmalignant conditions operated on in England, varicose veins recur most commonly. Recurrence rates for two other common surgical conditions, inguinal hernia and cholecystectomy, have both been reduced greatly by attention to technical operative detail. We feel that recurrence rates following treatment of varicose veins could similarly be reduced. Although an adequate dissection is probably the most important factor in reducing recurrence rates, diagnostic failures represent one area requiring further improvement.

Only long-term follow-up will show whether a significant reduction in recurrence is achieved, and perhaps help in the understanding of the reasons for recurrence after what appears to be an adequate operation.

ACKNOWLEDGMENTS

Our grateful thanks to Dr. R. Godwin and the staff of the X-ray Department, West Suffolk Hospital, and to the Photographic Department Ipswich Hospital.

REFERENCES

1. Doran FSA, White M: A clinical trial designed to discover if the primary treatment of varicose veins should be by Fegan's method or by an operation. Br J Surg 62:72, 1975
2. Hobbs JT: A random trial of the treatment of varicose veins by surgery and sclerotherapy, in Hobbs JT (ed): Treatment of Venous Disorders. Edinburgh, R&R Clark, 1977, p 195
3. Wesolowski SA, Greenfield H, Sawyer PN, et al: Diagnostic value of phlebography in venous disorders of the lower extremity. Cardiovasc Surg (Suppl) 133, 1965
4. Doran FSA, Barkat S: The management of recurrent varicose veins. Ann R Coll Surg Engl 63:432, 1981
5. Corbett CR, McIrvine AJ, Aston NO, et al: The use of varicography to identify the sources of incompetence in recurrent varicose veins. Ann R Coll Surg Engl 66:412, 1984
6. Craig O, Hobbs JT: Vulval phlebography in the pelvic congestion syndrome. Clin Radiol 25:517, 1974
7. Hobbs JT: Peroperative venography to ensure accurate sapheno-popliteal vein ligation. Br Med J 280:1578, 1980
8. Townsend J, Jones H, Williams JE: Detection of incompetent perforating veins by venography at operation. Br Med J 3:583, 1967
9. Royle JP: Operative treatment of varicose veins, in Greenhalgh RM (ed): Vascular Surgical Techniques. London, Butterworths, 1984, p 255
10. Haeger K: Technique of high ligation of the long saphenous vein. Acta Chir Scand 122:85, 1961
11. Rivlin S: Recurrent varicose veins. Med J Aust 1:1097, 1966
12. Ducimetiere P, Richard JL, Pequignot G, et al: Varicose veins: A risk factor for atherosclerotic disease in middle-aged men? Int J Epidemiol 10:329, 1981
13. Munn SR, Morton JB, Macbeth WAAG, et al: To strip or not to strip the long saphenous vein? A varicose veins trial. Br J Surg 68:426, 1981
14. Bettman MA, Paulin S: Leg phlebography: The incidence, nature and modification of undesirable side effects. Radiology 122:101, 1977

David Negus

38

Assessment of the Deep Venous System

The past fifteen years have seen an explosion in both invasive and noninvasive methods of investigating the peripheral vascular system and the introduction of comprehensively equipped vascular laboratories to most major centres of vascular surgery. These developments have largely been directed towards the investigation of peripheral arterial disorders, in particular the cerebral and lower limb circulation. Disorders of the peripheral veins are less often treated in highly specialised units and the investigation and management of deep venous thrombosis also comes within the province of the general surgeon as well as the peripheral vascular specialist. The same applies to the investigation and management of venous ulceration and the post-thrombotic syndrome.

This chapter is not intended to be an exhaustive account of the assessment of the deep venous system; rather it is a working handbook indicating which of the many investigations have been found to be most useful.

Patients presenting with acute deep vein thrombosis are best investigated at the bedside and investigation of the post-thrombotic syndrome can be conveniently carried out by the vascular technician and surgeon working together in the consulting room. Equipment is therefore mobile, being mounted on a trolley. In addition to the equipment, one or more "laboratory bench books" are important. There are now a number of excellent textbooks available, including the present one, and although references have been included in this account where appropriate, I have also added a bibliography in which these books are listed.

EQUIPMENT

A bewildering variety of instruments is available, for both invasive and noninvasive evaluations, including Doppler ultrasound, photoplethysmography, plethysmography (by which volume changes of the limb may be measured by water displacement, changes in electrical conductivity (impedance), air, or strain gauge), direct measurement of dorsal foot vein pressure, thermography, ^{125}Iodine fibrinogen uptake, and finally venography.

DIAGNOSTIC TECHNIQUES AND ASSESSMENT
PROCEDURES IN VASCULAR SURGERY

© 1985 Grune & Stratton
ISBN 0-8089-1721-8 All rights reserved

Doppler Ultrasound

Though a simple hand-held instrument, such as that manufactured by Sonicaid, is adequate for most investigations, zero crossing detection circuitry helps more precise evaluation and a number of instruments are listed by Needham.[1] Frequency analysis, though more accurate than zero crossing, is not necessary in studying the venous system. We use the Medasonics D10 instrument with two bidirectional pencil probes working at 5 and 10 MHz. The former is suitable for venous investigations. These probes are "bidirectional"; a button on the probe allowing either forward or reverse flow to become dominant on the amplifier or in the headphones, though this does not affect the zero-crossing recorder.

Photoplethysmograph (PPG)

The Medasonics instrument (PPG 13) is designed to "stack" with the Doppler ultrasound instrument and strain gauge plethysmograph and its output can be fed into the same recording system (Fig. 38-1).

Although PPG was first reported in the 1930s,[2,3] its use in investigating the venous system is of more recent introduction.[4] The instrument consists of a light-weight probe that contains both the light source and light detector, and this is attached to the skin by double-backed transparent adhesive tape. Light from the emitter is directed into the skin and the detector records changes in the intensity of the light that emerges from the adjacent skin. In the a.c. mode, changes of blood flow enables the instrument to be used as a pulse recorder. For venous assessment a slow changing d.c. signal is used and this reflects total blood value of the underlying skin rather than pulsation. The ideal wavelength is 805 nm.

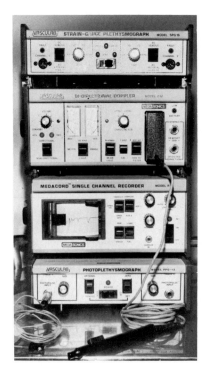

Fig. 38-1. The instruments: Strain-gauge plethysmograph, bidirectional Doppler ultrasound, chart recorder, and photoplethysmograph.

Strain-Gauge Plethysmography

Limb volume changes can be used to evaluate limb blood flow, or in the presence of a constant arterial input, venous obstruction. Inflation of a proximal cuff to 60 mmHg produces venous distension; normally sudden release of this cuff leads to rapid "deflation" of the limb with a steep down-slope on the recording system. Varying degrees of venous obstruction, whether chronic or from acute thrombosis, will flatten this slope to variable extent. Impedance plethysmography has been shown to increase the specificity and sensitivity of Doppler ultrasound examination in the detection of acute deep-vein thrombosis[5] and strain-gauge plethysmography also has strong advocates.[6] We use the Medasonics Indium-Gallium strain gauge (SPG 16), which is simple and reliable. The Indium-Gallium strain-gauges are long lasting, unlike the mercury-in-rubber type.

Recording

A variety of chart recorders are available. At present we use a single-channel instrument with a constant speed of 25 mm/sec (Medasonics R11). A twin channel chart recorder is not essential for day to day clinical work, but the Medasonics model (R12 A) has the advantage of variable speed (1–5–25 mm/sec) and a speed of 5 mm/sec is more appropriate to PPG recording.

An oscilloscope is useful and saves unnecessary waste of paper by the chart recorder while appropriate adjustments are made to obtain a satisfactory trace.

Computerised record keeping is now available and IBM has designed a system to link with the Medasonics instruments. This is expensive and unlikely to be necessary except in highly specialised vascular laboratories. PMS Instruments have developed a simpler and cheaper system incorporating a BBC micro-computer. A single oscilloscope will show both the trace being recorded and is available for computer data. This system will obviate the need for a chart recorder as the print out provides this facility and a programme is being developed that will enable individual patient data to be recorded and kept in the clinical records and also series of data to be stored for subsequent retrieval.

Sphygmomanometer Cuffs

A series of Hokanson cuffs are essential to any noninvasive vascular assessment system. The small finger and toe cuffs are not necessary in investigations of venous disorders, but thigh, calf, and ankle cuffs are essential. Medasonics have developed an automated system of cuff inflation. While this may save time and effort in a busy vascular laboratory, it is not necessary.

Ultrasound

B mode ultrasound imaging is often useful in detecting a Baker's cyst of the knee which may mimic deep vein thrombosis.

Other Available Methods

A relatively small selection of the many methods currently available is required. Other noninvasive systems include the Thulesius water-bath[7,8] which is an accurate method of measuring volume changes in the lower leg and foot and is particularly useful in research into compression stockings. We have been deterred from using it in a clinical situation by the problems associated with changing the water and the possible risk of cross-infection. Infrared thermography[9-11] has been shown to compare well with venography in the diagnosis of deep-vein thrombosis. At present its disadvantage is expense, though cheaper pencil probes are being developed. Valuable isotope methods include the ^{125}I-fibrinogen uptake test[12,13] and the 99m Tc-plasmin test.[14,15] The former continues to be used as a research tool in the diagnosis of established deep-vein thrombosis. It has the considerable disadvantage in clinical practice of delay in obtaining the final result; the 99m Tc-plasmin test has been developed to overcome this problem. Like the ^{125}I-fibrinogen test, the 99m Tc-plasmin test correlates well with venography.

Two other invasive tests should be mentioned for completeness. Foot venous pressure measurement[16,17] has a long and distinguished history and is a most useful method of assessing the function of the "calf muscle pump." However, its good correlation with PPG[18] makes the latter, which is truly noninvasive and far less time-consuming, much preferable for routine clinical use. Venography has the disadvantage of pain and thrombogenicity of the original contrast media.[19,20] The development of the new low osmolality contrast media, which include medrizamide and iopamidol are improvements[21,22] and an experienced radiologist can complete the examination in only a few minutes, which makes this method more acceptable than it previously was.

ACUTE DEEP-VEIN THROMBOSIS

The patient may present with obvious physical signs in the leg; oedema, tenderness, and increased temperature; with doubtful signs in the leg; or with pulmonary embolism. Although Doppler ultrasound can be used for rapid assessment where pulmonary embolism has occurred or is suspected, the safest approach for these patients is to perform immediate bilateral ascending venography, for only this investigation can show whether there is further loose thrombus with a risk of further embolisation. Patients presenting with a grossly swollen thigh and lower leg require immediate and full anticoagulation.

Noninvasive investigation is most useful in patients who present with doubtful physical signs and Doppler ultrasound is the most useful single investigation.

Doppler Ultrasound

The patient is positioned sitting up in bed at an angle of 45° with the ankle resting on a pillow so that the calf hangs free (Fig. 38-2).[23] The probe is placed over the common femoral artery, which is easily identified by its pulsation, and then

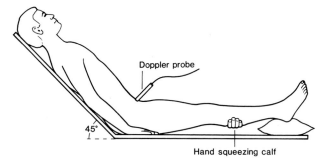

Fig. 38-2. The investigation of suspected deep-vein thrombosis; to show patient position; the Doppler probe over the common femoral vein and calf compression.

moved a little medially to lie over the femoral vein. The patient is asked to breathe deeply and, if the iliac system is patent, respiratory swings in venous flow can easily be heard. The bidirectional instrument is ideal, as arterial pulsations can be damped out. With the probe in the same position, the calf muscles are firmly compressed and a patent popliteal and femoral vein will transmit the pulse wave to produce a signal at the femoral vein (Fig. 38-3). Doppler ultrasound is accurate in detecting obstructive thrombi from the popliteal vein to the vena cava, but cannot detect small calf thrombi. Its accuracy can be improved by the use of plethysmography.[24]

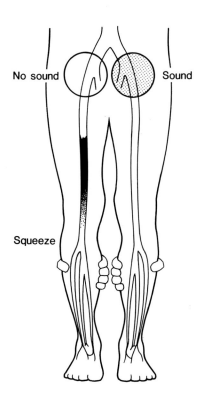

Fig. 38-3. Doppler ultrasound assessment of deep-vein patency.

Plethysmography

Plethysmography is time consuming and so undesirable. Venography is preferable in cases of doubt, reserving strain-gauge plethysmography for those few patients with a history of iodine reaction or who refuse to undergo radiologic investigation. The patient is positioned with the legs elevated, in order to empty the veins as much as possible and, after positioning the strain gauges round the calf, a thigh sphygmomanometer cuff is inflated to 60 mmHg. This venous occlusion produces gradual distension of the calf and when this has become stable after about two minutes, the thigh cuff is suddenly released. A rapid fall in the plethysmograph trace indicates patent veins. As an alternative, the ^{125}I-fibrinogen uptake test or the 99 mTc-plasmin test may be used if either of these is available.

VENOUS ULCERATION AND THE POSTTHROMBOTIC SYNDROME

After clinical investigation, noninvasive assessment of these patients is carried out in the out patient clinic. The following account describes our routine for examining a patient presenting with oedema and/or ulceration.

The patient is examined lying and standing in a good light, looking for abdominal pathology and the "Caput Medusae" veins indicative of vena caval obstruction. Similarly the groins are inspected for the presence of collateral veins that indicate iliac venous obstruction. Leg circumference is measured; an increase in circumference indicates gross deep venous incompetence or proximal obstruction. Peripheral pulses are examined. It is important to exclude arterial insufficiency in all patients presenting with ulceration, and oedematous ankles may make ulcers impossible to feel. Doppler ultrasound, using an arterial probe, must be used in cases of doubt in combination with an ankle sphygmomanometer cuff, and the ankle pulse pressures recorded. The patency of the iliac and femoropopliteal veins is assessed with Doppler ultrasound as has been described.

A history of "venous claudication" is strongly suggestive of iliac venous obstruction and this should be further investigated by a "stepping test"; a patient with significant obstruction to venous return develops severe congestive aching in the calves on marking time at one step a second and this usually prevents further exercise after two or three minutes.[25] Confirmation of iliac venous obstruction is by measurement of femoral venous pressures, both at rest and on exercise, which can conveniently be performed at the same time as perfemoral iliac phlebography. Normal femoral venous pressure, in the horizontal position, is <9 mmHg and on exercise the rise in venous pressure is <2 mmHg.[26]

The remainder of the examination and investigations are performed with the patient either standing or sitting. With the patient standing on a "mounting block," the legs are examined for the presence of superficial varicose veins and saphenous incompetence. Simple detection of a tapping impulse is usually sufficient for accurate diagnosis of the latter, but in cases of doubt Doppler ultrasound can be used in a modification of the Trendelenberg test.[27] A prominent calf varix is marked; the leg is elevated and a high thigh occluding cuff positioned; the patient then stands and the Doppler probe is placed over the prominent varix; finally the cuff is released and venous incompetence detected by audible reflux.

Dilated supramalleolar venules, "the ankle venous flare," are indicative of direct calf perforating vein incompetence, the "ankle blow outs," which are responsible for the most venous ulcers.[28] Finally foot and ankle cyanosis in the erect position may indicate deep venous incompetence.

PPG

If the presenting symptom is oedema, rather than ulceration, then lymph-oedema must be excluded. The patient sits on the edge of the examination couch or on an appropriately high stool with the leg hanging down and the PPG probe is attached to the ankle with double-backed adhesive tape either behind or in front of the long saphenous vein, not over it, as this will give a false reading (Fig. 38-4a). The

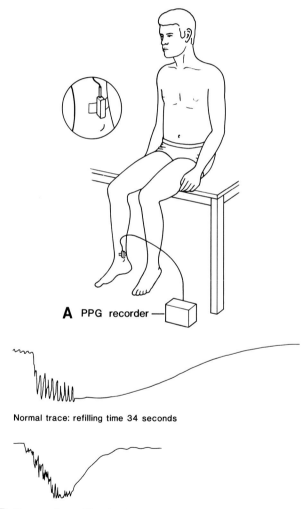

A PPG recorder

Normal trace: refilling time 34 seconds

B Venous reflux: refilling time 9 seconds

Fig. 38-4. (A) Photoplethysmograph (PPG): Patient position and probe attachment by double-backed transparent adhesive tape. (B) PPG: Normal vein refilling and reflux.

instrument is set to the d.c. mode and the gain and stylus positions are adjusted with the patient's leg hanging motionless. The patient is then asked to move the ankle briskly up and down thus activating "the calf muscle pump." Normally this produces a fall in subcutaneous venular volume after five or six pumps of the calf muscles.

When the PPG trace has stabilised at its lowest point, the patient is asked to stop moving and to relax and the recovery time is noted. This should normally be more than 21 seconds,[29] a more rapid recovery time indicating some degree of venous incompetence (Fig. 38-4b). PPG can be used for more precise evaluation of the cause of such incompetence by placing venous occlusion cuffs in varous positions to occlude either saphenous or perforating veins or both. Although this is sometimes useful, the results can be more difficult to interpret than Doppler ultrasound, and the latter is preferable for detailed examination of venous incompetence.

If the patient with oedema has no visible varicose veins or venous flare and a normal PPG recovery time, it can confidently be stated that the oedema is not of venous origin. In the absence of cardiac or renal causes and in a normally nourished patient, lymphoedema can then be diagnosed by exclusion and confirmed by lymphography if this is felt necessary.

Doppler Ultrasound Examination

With the patient erect the Doppler probe can be used to assess competence of each of the important systems: saphenous veins, the direct calf and ankle perforating veins, and the popliteal and femoral veins.

Saphenous Veins

Examination of long saphenous incompetence by the modified Trendelenberg test using Doppler ultrasound has already been described. Examination for short saphenous reflux is carried out at the same time as examination for popliteal reflux and will be described under that heading.

Direct Calf and Ankle Perforating Veins

The fascial defects where these veins penetrate the deep fascia may be palpable in a thin leg, and sometimes a small varix is visible at this point. Often there is no obvious physical sign, and it is then that Doppler ultrasound is most useful. A rough

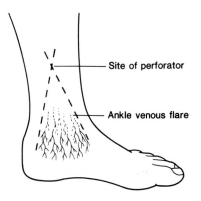

Site of perforator

Ankle venous flare

Fig. 38-5. "Ankle venous flare." Lines extended from anterior and posterior borders will meet at the site of perforating vein incompetence.

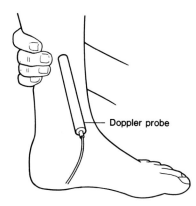

Fig. 38-6. Doppler ultrasound examination for perforating vein incompetence.

approximation of the site of an incompetent perforating vein can be obtained by
observing the anterior and posterior borders of the "ankle venous flare" and extending these proximally to the point where the lines cross ("the coastal navigation
sign") (Fig. 38-5). The Doppler probe is then placed over this point and the observer's other hand repeatedly squeezes and releases the calf muscles while the probe is
moved slowly (Fig. 38-6). The perforating vein incompetence is detected by the characteristic "in and out" signal which is both audible and can be recorded (Fig.
38-7).[30] Examination is usually only necessary on the medial side of the leg; the
presence of a lateral ulcer or venous flare indicates examination of the lateral surface
in the same way. It should be emphasised that it is only rarely possible to carry out
this examination satisfactorily in the presence of an infected ulcer. Several weeks of
ulcer cleaning and dressing may be necessary before examination is possible.

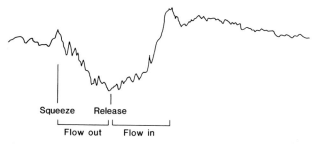

Fig. 38-7. Doppler ultrasound recording: a typical "out and
in" trace indicating perforating vein incompetence when the
calf muscles are squeezed and released.

Popliteal and Femoral Veins

The valvular competence of the superficial femoral and popliteal veins is assessed in similar manner by placing the Doppler probe over the vein in the popliteal
fossa. Maximal arterial pulsation is first found and the probe is then moved a little
laterally. A narrow cuff is placed just below the popliteal fossa to occlude the short
saphenous vein if this is incompetent. The calf is squeezed firmly (Fig. 38-8) and
proximal flow can be heard and observed on the oscilloscope or chart recorder. In
the presence of normal valves, no retrograde flow is seen or observed on release of

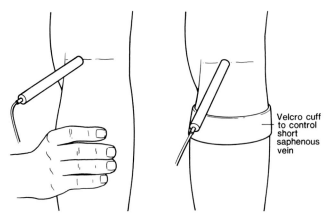

Fig. 38-8.   Doppler ultrasound examination for popliteal or short saphenous incompetence.

calf pressure (Fig. 38-9). Valvular incompetence produces a distinct and prolonged back-flow signal (Fig. 38-10).[31] The examination is much easier with the bidirectional probe, by means of which arterial pulsation can first be easily heard, then by pressing the switch the flow along the femoral vein away from the probe, and finally by pressing the switch again, reflux towards the probe.

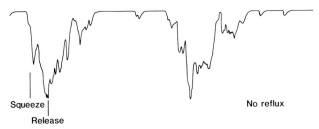

Fig. 38-9.   Doppler ultrasound trace of a normal popliteal vein; no reflux.

These simple investigations allow rapid assessment of the overall function of the calf muscle pump and of the sites of incompetence whose correction is necessary for the successful management of venous ulceration.[28] By combining clinical examination and noninvasive investigation in the manner described, a definitive diagnosis can usually be made within 10 minutes and venography is only necessary in a very few cases of doubt, usually where femoral or iliac obstruction is suspected.

ACKNOWLEDGEMENTS

I am grateful to Mr. Eamonn Nicholson for his continued help in carrying out the investigations described in this chapter. The Medasonics equipment was supplied, and has been serviced by PMS (Instruments), 107/109 King Street, Maidenhead, Berkshire and I thank them for providing a first class service and much good

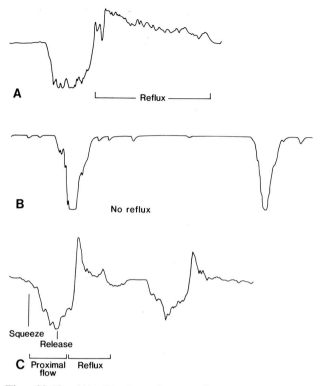

Fig. 38-10. (A) Short saphenous incompetence; reflux without cuff. (B) Short saphenous incompetence; reflux control by cuff compressing short saphenous vein. (C) Popliteal incompetence; reflux in spite of cuff controlling short saphenous vein.

advice. The manuscript was typed at extremely short notice by Mrs. Anneliese Berry and I am most grateful for her speed and accuracy and for considerable secretarial help from Miss Jill Wallace. Illustrations have kindly been undertaken by Mrs. Alison George, Department of Surgery, Charing Cross & Westminster Medical School. Finally, I am indebted to those many surgeons and vascular laboratory technicians, both in the UK and the USA, who have so kindly taken time and trouble to show me their methods.

BIBLIOGRAPHY

Noninvasive Diagnostic Techniques

Bernstein EF (ed): Non-invasive Diagnostic Techniques in Vascular Disease. St. Louis, Mosby, 1983.

Nicolaides AN, Yao JST (eds): Investigation of Vascular Disorders. New York, Churchill Livingstone, 1981

Bergan JJ, Yao JST (eds): Surgery of the Veins. Orlando, Fla, Grune & Stratton, 1984

Vascular Surgery Including Noninvasive Investigation

Rutherford RB (ed): Vascular Surgery. Philadelphia, Saunders, 1977
Moore WS (ed): Vascular Surgery, a Comprehensive Review. Orlando, Fla, Grune & Stratton, 1983

Investigation and Surgery of the Perforating Veins

May R, Partsch H, Staubsand J (eds): Perforating Veins. Baltimore, Urban & Schwarzenberg, 1981

Phlebography

Thomas ML: Phlebography of the Lower Limb. New York, Churchill-Livingstone, 1982

REFERENCES

1. Needham T: Directional Doppler ultrasonic blood velocity detectors: Available facilities, in Nicolaides AN, Yao JST (eds): Investigation of Vascular Disorders. New York, Churchill Livingstone, 1981
2. Hanzlik PJ, Deed F, Terada B: A simple method of demonstrating changes in blood supply of the ear and effects of some measures. J Pharmacol Exp Ther 56:194, 1936
3. Molitor H, Kniajuk M: A new bloodless method for continuous recording of peripheral circulatory changes. J Pharmacol Exp Ther 57:6, 1936
4. Barnes RW, Garrett WV, Hummel BA, et al: Plethysmographic assessment of altered cutaneous circulation in the postphlebitic syndrome. Technology in diagnosis and therapy. AAMI 13th Annual Meeting, Washington, DC, March 28–April 1, 1978, p 25
5. Yao JST, Hentin RE, Bergan JJ: Venous thromboembolic disease. Arch Surg 109:664, 1974
6. Barnes RW, Ross EA, Strandness E: Differentiation of primary from secondary varicose veins by Doppler ultrasound and strain-gauge plethysmography. Surg Gynecol Obstet 141:207, 1975
7. Norgren L: Foot volumetry before and after surgical treatment of varicose veins. Acta Chir Scand 141:129, 1975
8. Lawrence D, Kakkar VV: Postphlebitic syndrome: A functional assessment. Br J Surg 67:686, 1980
9. Cooke ED, Pilcher MF: Thermography in diagnosis of deep vein thrombosis. Br Med J 2:523, 1973
10. Cooke ED, Pilcher MP: Deep vein thrombosis. Preclinical diagnosis by thermography. Br J Surg 61:971, 1974
11. Cooke ED: The fundamentals of thermographic diagnosis of deep vein thrombosis. Acta Thermographica (Supp. 1): 1978
12. Atkins P, Hawkins LA: Detection of venous thrombosis in the legs. Lancet 2:1217, 1965
13. Negus D, Pinto DJ, LeQuesne LP, et al: ^{125}I-labelled fibrinogen in the diagnosis of deep vein thrombosis and its correlation with phlebography. Br J Surg 55:835, 1968
14. Persson RBR, Darte L: Int J Appl Radiol Isotopes 28:97, 1977
15. Olsson C-G: ^{99m}Tc-Plasmin: Development and current status, in Nicolaides AN, Yao JST (eds): Investigation of Vascular Disorders. New York, Churchill Livingstone, 1981
16. Beecher HH, Field ME, Krogh A: The effect of walking on the venous pressure at the ankle. Scand Arch Physiol 73:133, 1936

17. Pollack AA, Wood EK: Venous pressure in the saphenous vein at the ankle in man during exercise and changes in posture. J Appl Physiol 1:649, 1949

18. Miles C, Nicolaides AN: Photoplethysmography: Principles and development, in Nicolaides AN, Yao JST (eds): Investigation of Vascular Disorders. New York, Churchill Livingstone, 1981

19. Harris WH, Athanasoulis C, Wattman AC, et al: Cuffimpedance phlebography and ^{125}I-fibrinogen scanning versus roentgenographic phlebography for diagnosis of thrombophlebitis following hip surgery. J Bone Joint Surg 58:939, 1976

20. Albrechtsson V, Olsson CG: Thrombotic side effects of lower limb phlebography. Lancet 1:723, 1976

21. Lea Thomas M, Walters HL: Metrizamide in ascending venography of the legs. Br Med J 2:1036, 1979

22. Lea Thomas M: Phlebography of the lower limb. New York, Churchill Livingstone, 1982

23. Holmes MCG: Deep venous thrombosis of the lower limbs diagnosed by ultrasound. Med J Aust 1:427, 1973

24. Flanigan DP, Goodreau JJ, Burnham SJ, et al: Vascular laboratory diagnosis of clinically suspected deep vein thrombosis: A diagnostic and operative schema. Lancet 2:331, 1978

25. Negus D: Calf pain in the postthrombotic syndrome. Br Med J 2:156, 1968

26. Negus D, Cockett FB: Femoral vein pressures in postphlebitic iliac vein obstruction. Br J Surg 54:522, 1967

27. McIrvine AJ, Corbett CRR, Aston HO, et al: The demonstration of saphenofemoral incompetence: Doppler ultrasound compared with standard clinical tests. Br J Surg 71:509, 1984

28. Negus D, Friedgood A: The effective management of venous ulceration. Br J Surg 70:623, 1983

29. Flinn WR, Queral LA, Abramowitz HB, et al: Photoplethysmography in the assessment of chronic venous insufficiency, in Nicolaides AN, Yao JST (eds): Investigation of Vascular Disorders. New York, Churchill Livingstone, 1981

30. Miller SS, Foote AV: The ultrasonic detection of incomplete perforating veins. Br J Surg 61:653, 1974

31. Sumner DS, in Rutherford RB (ed): Vascular Surgery. Philadelphia, Saunders, 1977

Larry D. Flanagan
and John J. Cranley

39

Real-Time B-Mode Ultrasound Imaging in the Diagnosis of Venous Diseases of the Extremities

The diagnosis of iliofemoral thrombosis and thrombosis in the superficial veins is possible on clinical examination of the patient. The more common variety of deep venous thrombosis in the lower extremity up to the common femoral vein is undiagnosed clinically in 50% of the patients.[1] The classic symptoms and signs of deep venous thrombosis are nonspecific. Similarly, a patient may be entirely asymptomatic and yet have extensive deep-venous thrombosis. In recognition of this fact, many noninvasive tests have been developed for the diagnosis of deep-venous thrombosis. These include I^{131} fibrinogen scanning,[2] venous Doppler survey,[3] impedance plethysmography,[4] strain-gauge plethysmography,[5] radionuclide venography,[6] and phleborheography.[7] Each of the noninvasive techniques has its advantages and disadvantages. All are more accurate than clinical examination but less accurate than phlebography in diagnosing deep-venous thrombosis. To estimate the efficacy of these tests, their results have traditionally been compared to phlebography, which is considered the "gold standard." Yet thrombi may be undetected and chemical phlebitis may be caused by the contrast media used in phlebography.

Real-time B-mode ultrasound scanning, a modality used for the past several years to study patients with extracranial carotid artery disease, has recently been used to evaluate patients suspected of having deep-vein thrombosis. The feasibility of applying this technique to the visualization of thrombi in the extremities was noted in 1982 by Steven Talbot, a technician working in the laboratory of Dr. Clynn Ford in Salt Lake City, Utah. Talbot reported on 13 extremities in which clot was visualized in the veins by this technique.[8] This experience provided the impetus for using real-time B-mode venous scanning of the extremities in our laboratory.[9]

DIAGNOSTIC TECHNIQUES AND ASSESSMENT
PROCEDURES IN VASCULAR SURGERY

© 1985 Grune & Stratton
ISBN 0-8089-1721-8 All rights reserved

473

METHODS

The instrumentation and principles applicable to arterial scanning are also applicable to venous scanning. Simply, an ultrasound probe (Fig. 39-1) containing a piezo-electric crystal and transducer is applied to the body part being studied. The crystal, made to oscillate in response to an energizing voltage, produces sound waves that are transmitted into the tissues. Returning ultrasound waves, back-scattered toward their source by tissue acoustic interfaces, revibrate the crystal. By timing the return of the echoes, recording their amplitude as proportional to shades of grey (brightness), and displaying the two-dimensional information on a screen several times per second, one obtains a real-time (movie-like) B-mode (brightness mode) image of the structures being studied (Fig. 39-2).[10]

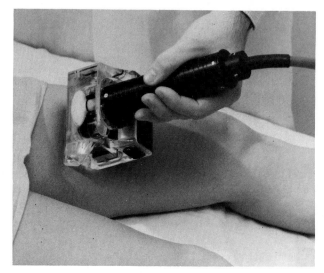

Fig. 39-1. Examination of the superficial femoral vein with the 4-MHz probe.

A pulsed Doppler attachment is frequently used in conjunction with real-time B-mode imaging. It is designed to detect blood flow selectively at a specific distance from the probe. The crystal emits bursts of ultrasound waves and receives back-scattered signals at specific time intervals. If the objects reflecting the ultrasound waves (eg, red blood cells) are moving, a frequency shift is produced that is proportional to the velocity of the objects relative to the sound beam. This information may then be represented as audible output for immediate analysis.

In our laboratory, a commercially available high-resolution ultrasound scanner (Biosound, Indianapolis) with two attached probes, a 4-MHz and an 8-MHz probe, is used. The 8-MHz probe, in addition, has an integrated 8-MHz pulsed Doppler attachment. The 8-MHz probe is utilized for visualization of the venous system in about 80% of the study time. The 4-MHz probe is used in about 20% of the study time.

The technique for examination of the lower extremities has undergone numerous changes over the past several months in our attempts to improve our visual-

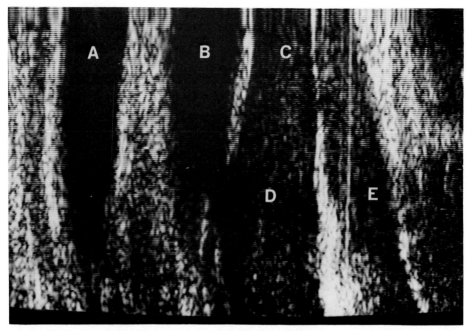

Fig. 39-2. Longitudinal view of vessels in the proximal thigh: (A) greater saphenous vein, (B) superficial femoral artery, (C) common femoral vein, (D) superficial femoral vein, and (E) deep femoral vein.

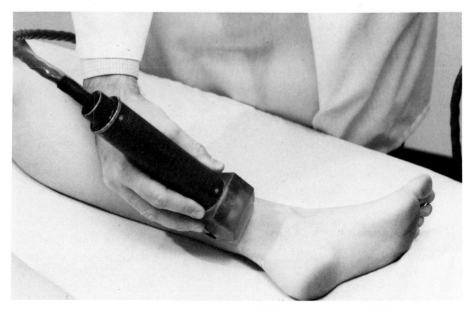

Fig. 39-3. Examination of the posterior tibial veins using the 8-MHz probe.

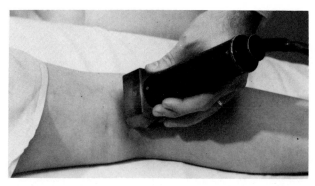

Fig. 39-4. Examination of the popliteal vein using the 8-MHz probe.

ization of the venous anatomy. At present the patient is placed in the reverse Trendelenburg position, with a tilt of 20 degrees. Copious acoustic gel is spread over the areas to be studied. The technician begins the study in the groin, using the 8-MHz probe to visualize in transverse and longitudinal views the common femoral, deep femoral, and superficial femoral veins. (Fig. 39-1). No attempt is made to study the venous anatomy above the inguinal ligament. The probe is moved down the leg to study the superficial femoral vein along the entire thigh and the greater saphenous vein from the saphenofemoral junction to the ankle. Next, the posterior and anterior tibial veins are visualized in the lower leg (Fig. 39-3). Depending on the

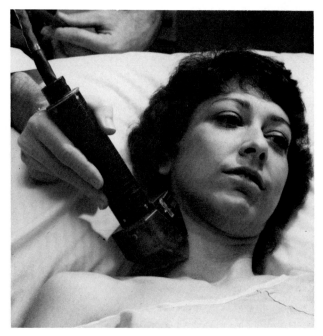

Fig. 39-5. Examination of the internal jugular vein using the 8-MHz probe.

extent of visualization of the venous anatomy at this time, the technician may restudy the veins in the thigh using the 4-MHz probe to visualize deeper structures. When this maneuver is completed, the opposite leg is studied in similar fashion. The patient is then turned to the prone position, remaining at 20 degrees of tilt. The popliteal and peroneal veins, as well as the lesser saphenous vein and soleal sinuses, are studied with the 4-MHz probe (Fig. 39-4).

Scans of the upper extremity are performed with the patient in the flat supine position. Acoustic gel is spread over the area to be studied and the technician begins by visualizing the internal jugular vein with the 4-MHz proble (Fig. 39-5). The subclavian vein is then visualized as it exits beneath the clavicle (Fig. 39-6). The study continues with visualization of the cephalic, axillary, and brachial veins, and also the veins of the forearm.

In every study an attempt is made to visualize the major named veins of the extremity. Each is evaluated with regard to its anatomy, physiology, and whatever pathology may be present.

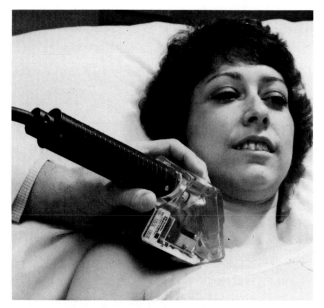

Fig. 39-6. Examination of the subclavian vein with the 4-MHz probe.

OBSERVATIONS

The common femoral vein is visualized nearly 100% of the time. In a very obese thigh, it may be seen only with the 4-MHz probe. A normal common femoral vein is slightly larger than the common femoral artery and is totally compressible when moderate pressure is applied with the probe. (Compressibility is defined as the ability to co-apt the blood vessel walls by means of external pressure). A valve may or may not be visualized within the common femoral vein. If a valve is seen, its function is assessed by pressing on the lower abdomen or by asking the patient to perform a Valsalva maneuver to determine whether the valve closes or permits reflux. Also, the vein should be seen to dilate with these maneuvers. Blood flow may be visualized in some veins, especially in the longitudinal view (Fig. 39-2).

The deep femoral vein is visualized in about two-thirds of patients. It is best seen in longitudinal view (Fig. 39-2). The deep femoral vein is sometimes difficult to compress because of surrounding structures. Inability to compress a normal deep femoral vein should not mislead one to assume that clot is present in the vessel. Blood flow is sometimes seen within the vessel. Valves are rarely seen.

The superficial femoral vein is seen along the entire length of the thigh in most patients, although on a large thigh it may be necessary to use the 4-MHz probe. The vessel is easily compressible throughout its length, except in the adductor canal—a region difficult to visualize and to compress. Valves are frequently seen and may be studied.

The posterior tibial veins, despite their small size, are visualized through much of their length in almost every patient (Fig. 39-7). Valves can be assessed even in these small veins, averaging 2–3 mm in diameter. Blood flow is not readily seen. It is difficult to assess valvular function and audible Doppler signals are difficult to obtain in these small veins.

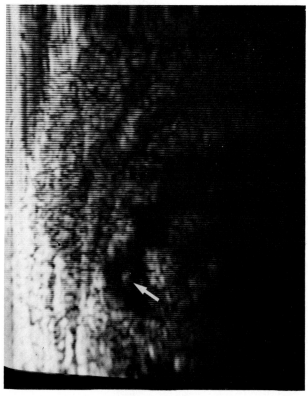

Fig. 39-7. Transverse view of posterior tibial veins with thrombosis (arrow).

The anterior tibial veins are visualized in 90% of patients, but can only be seen in the distal one-half of the lower leg. Valves are also seen in these small veins but their function is difficult to assess.

The popliteal vein is one of the easiest vessels to evaluate because of its large size and proximity to the skin (Fig. 39-8). Valves are seen over 50% of the time and their function can be easily assessed by using compression maneuvers on the calf and thigh with direct visualization of valvular movement and also by audible Doppler signals.

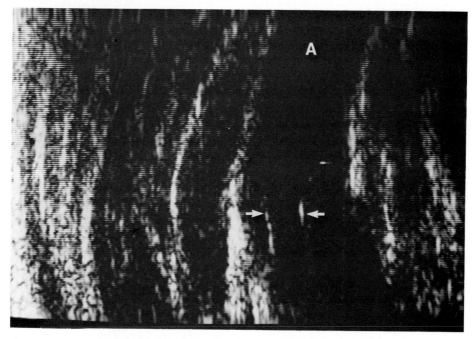

Fig. 39-8. Longitudinal view of popliteal vein with 8-MHz probe (A) popliteal vein. Arrows demonstrate cusps of a popliteal valve.

Soleal sinuses are seen in about 30% of patients. They can be shown to empty with active plantar flexion or passive dorsiflexion of the foot. Valves, of course, are not present in soleal sinuses. Peroneal veins are seen with difficulty; their small size makes evaluation and assessment hard.

Communicating veins in the thigh and calf can be found in the majority of patients when actively sought (Fig. 39-9). Direction of flow can be ascertained by compressing the thigh or calf. Valves can be seen within the communicating veins in some patients and their function can be assessed.

The greater saphenous vein is easily studied along its entire course and valvular function can be noted. The lesser saphenous vein is observed regularly, but is small in size and difficult to evaluate in some patients.

The need to diagnose deep venous thrombosis by noninvasive methods has been the primary reason for utilizing real-time B-mode venous imaging in our laboratory. In studying several hundred patients, those with normal veins and those with

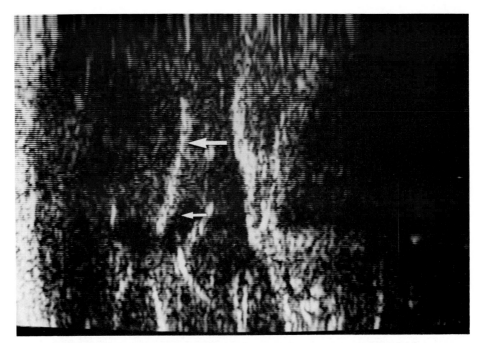

Fig. 39-9.   Calf perforator vein (small arrow). Large arrow denotes fascia.

deep-venous thrombosis, we have identified many of the ultrasound characteristics of normal veins as well as of those which are occluded with acute or chronic thrombus. The most important of these are discussed.

Compressibility

Compressibility of the veins using moderate pressure exerted on the probe handle while visualizing the vein in transverse view is one of the most important indicators of a normal vein. Because of the low venous pressure and the small size of the 8-MHz probe (4 cm) it is possible to co-apt the walls of most of the named veins in the upper and lower extremities with ease. Inability to do so suggests the presence of intraluminal thrombus. It bears noting, however, that the posterior tibial veins at the malleolus, the superficial femoral vein at the adductor canal, the deep femoral vein at its juncture with the common femoral vein and the subclavian vein beneath the clavicle are regions that are normally not compressible. Inability to compress the vessels at these anatomic points should not be mistaken for the presence of intraluminal clot.

Direct Visualization

In most cases of venous thrombosis, the intraluminal clot can be directly visualized using the real-time B-mode scanner (Fig. 39-10). Unlike fresh clot in the arterial system, which is difficult to visualize because of its homogeneity and light echogenicity, the thrombus within veins, whether it be acute or chronic, is visible. This is true because venous clot is usually laminar and contains many acoustic interfaces, whereas fresh intraarterial clot is usually of the non-laminar variety and is not a good reflective medium for ultrasound waves.

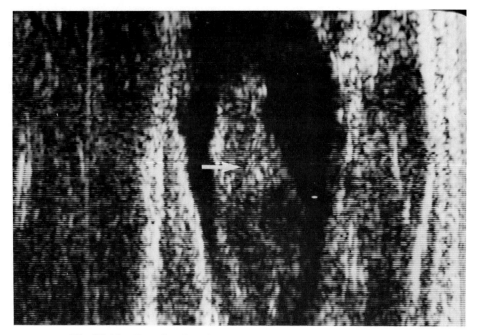

Fig. 39-10.   Free-floating clot in the greater saphenous vein (arrow).

Blood Flow

In the large veins of the extremities, especially the common femoral, the internal jugular and subclavian veins of the extremities, especially the common femoral, the internal jugular and subclavian veins, it is many times possible to visualize blood flow. Visualization is indirectly related to blood velocity. Thus, if one can slow the rate by such maneuvers as proximal compression, tilting, or the Valsalva maneuver, it may be easier to visualize flow. The visualization of flowing blood in veins is thought in some way to be due to rouleaux formation, but the exact events that occur between ultrasound waves and blood to make this phenomenon possible have not yet been clarified.[11] If flow is not seen in a large blood vessel, no useful information regarding the presence or absence of clot has been obtained.

Audible Doppler

A fourth method of determining whether a vessel contains clot is utilization of the audible Doppler attachment of the 8-MHz probe. This instrument is very similar in use to the familiar hand-held Doppler for identifying venous disease. When viewing the vessel in the cross-section plane, one should be able to obtain an audible Doppler signal which is phasic with respiration and which increases in pitch and intensity with compression of the distal extremity. Failure to detect signals that are normal in pitch, phasic with respiration, and that can be augmented with distal compression is indicative of disease.

The ability to differentiate acute from chronic thrombus, which is of obvious clinical value, has been explored intensively in our laboratory. As noted above, the direct visualization of thrombus in arteries may be difficult. However, much as the thrombus in a chronically occluded carotid artery is easier to visualize than that in an acutely occluded carotid artery, so also is the chronic thrombus in veins more easily visualized than acute thrombus. As noted in our earlier publications,[9,12] this is the direct result of increased echogenicity of the chronic thrombus as compared to the acute thrombus. Since those reports, we have done additional studies in our laboratory on the echogenicity of blood clot as related to its age. In both in vitro and in vivo studies we have noted little change in the echogenicity of clot in the first 32 days.[13] Observations have not been extended further, but it remains our clinical impression that chronic thrombus of several months' duration is more highly echogenic than acute thrombus.

As noted above, compressibility of a vein is an important criterion of the patency of that vessel. A vessel that is difficult to compress may indicate venous hypertension that may indeed be due to acute or chronic thrombus, but may also result from extrinsic compression or from some other cause, such as congestive heart failure. Thus, compressibility of the vessel per se is not a useful method of dating clot.

Compressibility of the clot itself, on the other hand, reflects the firmness of that thrombus and therefore, its age. Acute clot is quite soft and compressible, whereas chronic clot is more firm and difficult to compress.

The surface characteristic of clot vary with age. Acute thrombus demonstrates a surface that is usually quite regular and smooth. As clot ages and contracts, the surface becomes more irregular.

Attachment of the thrombus to the blood vessel wall is thought to be an accurate indicator of thrombus age. A free-floating thrombus that is totally unattached to the surrounding vessel is presumed to be an acute thrombus (Fig. 39-11);

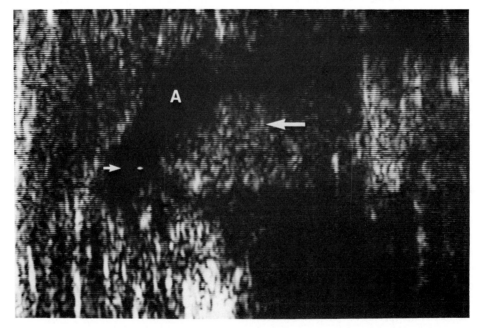

Fig. 39-11. Acute free-floating clot within the common femoral vein (large arrow). (A) Venous lumen, Small arrow shows saphenous vein origin.

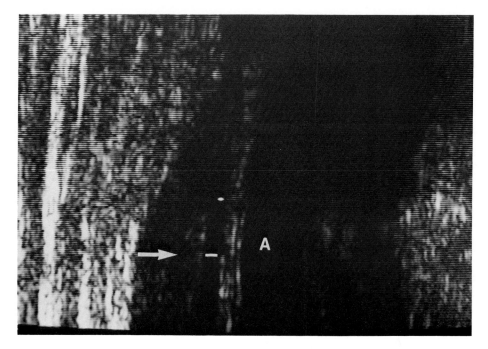

Fig. 39-12.   Longitudinal view of the popliteal vein with 75% obstruction by acute thrombus (arrow). Residual lumen is denoted by the spacer, (A) Popliteal artery.

however, one which demonstrates attachment to the venous wall may be chronic or acute.

The texture of the clot is variable. Acute thrombus is usually somewhat homogeneous in appearance, whereas chronic clot is heterogeneous (Fig. 39-12, 39-13).

The size of the blood vessel studied has been noted above to be an indicator of the presence of clot. In addition, the size of the vessel gives some clue as to the age of the clot. Acute thrombi may cause venous dilatation as a consequence of the clot itself, or as a result of increased venous pressure due to clot located more cephalad. Obstruction may preclude the normal response to the Valsalva or compression maneuvers. Chronic thrombosis, with collateral formation and damaged vein walls, may be seen as veins that are normal or small in size. Again, the normal response to Valasalva or compression maneuvers may be absent. In this case, however, it is because the veins are noncompliant or have diseased valves.

As noted above, visualization of blood flow is an important phenomenon in making the diagnosis of deep-venous thrombosis. If present, it is evidence that the vein is open. Flow is usually seen in the presence of chronic disease, but is not seen if obstruction is total.

The audible Doppler signals are usually heard in the presence of chronic disease but may be high-pitched and may reveal incompetence of veins when distal compression is performed. With acute obstruction, the signals will simply not be heard within the vein.

Collateral vessels are seen with chronic obstruction, whereas they are not seen with acute obstruction.

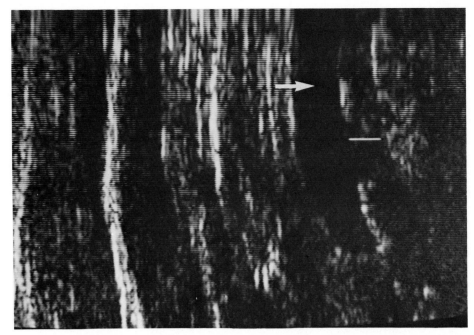

Fig. 39-13. Longitudinal view of the superficial femoral vein with partial obstruction by chronic clot (spacer). Large arrow denotes venous lumen.

We have used real-time B-mode ultrasound scanning primarily as a method of diagnosing deep venous thrombosis. In addition, early in the experience we began to visualize valves in the larger veins, such as the subclavian, common femoral, and superficial femoral as well as in the popliteal and smaller veins. For example, the popliteal vein exhibits a valve that can be studied in over 50% of patients.

The ability to visualize valves has enabled us to make some interesting observations. In the tilt position, the normal valve in the lower extremity remains partially open (Fig. 39-14). Compression of the leg distal to the valve causes opening while compression of the proximal leg causes closure (Fig. 39-15). A Valsalva maneuver causes closure of a common femoral valve but usually has no effect on a popliteal valve if valves in the more cephalad venous system are normal. In those veins in which blood flow can be directly visualized, this flow will be seen to cease in response to compression maneuvers in the proximal portion of the leg. This phenomenon is due to the presence of functioning valves. Likewise, as explained above, the audible Doppler instrument can be used to validate these findings.

Diseased valves may have one of several characteristics. If the valve is totally destroyed, then it is not visible. If the vein is dilated, the valve may appear normal but reflux can be demonstrated with the audible Doppler attachment, by hearing reverse blood flow, or by simply noting that the valve does not close, as would be expected when compression of the leg is done. The valve cusps may be "frozen" in the open position by thrombus lying behind the valves themselves (Fig. 39-16). Although previously described, true prolapse of valves is rarely seen.

A remarkable finding has been noted in regard to normal valves which has been described in a previous publication.[12] In brief, this consists of a rhythmic

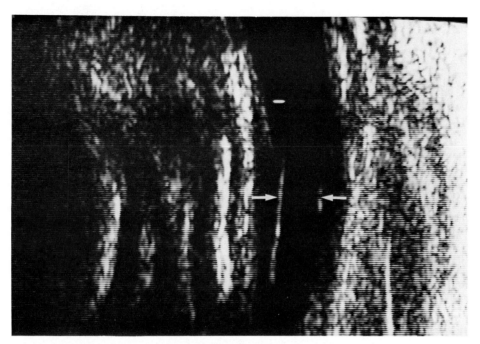

Fig. 39-14. Open valve, superficial femoral vein. Arrow denotes valve cusps.

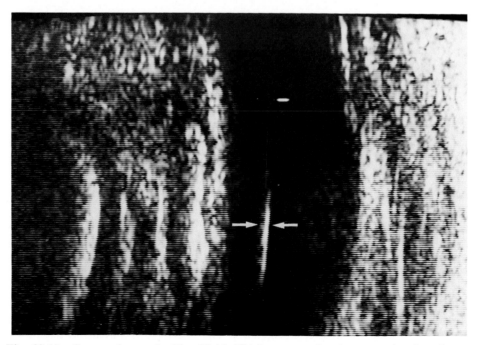

Fig. 39-15. Same valve as in Fig. 39-14. Thigh compression has caused valve closure (arrows).

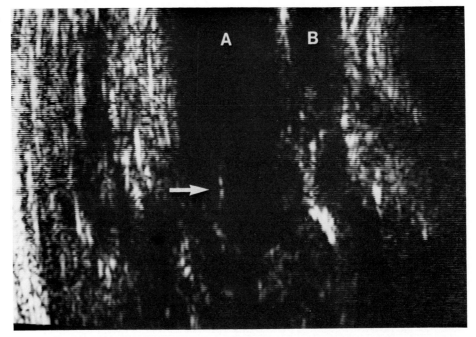

Fig. 39-16. Longitudinal view of "frozen" popliteal vein valve: (A) vein, (B) artery. Arrow denotes immobile valve.

opening and closing of venous valves in the upper and lower extremities which occurs with each heart beat. The venous valve remains closed during diastole and opens during systole. Synchronous with the observed opening of the valve, the diameter of the pulsating artery is seen to abruptly increase. This suggests that the pulsation of the artery against the vein wall is directly responsible for propelling blood distally in the venous system and causing the valves to open. However, it is very possible that the events are occurring so rapidly that what one really is seeing is vis a tergo. In other words, one may be seeing the arterial pulsation and noting simultaneously the increased venous flow which has been caused by the propulsion of blood from the arterial to the capillary to the venous system. We believe that the opening and closing of the valves synchronously with the arterial pulsations is probably a combination of these and perhaps other as yet unclarified factors.

RESULTS

Between August 1, 1982 and October 15, 1984, we have used real-time B-mode venous scanning to study 800 patients. A total of 1,667 scans were performed, 1,345 of the lower and 342 of the upper, extremities. Fifty-nine phlebograms have been obtained. In all, we have noted five errors, four of which were interpretational and one of which was a true miss (Table 39-1). The three false positives included misinterpretation of visualized bowel above the inguinal ligament as representing clot before it was realized that our probes do not permit study of the iliac veins; interpretation of lack of compressibility of the deep femoral vein as caused by clot, when

Table 39-1
B-Mode Venous Scan "Misses"

Type of Miss	Type
False positives	Iliac vein clot*
	Deep femoral vein clot*
	Calf vein clot*
False negatives	Innominate vein clot*
	Calf vein clot‡

* Interpretational error.
‡ True miss.

in fact this vein is frequently noncompressible in the normal limb; and interpretation of structures deep within the calf as thrombi, when in fact they were not. The fourth interpretational error was a false-negative scan in a patient with clot in the innominate vein, a region that cannot be seen with this technique. The only true error is a false-negative scan in a patient with calf vein thrombi that were demonstrated phlebographically in the posterior tibial and the greater saphenous veins just below the knee.

It is worthy of note that we have found what we believe to be a false-negative phlebogram in this group of 59 patients. Thrombus clearly visible in one of the posterior tibial veins on the B-mode scan was not diagnosed phlebographically by the radiologist.

The relatively small number of phlebograms, compared to the more than 1,600 scans we have performed to date, is rather striking. Reasons for our inability to obtain phlebograms include our heavy reliance on the phleborheograph in the past as well as now; the reluctance of staff physicians to order roentgenogram confirmation when the B-mode scan appears to be clearly positive; and the early realization that B-mode venous scanning in combination with phleborheography affords a high degree of accuracy in the diagnosis of deep-venous thrombosis. Many of the 59 phlebograms that have been obtained were of patients in whom the B-mode scan was difficult to interpret.

The overall specificity of this study, based on the 59 phlebographic correlations, is 88%. The sensitivity is 94%, the negative predictive value 91%, and the positive predictive value, 92% (Table 39-2).

Follow-up scans have been obtained on more than 100 extremities. On many occasions we have observed proximal and distal propagation of clot, and at least

Table 39-2
Phlebographic Correlations

		Phlebography		
		Normal	Abnormal	Total
B-Mode	Normal	21	2	23
Ultrasound	Abnormal	3	33	36
	Total	24	35	59

Note. The specificity was 88%, the sensitivity was 94%, the positive predictive value was 91%, and the negative predictive value was 92%.

once have performed thrombectomy and ligation of the superficial femoral vein because of clot propagation while the patient was being treated with full-dose heparin. We have been able to demonstrate disappearance of large free-floating clots in the common femoral vein in a patient with pulmonary embolism as documented by ventilation perfusion scan.

We have identified over 100 free-floating clots in the veins of the lower extremity. In our initial experience, we had no first-hand knowledge of the natural history of free-floating thrombus and performed thrombectomy on such patients. Over the past year, however, we have observed large free-floating clots frequently and with regularity. Many of them have been scanned in follow-up and have been noted to lyse or to become attached to the vein wall. This evidence has convinced us that it is unnecessary to subject patients with free-floating clots, diagnosed by B-mode scanning, to thrombectomy or venous interruption merely on the basis of this finding.

Table 39-3 lists the major ultrasonographic parameters that must be evaluated when studying the venous system with real-time B-mode ultrasound.

Table 39-3
Major Ultrasound Parameters of
Venous B-Mode Imaging

Vessel	Thrombus
Visibility	Visibility
Compressibility	Compressibility
Size	Texture
Flow	Adherence to vessel
Collaterals	Surface character
Valves	Audible Doppler
Anatomy	Spontaneity
Reflux	Phasicity
	Augmentation
	Reflux

DISCUSSION

The development of noninvasive techniques for making the diagnosis of deepvenous thrombosis has evolved primarily because of the inaccuracy of clinical diagnosis and the need to study the patients using a method that is less expensive, less thrombogenic, and simpler than phlebography. These criteria are met by several modalities: venous Doppler survey, fibrinogen scanning, impedance plethysmography, phleborheography, and others. All these tests are indirect methods of gaining knowledge of the physiology of an extremity. On the other hand, B-mode venous imaging is a unique test that provides an unmediated, movie-like projection of the anatomic structures as well as physiologic data. Not only can the presence of clot be confirmed, but the location and nature of the clot can often be precisely defined, eg, free-floating, attached, totally obstructing v partially obstructing, chronic v acute, etc). In addition, valvular structures can be studied, reflux noted, and other physiologic data accumulated. Structures surrounding the veins that might compress the venous system can be noted. It is not uncommon when using this technique to make an unexpected diagnosis while ruling out the possibility of deep venous thrombosis. For example, we have seen external compression by thigh musculature, Baker's cyst, and popliteal aneurysms. We have diagnosed subfascial and intramuscular haemorrhage, which was mistaken for deep-venous thrombosis. Another surprising finding was the identification of oedema fluid in the calf which was loculated rather than diffuse (Fig. 39-17).

Phleborheography was developed in our laboratory in the early 1970s and has been used continuously to diagnose deep-venous thrombosis. This method has yielded excellent results in our hands, with a sensitivity and specificity for above-knee clots of >90% respectively.[14] The equipment is relatively inexpensive and the cost of performing the test on a routine basis is quite moderate. Its disadvantages are that is requires a high degree of technical training and that there are several conditions under which it cannot be performed, ie, on patients with an amputation, a cast, uncontrollable tremors, or who are uncooperative. Real-time B-mode ultrasound can be used to study many of these patients. This technique requires little patient cooperation, is not affected by extrinsic compression, can be performed on amputees patients with uncontrollable movements.

Over the last several months we have expanded the use of real-time B-mode ultrasound to the study of patients with chronic venous insufficiency. These patients

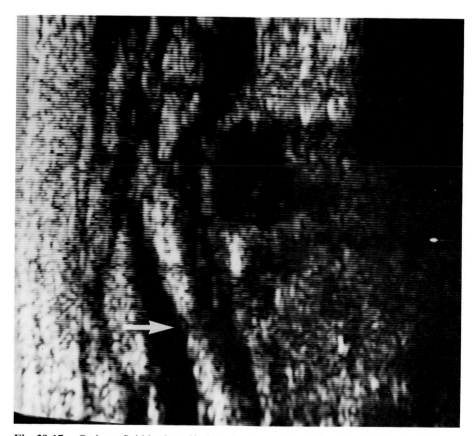

Fig. 39-17. Oedema fluid in the calf which is observed to be loculated rather than diffuse.

have been classically studied using methods such as venous Doppler survey, direct pressure measurements, and ascending and descending phlebography. To date, we have studied more than 100 of these patients with particular emphasis on evaluating the presence of outflow obstruction and valvular function. We are able to diagnose outflow obstruction up to the level of the inguinal ligament, to evaluate valves for reflux, and to evaluate reflux in communicating veins as well.

The disadvantages of real-time B-mode ultrasound scanning for studying patients with acute and chronic venous diseases include initial cost of the instrumentation, increased cost of each individual study, and technical expertise that is required for performing the test and for its interpretation. We believe that the extra cost is warranted in that it affords a high degree of accuracy and a large amount of useful information that could not otherwise be obtained, except by phlebography. The cost is off-set somewhat, because in many cases it eliminates the need for a phlebogram. Furthermore, most laboratories that are involved in the diagnosis of vascular problems already have a real-time B-mode scanner and in most cases can utilize the instrument for studying the venous system. Technicians who perform carotid artery scans can in most cases learn to perform venous scans with additional training and physicians can learn to interpret venous scans with proper supervision. Admittedly, the method is technically sophisticated and in our opinion it is somewhat more difficult to study the venous system than the carotid arteries.

SUMMARY

Based on our experience with over 1600 real-time B-mode venous scans, we believe that this technique equals or surpasses other noninvasive techniques in accuracy. In most cases, it obviates the need for phlebography in the diagnosis of acute deep venous thrombosis and in the evaluation of patients with chronic deep venous insufficiency.

REFERENCES

1. Cranley JJ, Canos AJ, Sull WJ: The diagnosis of deep venous thrombosis. Fallibility of clinical symptoms and signs. Arch Surg 111:34, 1976
2. Palko PD, Nanson EM: Early detection of deep venous thrombosis using iodine-131 tagged fibrinogen. Surgical Forum 14:303, 1963
3. Sumner DS, Baker DW, Strandness DE: The ultrasonic velocity detector in a clinical study of venous disease. Arch Surg 75:97, 1968
4. Mullick SG, Wheeler HB, Songster GF: Diagnosis of deep venous thrombosis by measurement of electrical impedance. Am J Surg 119:417, 1970
5. Barnes RW, Collicott PE, Mozersky DJ: Noninvasive quantification of maximum venous outflow in acute thrombophlebitis. Surgery 72:971, 1972
6. Barnes RW, McDonald GB, Hamilton GW, et al: Radionuclide venography for rapid dynamic evaluation of venous disease. Surgery 73:706, 1973
7. Cranley JJ, Gay, AY, Grass AM, et al: A plethysmographic technique for the diagnosis of deep vein thrombosis of the lower extremities. Surg Gynecol Obstet 136:385, 1973
8. Talbot SR: Use of real-time imaging in identifying deep venous obstruction: A preliminary report. Bruit 6:41, 1982

9. Sullivan ED, Peter DJ, Cranley JJ: Real-time B-mode ultrasound J Vasc Surg 1:465, 1984

10. Wicks DJ, Howe KS: Fundamentals of Ultrasonographic Technique. Chicago, Year Book Medical, 1983

11. Machi J, Sigel B, Beitler JC, et al: Relation of in vivo blood flow to ultrasound echogenicity. J Clin Ultrasound 11:3, 1983

12. Flanagan LD, Sullivan ED, Cranley JJ: Venous imaging of the extremities using real-time B-mode ultrasound, in Bergan JJ, Yao JST (eds): Surgery of the Veins. Orlando, Fla, Grune & Stratton, 1985, pp 89–98

13. Peter DJ Flanagan LD, Cranley JJ: Quantitative analysis of blood clot echogenicity. (Submitted for publication.)

14. Cranley JJ: Diagnosis of deep venous thrombosis by phleborheography, Bernstein EF (ed): Noninvasive Diagnostic Techniques in Vascular Disease. St. Louis, Mosby, (in press)

PART IX

Practical Developments

Denton A. Cooley

40

Development of Vascular Prostheses to Meet the Surgeon's Requirements

As vascular surgery has developed through the past few decades, the needs of the surgeon for prosthetic grafts and materials has changed accordingly.[1] With a growing emphasis on the direct versus an indirect approach and a curative versus a palliative concept of therapy, tools of the trade have assumed increasing importance. For occlusive lesions, restoration of pulsatile flow to the vessels located distally is the goal, while for aneurysms, removal or repair with intervening grafts has become the prime objective.

As new instrumentation for the vascular surgeon became necessary, instrument providers cooperated to supply these needs (Fig. 40-1). Fabrication of the implantable prostheses required a close and more critical participation between supplier and consumer. Thus, a combined effort has been necessary to develop materials for the modern vascular surgeon under the scrutiny of regulatory agencies such as the Food and Drug Administration and cardiovascular societies.

Prostheses for vascular surgery must possess certain characteristics, including compatibility between the synthetic materials and the surrounding tissue. Among the synthetic materials tested clinically are nylon, Vinyon-N, Teflon, and polyesters.[2-5] Nylon, which is hydrophilic, has been discarded since degeneration occurs in this material after six to twelve months, and Vinyon-N had limited durability.[6] Because Teflon and polyester are more durable, these materials are now preferred for prosthetic grafts.[7]

FABRICATION OF VASCULAR GRAFTS

Fabric Grafts

Fabrication of grafts has presented a variety of problems. Textile engineers have cooperated with the surgeon to develop fabrics of known porosity and durability (Fig. 40-2). Early attempts to make the grafts more delicate and pliable

DIAGNOSTIC TECHNIQUES AND ASSESSMENT PROCEDURES IN VASCULAR SURGERY

© 1985 Grune & Stratton
ISBN 0-8089-1721-8 All rights reserved

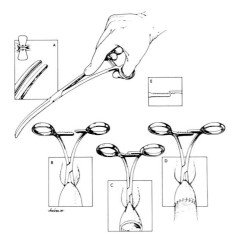

Fig. 40-1. Atraumatic vascular clamps developed for use in vascular surgery. The handles are long and sufficiently strong while remaining flexible to apply varying degrees of pressure to the blood vessel. The jaws have a double row of serrations to hold securely without crushing or cutting the vessel walls. As the clamp is gradually released, the long ratchet permits adjustment in the proximal blood pressure as the blood volume is redistributed. Bleeding through the graft is also minimized. More recently, vascular clamps for aortic occlusion have been made with 12 stops, giving an even wider range of control for both occlusion and release.

Cardiovascular Fabrics

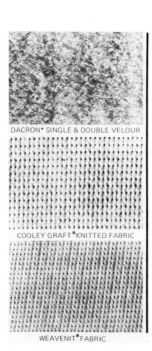

DACRON* SINGLE & DOUBLE VELOUR

COOLEY GRAFT*KNITTED FABRIC

WEAVENIT*FABRIC

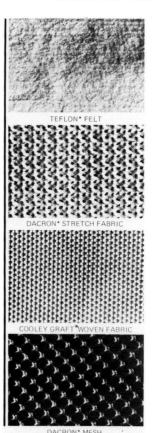

TEFLON* FELT

DACRON* STRETCH FABRIC

COOLEY GRAFT*WOVEN FABRIC

DACRON* MESH

Fig. 40-2. Fabrics that have been available for use in vascular grafts. Both knitted and woven textures are shown.

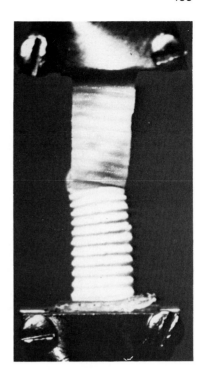

Fig. 40-3. Grips of an Instron machine (fixed, upper; moving, lower) used in this instance to determine the tensile strength of a vascular graft.

resulted in late aneurysmal formation when the grafts were subjected to prolonged pulsatile circulation (Fig. 40-3).[8-12] Thus, when finer diameter threads are used, durability may be sacrificed.[13] Graft porosity is important to the clinical surgeon since curtailment of blood loss at the operating table is essential to success.[14-16] In general, two types of textile grafts are being fabricated, namely the knitted and woven. The principal advantage of the woven graft over the knitted one is its provision for low porosity. Unfortunately, the lower the porosity, the less is the tendency for surrounding tissues to grow firmly into the graft. This tendency can be tested in experimental animals by implanting several types of grafts into the aorta, removing them at specified intervals, and determining the amount of force necessary to peel off the surrounding tissue and fibrous ingrowth. The greater the peeling force required to separate the graft from the tissues, the greater the degree of healing between the graft and tissue. Knitted grafts permit fibroblastic and tissue ingrowth into the graft that provides a basis for development of a pseudoendothelial lining. Thus, these grafts have greater healing capabilities and are more favorable for long-term use and prevention of infection.[16] Velour grafts, which are fabricated from texturized fiber and have small tufts or hooklets on the surface, provide even greater tissue compatibility and ingrowth.[17-19] In fact, in some instances the strong tissue adherence to the graft has been considered a disadvantage if the graft requires subsequent removal.

Also evident in velour grafts is resistance to subsequent thrombosis. The internal lining of the velour grafts adheres firmly to surrounding tissues, while fibrin deposition in woven grafts is loosely attached.[20,21] Thus, embolization of the fibrinous lining can be a problem if woven grafts of small diameter or fabricated from Teflon are used in femoral and popliteal reconstructions. This disadvantage,

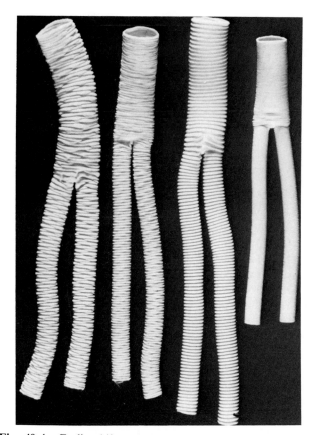

Fig. 40-4. Earlier bifurcation grafts showing variations in size and degree of crimping.

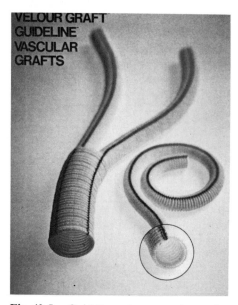

Fig. 40-5. Guideline velour vascular grafts.

however, is not important in large-caliber vessels, particularly in the thoracic aorta. Thus, woven grafts have become standard in replacement of the thoracic aorta, especially in those cases where cardiopulmonary bypass and full heparinization are standard. One may conclude, therefore, that for grafts placed in the thoracic and perhaps the abdominal aorta, woven grafts serve the purpose well. For more peripheral arteries, however, knitted grafts should be used.

Additional considerations are important in the fabrication of vascular prostheses. The construction of bifurcation grafts, for example, has been modified through the years (Figs. 40-4, 40-5).[22,23] Previously, bifurcated grafts were constructed to make the diameter of the proximal vessel twice the diameter of the branches. This, however, does not conform to human anatomy, in which the proximal vessel should have twice the area rather than twice the diameter of the distal vessel. Thus, for an aortic bifurcation graft, instead of a 16 to 8-mm relationship, there should be a correlation of approximately 16 mm to 9–10 mm distally. To develop a lumen of appropriate size for the distal vessels, the formula used to calculate the area of a circle, πr^2, should be used rather than the standard diameter. Most manufacturers have now incorporated this concept in the fabrication of bifurcated grafts. A major need remains, however, for a small graft (<4 mm in diameter) which is functional and resists thrombosis. Research is currently underway to develop such a prosthesis which would be extremely useful, particularly for myocardial revascularization.

Clinical Considerations

Certain practical considerations are necessary for the surgeon, including the ease with which sutures are passed through the graft. Some tightly woven grafts, for example, present true obstacles, since disposable round needles do not easily penetrate these grafts. A cutting-edge needle might split the graft and lead to bleeding from the suture line. Needle holes are also a concern with certain graft materials, particularly expanded microporous polytetrafluoroethylene (PTFE) or Gore-Tex (Gore and Associates, Elkton, Md) grafts. In our early experience with PTFE grafts, when 3-0 and 4-0 monofilament sutures were used for aortic anastomoses, the splits caused by passage of the needle bled excessively. Therefore, we reserved these grafts for reconstruction of vessels where 5-0 and 6-0 sutures were appropriate. Manufacturers have recently modified the grafts to make bleeding less of a problem.[24,25] Knitted grafts, however, are stronger at the suture lines, and they do not cause fraying of the edges as occurs in some instances with woven grafts. Another consideration is the tendency of grafts to kink as they pass over fixed points or over joints where flexion occurs. To overcome this problem, crimping has been widely used in the fabrication of fabric grafts and has proved to be satisfactory.[26] For PTFE grafts, the problem may be alleviated either by a crimping process (Vitagraft, Extracorporeal, King of Prussia, Pa) or by external reinforcement (Impra graft, Impra, Tempe, Ariz).[27]

The problem of porosity has diminished with the availability of tightly woven grafts of polyester, Dacron, or Teflon, making bleeding through the interstices minimal. Perhaps the most impervious is the woven Teflon graft; however, since Teflon does not adhere to surrounding tissues, in our opinion, the long-term performance has not been acceptable, and we no longer use grafts made of this fiber clinically. The polyester fiber, however, has been satisfactory, and the degree of porosity of the woven graft is clinically acceptable. To enhance the nonpermeability of grafts, particularly the knitted and velour, it is now standard to preclot with the patient's unheparinized blood. In patients undergoing cardiopulmonary bypass with full heparinization, heparin may be absorbed into the fabric and produce troublesome and sometimes serious bleeding intraoperatively. To prevent and overcome this problem, we have introduced a method of preclotting woven Dacron grafts in which autologous plasma is obtained at the operating table and then applied to the graft (Fig. 40-6).[28] Placing the saturated graft in the autoclave for three to five minutes renders the graft virtually impervious to bleeding. Modifications of this method are employed by others and include the use of human albumin, homologous plasma, biologic glue, or autologous whole blood.

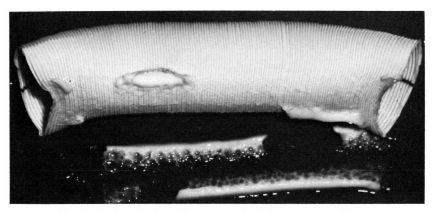

Fig. 40-6.   Preclotting of Dacron graft with autologous plasma.

Manufacturers are now busy developing grafts that have been "preclotted" prior to delivery. A number of substances are being studied, and bovine collagen suspensions impregnated into the graft and freeze-dried are undergoing investigational application. A final solution to this problem is imminent. For patients undergoing only mild heparinization for operations below the diaphragm, simple preclotting with autologous unheparinized blood gives sufficient protection against intraoperative bleeding.

Biologic Grafts

Biologic tissue grafts have been used from the beginning of the modern surgical era. Homologous and heterologous grafts were used during the early years of direct vascular surgery. Preparation and preservation of these grafts ranged from using nutrient solutions to various fixatives and even freeze-drying, but in most instances the long-term results were unsatisfactory due to degeneration, calcification, and fragmentation. Yet the need for a biologic substitute has been evident, and the most practical and satisfactory substance found to date has been the preserved human umbilical artery (Dardik-Meadox, Meadox Medicals, Oakland, NJ).[29,30] In this process, the umbilical cord is detached from the human placenta. An intricate strip-

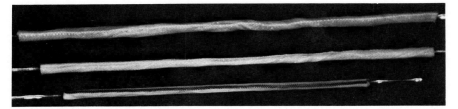

Fig. 40-7. Preserved human umbilical vein.

ping of the graft down to the contained umbilical vein follows, and the vein is placed on a glass rod or stent to overcome the tortuosity and increase the diameter, with the end result being a straight graft of some 30–40 cm (Fig. 40-7). The graft is then preserved in glutaraldehyde solution. Because the grafts do not have sufficient inherent strength to resist aneurysmal formation, a Dacron mesh is applied externally to prevent late aneurysmal formation (Fig. 40-8). Umbilical grafts have proved to be effective in two principal situations, ie, the revascularization of popliteal and tibial arteries of small diameter, where synthetic grafts have a high tendency to develop fibrosis and stenosis of the distal anastomoses, and the development of access loops for renal dialysis, where an arteriovenous communication is necessary.[31] At present, for example, the choice of grafts for these procedures is either the Dardik umbilical vein or a PTFE graft.

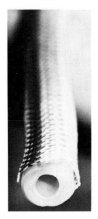

Fig. 40-8. View of Dardik-Meadox umbilical vein showing the external Dacron mesh used to prevent late aneurysmal formation.

A recent example of the cooperation between the fabricator and the surgeon is the intraluminal graft for aortic replacement reported independently in 1978 by Ablaza et al[32] and Dureau et al,[33] and in 1982 by Lemole et al[34] (Fig. 40-9). Since the period of circulatory interruption necessary for replacement by the customary suture technique may be prolonged causing ischemic complications in distal organs, this sutureless device has found some advocates. The graft is inserted into the open lumen of the aorta proximally and distally and held secure by a tape ligature around the aorta. Some surgeons report success with this graft, but all still adhere to the standard suture technique.

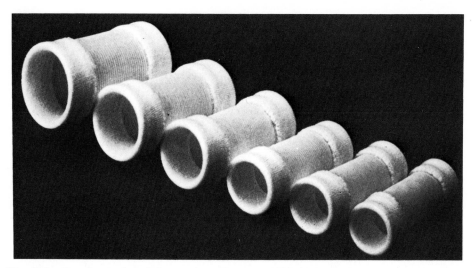

Fig. 40-9. Intraluminal graft for aortic replacement. This low porosity Dacron graft (USCI, Division of C.R. Bard, Inc, Billerica, Ma) has rigid support rings attached to each end, which can be inserted into the proximal and distal aorta and tied in place with a heavy ligature.

SUMMARY

Finally, the surgeon must use his own judgment in selecting a prosthesis for a particular need, since no single one appears to provide for all circumstances that might be encountered. In regard to materials, we use Dacron or polyester grafts because of the improved healing properties, durability, ease of handling, and control of intraoperative bleeding (Fig. 40-10). PTFE grafts are used in the smaller sizes and configurations. They provide for satisfactory healing with adequate tissue ingrowth and the blood loss at operation is confined only to the suture lines, where the needle holes may still be troublesome. We have not as yet used the larger diameter Teflon grafts because of certain disadvantages outlined above. For bypass grafts in the lower extremities and for access grafts, PTFE in various forms offers distinct advantages. The umbilical vein graft is reserved for distal anastomoses into the popliteal and tibial arteries, although it is still used widely for patients undergoing renal dialysis.

The development of vascular prostheses is undergoing constant change and improvement. Almost daily new materials and prostheses appear, and with each the ideal graft becomes more nearly available. Continued cooperation between surgeons and suppliers is necessary, and this close relationship should not be disrupted by

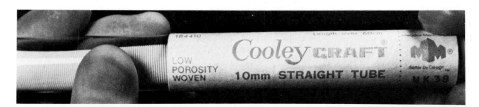

Fig. 40-10. Cooley-Meadox low porosity Dacron graft used in vascular surgery.

excessive regulations that place obstacles to future research and development. While the protection of the beneficiary, namely the patient, is the objective of such regulations, the opposite result may occur if he is denied the use of an improved product.

REFERENCES

1. Voorhees AB, Jaretski A, Blakemore A: Use of tubes constructed of Vinyon-N cloth in bridging arterial defects. Ann Surg 135:332, 1952
2. Blakemore A, Voorhees AB Jr: The use of tubes constructed from Vinyon-N cloth in bridging arterial defects. Experimental and clinical. Ann Surg 140:324, 1954
3. Edwards WS: Arterial grafts, past, present and future. Arch Surg 113:1225, 1978
4. Wesolowski SA, Fries CC, Martinez A, et al: Arterial prosthetic materials. Ann NY Acad Sci 145:325, 1967
5. Lidenauer SM, Weber TR, Miller TA, et al: Velour vascular prosthesis. Trans Am Soc Artif Intern Organs 20:314, 1974
6. Dale WA: Arterial grafts: 1900–1978, in Dardik H (ed): Graft Materials in Vascular Surgery. Chicago, Year Book, 1978, pp 3–15
7. Lindenauer SM: The fabric vascular prosthesis, in Rutherford RB (ed): Vascular Surgery, 2 ed. Philadelphia, Saunders, 1984, pp 382–394
8. Kim GE, Imparato AM, Nathan I, et al: Dilation of synthetic grafts and junctional aneurysms. Arch Surg 114:1296, 1979
9. Knox WG: Aneurysm occurring in a femoral artery Dacron prosthesis five and one-half years after insertion. Ann Surg 156:827, 1962
10. Komoto Y, Kawakami S, Uchida H: Prosthetic aneurysm in an axillo-femoral Dacron bypass graft. Vasc Surg 12:274, 1978
11. Kinley CE, Marble AE: Compliance: A continuing problem with vascular grafts. J Cardiovasc Surg 21:163, 1980
12. Cooley DA, Subram A, Houchin DP: Clinical experience in 1040 patients with double-velour knitted Dacron vascular prostheses: with particular reference to dilatation and aneurysm formation. Cardiovasc Dis Bull Texas Heart Institute 8:320, 1981
13. Ottinger LW, Darling RC, Wirthlin LS, et al: Failure of ultralightweight knitted Dacron grafts in arterial reconstruction. Arch Surg 111:146, 1976
14. Fry WJ, DeWeese MS, Kraft RO, et al: Importance of porosity in arterial prostheses. Arch Surg 88:836, 1964
15. Sauvage LR, Berger K, Wood SJ, et al: A very thin, porous, knitted arterial prosthesis: Experimental data and early clinical assessment. Surgery 65:78, 1969
16. Wesolowski SA, Fries CC, Karlson KE, et al: Porosity: Primary determinant of ultimate fate of synthetic vascular grafts. Surgery 50:91, 1961
17. Bennett JG, Trono R, Norman JC, et al: Experimental comparisons of vascular grafts. Cardiovasc Dis Bull Texas Heart Institute 4:18, 1977
18. Cooley DA, Wukasch DC, Bennett JG, et al: Double velour knitted Dacron grafts for aorto-iliac vascular replacement, in Sawyer PN, Kaplitt MJ (eds): Vascular Grafts: Current Status and Future Trends. New York, Appleton-Century-Crofts, 1978, pp 197–207
19. Wukasch DC, Cooley DA, Bennett JG, et al: Results of a new Meadox-Cooley double velour Dacron graft for arterial reconstruction. J Cardiovasc Surg 20:249, 1979
20. Holub DA, Trono R, Klima T, et al: Macroscopic, microscopic, and mechanical analyses of prototype double velour vascular grafts. Cardiovasc Dis Bull Texas Heart Institute 5:365, 1978
21. Ghidoni JJ, Liotta D, Hall CW, et al: Healing of pseudointimas in velour-lined impermeable arterial prostheses. Am J Pathol 53:375, 1968

22. Buxton BF, Wukasch DC, Martin C, et al: Practical considerations in fabric vascular grafts: Introduction of a new bifurcated graft. Am J Surg 125:288, 1973

23. Cooley DA, Wukasch DC: Techniques in Vascular Surgery. Philadelphia, Saunders, 1979, pp 8–10

24. Campbell CD, Brooks DH, Webster MW, et al: The use of expanded microporous polytetrafluoroethylene for limb salvage: A preliminary report. Surgery 79:485, 1976

25. Veith FJ, Gupta SK: Expanded Polytetrafluoroethylene Vascular Grafts, in Rutherford RB (ed): Vascular Surgery, 2 ed. Philadelphia, Saunders, 1984, pp 394–404

26. Crawford ES, DeBakey ME, Cooley DA, et al: Use of crimped, knitted, Dacron grafts in patients with occlusive disease of the aorta and of the iliac, femoral, and popliteal arteries, in Wesolowski SA, Dennis C (eds): Fundamentals of Vascular Grafting. New York, McGraw Hill, 1963, pp 356–364

27. Campbell CD, Brooks DH, Webster MW, et al: Aneurysm formation in expanded polytetrafluoroethylene prostheses. Surgery 79:491, 1976

28. Cooley DA, Romagnoli A, Milam JD, et al: A method of preparing woven Dacron aortic grafts to prevent interstitial hemorrhage. Cardiovasc Dis Bull Texas Heart Institute 8:48, 1981

29. Dardik H, Ibrahim IM, Dardik I: The role of the peroneal artery for limb salvage. Ann Surg 189:189, 1979

30. Dardik H: Modified human umbilical cord vein allograft, in Rutherford RB (ed): Vascular Surgery 2 ed. Philadelphia, Saunders, 1984, pp 405–412

31. Anderson CB, Etheredge EE, Sicard GA: One hundred polytetrafluoroethylene vascular access grafts. Dialy Transplant 9:237, 1980

32. Ablaza SGG, Ghosh SC, Grana VP: Use of a ringed intraluminal graft in the surgical treatment of dissecting aneurysms of the thoracic aorta. J Thorac Cardiovasc Surg 76:390, 1978

33. Dureau G, Villard J, George M, et al: New surgical technique for the operative management of acute dissections of the ascending aorta. J Thorac Cardiovasc Surg 76:385, 1978

34. Lemole GM, Strong MD, Spagna PM, et al: Improved results for dissecting aneurysms: Intraluminal sutureless prosthesis. J Thorac Cardiovasc Surg 83:249, 1982

Index